# Advancing the Frontiers of Cardiopulmonary Rehabilitation

**Jean Jobin, PhD**
Hôspital Laval
Québec, Canada

**François Maltais, MD**
Hôspital Laval
Québec, Canada

**Paul Poirier, MD**
Hôspital Laval
Québec, Canada

**Pierre LeBlanc, MD**
Hôspital Laval
Québec, Canada

**Clermont Simard, PhD**
Physical Education Department
Laval University
Québec, Canada

**Human Kinetics**

BS

**Library of Congress Cataloging-in-Publication Data**

Advancing the frontiers of cardipulmonary rehabilitation / editors Jean
Jobin . . . [et al.].
     p. cm.
Includes bibliographical references
   ISBN 0-7360-4216-4
   1. Cardiopulmonary system--Diseases--Patients--Rehabilitation.   I.
Jobin, Jean, 1949-
   RC669 .A385 2002
   616.1'06--dc21              2002003620

ISBN: 0-7360-4216-4

**Acquisitions Editor:** Loarn D. Robertson, PhD; **Managing Editor:** Lee Alexander; **Graphic Artists:** Yvonne Griffith and Dawn Sills; **Cover Designer:** Kristin A. Darling; **Printer:** Versa Press

Printed in the United States of America

10  9  8  7  6  5  4  3  2  1

**Human Kinetics**
Web site: www.humankinetics.com
*United States:* Human Kinetics
P.O. Box 5076
Champaign, IL 61825-5076
800-747-4457
e-mail: humank@hkusa.com

*Canada:* Human Kinetics
475 Devonshire Road Unit 100
Windsor, ON N8Y 2L5
800-465-7301 (in Canada only)
e-mail: orders@hkcanada.com

*Europe:* Human Kinetics
Units C2/C3 Wira Business Park
West Park Ring Road
Leeds LS16 6EB, United Kingdom
+44 (0) 113 278 1708
e-mail: hk@hkeurope.com

*Australia:* Human Kinetics
57A Price Avenue
Lower Mitcham, South Australia 5062
08 8277 1555
e-mail: liahka@senet.com.au

*New Zealand:* Human Kinetics
P.O. Box 105-231, Auckland Central
09-523-3462
e-mail: hkp@ihug.co.nz

5-20-03

# Contents

# List of Contributors

**Kathy Berra:** SCRDP, 730 Welch Road, Palo Alto, California 94303, United States of America. **kberra@scrdp.standford.edu.** Fax: (650) 725-6247.

**Peter Bogaty:** Institut universitaire de cardiologie et de pneumologie, Hôpital Laval, 2725 chemin Ste-Foy, Sainte-Foy, Québec, Canada, G1V 4G5. Fax: (418) 656-4562

**Bartolome R. Celli:** St. Elizabeth's Medical Center, 736 Cambridge Street, Boston, Massachusetts 02135, United States of America. **bcelli@cchcs.org.** Fax: (617) 789-2893.

**Richard Debigaré:** Institut universitaire de cardiologie et de pneumologie, Hôpital Laval, 2725 chemin Ste-Foy, Sainte-Foy, Québec, Canada, G1V 4G5.

**Marc Decramer:** Respiratory division, Katholieke University Hospital, HERESTRAAT 49, 3000 Leuven, Belgium. **marc.decramer@uz.kuleuven.ac.bc.** Fax: 011 32 16 346803.

**Adam de Jong:** Beaumont Rehabilitation and Health Center, Cardiac Rehabilitation Department, 746 Purdy Street, Birmingham, Missouri 48009, United States of America. **adejong@beaumont.edu.** Fax: (248) 258-1392.

**Jean Deslauriers:** Centre de pneumologie de l'Hôpital Laval, Division of Thoracic Surgery, 2725 chemin Ste-Foy, Sainte-Foy, Québec, Canada, G1V 4G5. Fax: (418) 656-4762

**Claudio F. Donner:** Fondazione Salavatore Maugeri, Clinica del Lavoro e Della Riabilitazione, Via per Revislate 13, 28010 Veruno, Italy. **cfdonner@fsm.it.** Fax: 39 0322 884776.

**Paul Dubach:** Kantonsspital Chur, Loestrasse 170, CH 7000, Chur, Switzerland. **paul.dubach@ksc.gr.ch.** Fax: 0041 81 256 66 61.

**Barry A. Franklin:** Beaumont Rehabilitation and Health Center, Cardiac Rehabilitation Department, 746 Purdy Street, Birmingham, Missouri 48009, United States of America. **bfranklin@beaumont.edu.** Fax: (248) 258-1392.

**Victor Froelicher:** Palo Alto Veterans Affairs Medical Center, Bldg 100, Room E2-441, 3801 Miranda Ave., Palo Alto, California 94304, United States of America. **vicmd@aol.com.** Fax: (650) 852-3473.

**Roger S. Goldstein:** West Park Hospital, 82 Buttonwood, Toronto, Ontario, Canada, M6M 2J5. **rgoldstein@westpark.org.** Fax: (416) 243-8947.

**Jean-Marie Grosbois:** CLEFAR, 69 rue de la Louvière, 59800 Lille, France. **jmgrosbois@nordnet.fr.** Fax: 03 20 55 02 50.

**Robert G. Haennel:** Faculty of Kinesiology and Health Studies, University of Regina, 3737 Wascana Parkway, Regina, Saskatchewan, Canada, S4S 0A2. **Bob.Haennel@uregina.ca.** Fax: (306) 585-4854.

**Dawn M. Hamilton:** Cardiovascular Research Unit, Pacemaker Clinic, Rm 3B 02.03, Regina General Hospital, 1440, 14th Ave., Regina, Sakatchewan, Canada, S4P 0W5. **DHamilton@ReginaHealth.sk.ca.** Fax: (306) 766-4177.

**William G. Herbert:** Department of Human Nutrition, Foods and Exercise, 213 War Memorial Hall, Virginia Tech, Blacksburg, Virginia 24061, United States of America. **wgherb@vt.edu.** Fax: (540) 231-8476.

**Jean Jobin:** Institut universitaire de cardiologie et de pneumologie, Hôpital Laval, 2725 chemin Ste-Foy, Sainte-Foy, Québec, Canada, G1V 4G5. Fax: (418) 656-4617

**Martin Juneau:** Institut de cardiologie de Montréal, 5000 rue Bélanger Est, Montréal, Québec, Canada, H1T 1C8. **juneau@icm.umontreal.ca.** Fax: (514) 376-7782.

**Mike King:** Biotronik Life Systems Canada Inc., Suite 201, 19292 60th Ave., Surrey, British Columbia, Canada, V3S 8E5. **MichaelKing2@compuserve.com.** Fax: (604) 514-3780.

**Yves Lacasse:** Institut universitaire de cardiologie et de pneumologie, Hôpital Laval, 2725 chemin Ste-Foy, Sainte-Foy, Québec, Canada, G1V 4G5. **Yves.Lacasse@med.ulaval.ca.** Fax: (418) 656-4762

**Marie-Hélène Leblanc:** Institut universitaire de cardiologie et de pneumologie, Hôpital Laval, 2725 chemin Ste-Foy, Sainte-Foy, Québec, Canada, G1V 4G5. **d.goulet@ssss.gouv.qc.ca.** Fax: (418) 656-4562.

**Pierre LeBlanc:** Institut universitaire de cardiologie et de pneumologie, Hôpital Laval, 2725 chemin Ste-Foy, Sainte-Foy, Québec, Canada, G1V 4G5. **Pierre.Leblanc@med.ulaval.ca.** Fax: (418) 656-4762

**François Maltais:** Institut universitaire de cardiologie et de pneumologie, Hôpital Laval, 2725 chemin Ste-Foy, Sainte-Foy, Québec, Canada, G1V 4G5. **medfma@hermes.ulaval.ca.** Fax: (418) 656-4762

**Dany Michel Marcadet:** 23 rue Georges Bizet, 75116 Paris. **dmarcadet@dial.oleane.com.** Fax: 01 47 20 17 67.

**Claudia Mosimann:** Kantonsspital Chur, Loestrasse 170, CH 7000, Chur, Switzerland.

**Jonathan Myers:** Palo Alto Veterans Affairs Medical Center, Bldg 100, Room E2-441, 3801 Miranda Ave., Palo Alto, California 94304, United States of America. **drj993@aol.com.** Fax: (650) 852-3473.

**Denis E. O'Donnell:** Queens University, 102 Stuart Street, Kingston, Ontario, Canada, K7L 3N6. **Odonnell@post.queensu.ca.** Fax: (613) 549-1459.

**Carmen Paquette:** Institut universitaire de cardiologie et de pneumologie, Hôpital Laval, 2725 chemin Ste-Foy, Sainte-Foy, Québec, Canada, G1V 4G5. Fax: (418) 656-4581.

**Lee M. Pierson:** Duke University Medical Center, DUMC Box 3119, Durham, North Carolina 27710, United States of America. **piers003@mc.duke.edu.**

**Bruno Pilote:** Institut universitaire de cardiologie et de pneumologie, Hôpital Laval, 2725 chemin Ste-Foy, Sainte-Foy, Québec, Canada, G1V 4G5. Fax: (418) 656-4617.

**Paul Poirier:** Institut universitaire de cardiologie et de pneumologie, Hôpital Laval, 2725 chemin Ste-Foy, Sainte-Foy, Québec, Canada, G1V 4G5. **Paul.Poirier@crhl.ulaval.ca.** Fax: (418) 656-4581.

**Christian Préfaut:** Hôpital Arnaud de Villeneuve, 371 Avenue du Doyen Giraud, 34295 Montpellier, Cedex 5, France. **c-prefaut@chu-montpellier.fr.** Fax: 011 33 04 67 33 59 23.

**Susan E. Quaglietti:** Palo Alto VA Health Care System, 3801 Miranda Avenue, Palo Alto, California 94304, United States of America. Fax: (650) 852-3473. **squaglietti@aol.com**

**Susan M. Revill:** Ashfield Community Hospital, Kirby-in-Ashfield, Nottinghamshire, NG17 7AE, United Kingdom. **sue.revill@ach.cnhc-tr.trent.nhs.uk** Fax: 011 44 1623 784782.

**Paul M. Ribisl:** Wake Forest University, Box 7868, Winston-Salem, North Carolina, NC 27109, United States of America. **ribisl@wfu.edu.** Fax: (910) 759-4680.

**Didier Saey:** Institut universitaire de cardiologie et de pneumologie, Hôpital Laval, 2725 chemin Ste-Foy, Sainte-Foy, Québec, Canada, G1V 4G5.

**Catherine T. Sharp:** Peace Arch Hospital Rehabilitation, 15521 Russell Ave., White Rock, British Columbia, Canada, V4B 2R4. **catherine.sharp@southfraserhealth.com** Fax: (306) 585-4854.

**Michael T. Sharratt:** Department of Kinesiology, University of Waterloo, Waterloo, Ontario, Canada, N2L 3G1. **sharratt@healthy.uwaterloo.ca.** Fax: (519) 746-6776.

**Katerina Shetler:** Palo Alto Veterans Affairs Medical Center, Bldg 100, Room E2-441, 3801 Miranda Ave., Palo Alto, California 94304, United States of America. Fax: (650) 852-3473.

**Sebastian Sixt:** Kantonsspital Chur, Loestrasse 170, CH 7000, Chur, Switzerland.

**Clermont Simard:** Département d'éducation physique, Université Laval, Québec, Québec, Canada, G1K 7P4. **Clermont.Simard@edp.ulaval.ca.** Fax: (418) 656-3020.

**Martin J. Sullivan:** Duke University Medical Center, 1300 Moreene Road, Box 3022, DUMC, Durham, North Carolina 27710, United States of America. **sulli003@mc.duke.edu.** Fax: (919) 681-8376.

**Pier Luigi Temporelli:** Division of Cardiology, Salvatorre Maugeri Foundation, IRCCS, Via Revisloate 13, 28010 Veruno, Italy. **pltemporelli@fsm.it.** Fax: 011 39 03 22 83 02 94.

**David R. Thompson:** Department of Health Sciences, University of York, Genesis 6, York Science Park, York Y01 5DQ, United Kingdom. **drt2@york.ac.uk.** Fax: 011 44 1904 434102.

**Katherine A. Webb:** Respiratory Investigation Unit, Kingston General Hospital, 76 Stuart Street, Kingston, Ontario, Canada, K7L 2V7. **kw2@post.queensu.ca.** Fax: (613) 548-1307.

**Philip K. Wilson:** 423 N. 24th Street, La Crosse, Wisconsin, WI 54601, United States of America. **pkwilson@centurytel.net.** Fax: (608) 788-1479.

# Acknowledgments

The editors wish to thank Dr. Jean Deslauriers for his outstanding work as ad hoc editor of the original manuscripts. We also want to acknowledge the excellent work of Mr. Réjean Lamontagne, MA, as coordinator and technical assistant in the preparation of this book.

PART I

# Introduction

Chapter 1

# Conceptualization and Evolution of Cardiopulmonary Rehabilitation— Toward a New Paradigm

Jean Jobin, PhD, François Maltais, MD, Paul Poirier, MD, Pierre LeBlanc, MD, Clermont Simard, PhD, Canada

## Introduction

Since the explosion of cardiac surgery around the second half of the 20$^{th}$ century, cardiopulmonary Rehabilitation has been defined by many institutions such as the World Health Organization (WHO) (1), and more recently, the American Association of Cardio-Vascular and Pulmonary Rehabilitation (AACVPR) (2,3), in the following words: *Rehabilitation is the sum of activities necessary to restore or maintain an optimal level of physiological, psychological, social, occupational, and emotional functioning* (4).

## Rehabilitation: A Systemic and Wholesome approach

This definition is usually interpreted in the light of the mechanistic paradigms of conventional medicine. In the mind of the authors of this paper, however, rehabilitation ought to be systemic and wholesome in its approach, implying that these activities must be integrated and coordinated together in a holistic way. Furthermore, and contrary to what is most often conceptualized, the object of rehabilitation should not be the patient's disease but rather the person, and the person as a whole. The main goal of rehabilitation is not only to reintegrate the individual into society and life in the most efficient possible way, but also to make him move forward because most human beings are always trying to reach higher levels of achievement. To reach these goals, the rehabilitation process must start with an integrated and coordinated plan of action around a "person", the "rehabilitatee" (main actor), and the plan must be coordinated by the "rehabilitator", which acts as a guide and companion to the main actor.

This implies that rehabilitation must integrate education, adaptive interventions, and medical care as they are needed by the patient. With this approach, rehabilitation envisions the person as a complex web made of a multitude of characteristics integrated in a unique fashion. Some of these numerous characteristics include age, sociocultural identity, physical, biological, psychological, and spiritual environments, health and morbidity statuses, gender, etc., emphazising the concept of complexity. The person (not the disease) to rehabilitate is not simply complicated, it is incredibly complex. It is not merely a juxtaposition of structures and functions as frequently envisioned by conventional mechanistic medical paradigms. In fact, cardiopulmonary rehabilitation would be a perfect fit for the approach promoted by the new integrative medicine paradigm now being developed all around the world (For more details, see chapter 9 by Sullivan).

It is in that perspective that we envision the new paradigm of cardiopulmonary rehabilitation. Unfortunately, rehabilitation is often reduced to one or few of its components or to a non-integrated mixture of multiple interventions, most often oriented toward the disease status of the patient. For example, we often reduce rehabilitation to interventions that we, as health care professionals, most often use and these often carry with them our specific and biased ways of seeing the world. These interventions, be it education, exercise, physical therapy, psychological counseling, pharmacological treatments, etc., are not rehabilitation if they are not integrated with other interventions. The person as a whole must remain its primary object in a context of an optimal reintegration in society with as much autonomy as possible.

## Rehabilitation is not Secondary Prevention Alone

Thus reducing the rehabilitation process to secondary prevention alone, (as often done in cardiac rehabilitation) disables the whole process. In this instance, the object of prevention is not the person but rather the disease as assessed through risk factors which are often taken as separate entities, or one or a few at the time. This does not mean that these actions are useless but that they are rather not done under the new rehabilitation paradigm. For us, these new concepts must be developed rapidly in order to widen the frontiers limiting the development and expansion of cardiopulmonary rehabilitation. Cardiopulmonary rehabilitation must be integrated under a new rehabilitation paradigm instead of under the traditional cardiovascular and pulmonary care paradigms.

This is even more important because the consequences of cardiovascular diseases, for instance, are not as easily observable as they used to. Indeed, medical and surgical treatments have improved in such a way over the past two decades that the physical consequences of the disease or of surgical interventions such as open heart surgery or PTCA have been reduced to almost none. Similarly, the psychosocial "side effects" of these interventions are often underestimated when not simply discarded. The evidence (5) and the day to day practice of cardiac rehabilitation teaches us however that these patients are clearly in great need of rehabilitation through physical, psychological, sociological and spiritual interventions. As secondary prevention programs tend to advocate, it can also be done through actions aiming at preventing relapses or evolution of the disease.

## Rehabilitation Should not be Limited to the Medical Community

Another problem limiting further developments of cardiopulmonary rehabilitation is that the medical community often uses some misunderstanding of the mechanisms of action to justify its limited involvement and inaction (4,6). It is often an excuse to cover up lack of knowledge, unconscious, more self serving motivations, and easiness. Contrary to conventional medical treatments where health professionals control the game, the patient is the main actor in a true rehabilitation process, as it should also be

the case in true prevention processes. The concept of the patient as a whole (physical, psychological, sociological and spiritual) is currently being developed in contemporary integrative medicine and in some non-conventional traditional medicines. Are the medical and allied health professions ready to let go of their control on diseases and let the patient take control of the healing process and of his health? In rehabilitation the "rehabilitator" is a guide to a human being who becomes complementary to the actor. Unfortunately, very few cardiopulmonary rehabilitation professionals currently share this wisdom. If the patient is to become the actor, he must be aware of his role and more information must be made available to him and to the public in general. This information must stress the possible impacts of rehabilitation on health status and healing process.

At the onset of the Third Millennium, the history and tradition of cardiopulmonary rehabilitation must be moved forward by highly dedicated individuals who will help to keep it in harmony with the novel orientations of health services and with the integrity of the human being in constant development. In cardiopulmonary rehabilitation, these two entities, history and tradition, have been both strongly dependant on the actions of the medical establishment which has served it very well so far. Consequently, they are primarily and largely structured around a more mechanistic (conventional) medical paradigm, oriented toward patient care and most often not taking into account the bio-psycho-socio-spiritual needs of individuals suffering from cardiopulmonary diseases or having received a surgical or other invasive procedure (5,7).

## Rehabilitation: A Way Toward Autonomy

Under the new rehabilitation paradigm, and complementary to the standard medical paradigm, cardiopulmonary rehabilitation would give better wholesome consideration to ill organs/systems. It would take into account the impact of the disease on other bodily components and personal characteristics, and its interaction with the psychosocial environment of the individual affected by this morbid state. One has to bear in mind that the rehabilitation candidate is in search not only of a new living balance so that he or she can compensate for the lost one, but also of a better functional secure autonomy. As the population of patients with cardiovascular and pulmonary diseases is getting older, autonomy has become a new societal goal that cardiopulmonary rehabilitation must embrace.

As cardiopulmonary rehabilitation specialists, we must refocus our professional ethics by revisiting some of our interventions. Even now, available services are seldom designed by people who have a wholesome vision of a person, and who could, through specific actions, respond to the well identified needs of that person. Evidently, cardiopulmonary rehabilitation is dependent on many different corpuses of knowledge, as well as on specialists from different disciplines, and it must try to reach multidimensional goals. One must try to develop pedagogical actions that will allow true interactions with patients through a medico-educative approach oriented primarily toward an individual in need of rehabilitation. All of this must be done in a given psychosocial, cultural and spiritual make up.

In both directions, whether it is a change from normal to morbid status, or back to a more healthy status, the individual is always searching for his own evolving self balance. Because this self balance is constantly changing, the rehabilitation team must work in reciprocity with the individual, acknowledging that factors determining morbidity and healing status are the prime responsibility of the patient and of the care giving and rehabilitative teams. The person in a rehabilitative process, as well as the acting team of health care professionals, must be sensibilized to this aspect. Through this sensibilization process, everyone's roles will be better defined, understood and organized and consequently, the eventual outcomes will be more valuable. Thus every one will feel more dynamically and totally involved in the normalization/developmental process. All of this should lead to changes in attitude, behavior, life style and moral values.

Even though we agree with the following principles often adopted by public health services (8), we are convinced that to restrain cardiopulmonary rehabilitation to secondary prevention is a mistake because it keeps the latter away from the new rehabilitation paradigm:

Preventive services must:

"1—Develop or improve mobilization of the community around intense and diversified actions on promotion of healthy life styles such as physical activity, nutrition, and non-smoking;

2—Put the emphasis on personal initiatives, self help, creation of environments leading to improved health, integration of prevention into clinical practices, reinforcing of inter-sector actions as well as the implications of partners". (ad lib translation)

Of course these goals must be part of any prevention program as well as of any rehabilitative interventions. Although, in an ideal world, health must embrace all components of the person and his environment, it must be underlined that prevention, as applied and usually thought of in contemporary medicine, concerns only the disease hosted by the body of the person involved or a disease affecting a cohort of people as in public health services. Ultimately, prevention does everything so that death is delayed as long as possible. More specifically, its main objective is that a given patient does not die from his current disease (cardiovascular, pulmonary, cancer etc.); it often considers only one disease at a time. Although these goals represent almost the whole spectrum of prevention, they are only a minor part of the rehabilitation paradigm.

Indeed, one must rehabilitate without doing any harm. One must also prevent progression of the disease as well as decrease the number of relapses. Even after having accomplish that much, one will have done very little to reintegrate the patient in his psycho-sociological-biological-spiritual-cultural-physical environment, which is one of the specific goals of rehabilitation.

In fact, these preventive objectives do not really address the issue of the person as a whole. They are too often based on the conventional mechanistic medical paradigm. It is therefore clear that the goals of prevention and more specifically of secondary prevention do not include the main objectives of rehabilitation. On the other hand, rehabilitation must include some level of prevention (primary or secondary) because it would make no sense to rehabilitate someone if we let the disease progress, or let the patient die prematurely while he is working so hard to reach some degree of optimization of a new self balance. This is why we do not believe that prevention, let alone secondary prevention, is a panacea and could replace rehabilitation altogether. Some even have the perception that, organizationally and financially, cardiopulmonary rehabilitation may lose significantly by being identified exclusively to prevention, be it secondary (9). We are further convinced that putting rehabilitation as a sub-unit of a prevention program would be dangerously reducing its own perspective and efficacy. Secondary prevention must however be an integrated part of any good rehabilitative intervention as recently described by Ades (10).

In the same vein, it does not make much sense to reduce cardiopulmonary rehabilitation to a single health discipline. When taken individually, for instance, physical therapy or psychology counseling do not consider the person as a whole. In cardiovascular rehabilitation, where physical and even musculo-skeletal interventions are now considered important components (11,12), it is difficult to envision that typical therapy will embrace the whole of the needs of the patient if we admit that many side effects other than physical may be experienced (5) following these interventions. The same reasoning can be applied to pulmonary patients. Because of what we currently know about the impact of cardiovascular and pulmonary diseases on skeletal muscle (11,12), psychological interventions alone would have a limited beneficial rehabilitative impact.

Thus, physical therapy, as well as prevention programs mostly aims at reducing disease specific symptoms or casualties, cannot be considered substitutes for rehabilitation. A cardiac rehabilitation program may be considered a secondary prevention program, but not the opposite, unless the former adopts all of the objectives of true rehabilitative interventions as we have tried to conceptualize them.

## Rehabilitation: Toward a New Integrated Approach

Because of these concepts, many experts now think that cardiopulmonary rehabilitation must be reoriented and re-developed around the new rehabilitation paradigm. Accordingly, our group has expressed interesting leads and thoughts on this matter (13). It appears essential that all institutions, supported by judiciously selected experts representing the broadest possible set of views, develop concerted efforts for the benefit of the largest number of individuals. This recommendation implies that we have no restriction on knowledge and practice and that knowledge flows freely between all types of health care professionals as well as to and from patients. This would help avoiding the pyramid like effect (knowledge flowing from the physician down to all others including the patient) (figure 1.1) that we most often see in the context of the conventional mechanistic medical paradigm. We should have a star like model, the patient

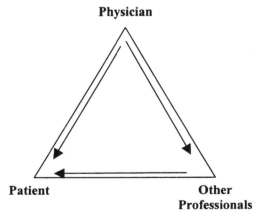

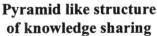

**Pyramid like structure
of knowledge sharing**

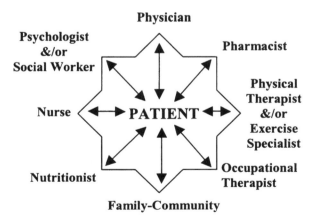

**Star like structure
of knowledge sharing
(number of arms unlimited)**

**Figure 1.1**   Schematic representation of the flow of knowledge-interactions in rehabilitation.

being the center of interest of all others (including health care professionals, and community-family members alike), and the information flowing in all directions. This concept does not mean that there should not be a leader, but only that the leadership may come from numerous potential sources. As an example, the scientific sessions of the Québec International Symposium on Cardiopulmonary Rehabilitation are presented side by side with public type informative sessions for the lay person (Le Salon de la Santé de Québec", "The Québec City Health Show"). Similarly, we can focus on some scientific subjects being presented in more popular events such as the VIII[th] World Congress of Sports for All held in Québec city in 2000 (14). This also implies that cardiopulmonary rehabilitation must be accessible to any person in need of it or willing to benefit from it. Any kind of patient selection or restriction as it is sometimes (15) suggested is unwarranted when one looks at the proven benefits of rehabilitation (4,6,10).

Researchers, scholars, and clinicians must unanimously support the obligation to improve the quality of life of the greatest possible number of people suffering from cardiopulmonary insufficiency. We hope that cardiopulmonary rehabilitation will become an essential service beginning as soon as the disease or multiple risk factors have been identified and that it will accompany patients along with other medical-health services in an integrated fashion.

The impacts of cardiopulmonary rehabilitation on the stabilization of quality of life as well as on its improvement are numerous (4,6,10). How to offer it without delay to as many patients as possible is still a contemporary preoccupation and answers will likely come from concertation between many different partners. In this matter, the United Kingdom (16) leads the way and although the numbers are still relatively small (from 10% in post-infarct to 56% in post CABG patients), the percentage of patients engaged in cardiac rehabilitation is higher than in any other location around the world including the Province of Québec (17). Because similar numbers are also characteristic of pulmonary rehabilitation, cardiopulmonary rehabilitation as a whole remains largely underused (4,6) world wide.

This enlarged vision implies that all specialists, like those from health services, education, communication, and leaders form the public and private sectors, including non profit charitable organizations to name a few, must work together under a new unified paradigm aiming at making cardiop-

ulmonary rehabilitation services available to all segments of the population. Further, and as illustrated by the Framingham study (18) where cultural factors have been recently considered, one must look forward to new research activities, as well as to increase the place of preventive approaches in rehabilitation.

Unfortunately, and this is our challenge, cardiopulmonary rehabilitation is and remains for many health care professionals and decision making people a reality that is still far away (4,6,17). The 30 chapters included in this volume present this ever evolving area of knowledge and practice as conceptualized by some of the most outstanding leaders in their fields.

## About This Book

In 2001, Québec City was for the second time, (the first being held in 1999) (13), the theatre of an international symposium involving a group of outstanding international experts in cardiopulmonary rehabilitation sciences. The main theme of this event, which regrouped over 500 participants from 23 different countries, was: *"Integrating Cardiopulmonary Rehabilitation to the Treatment of the Disease"*. Thirty experts presented their thoughts in 9 different colloquia. This book includes selected papers prepared by the speakers and for most of them, the contents are more extensive than what was actually presented at the Symposium. All these 30 papers are original. The great majority are review articles, and a few are the presentation of original research work. Chapters have been regrouped in 11 sections representing the 9 colloquia of the Symposium, plus the opening statement presented in section 1 (Introduction). In the spirit of the symposium, the editors have prepared two challenging papers to introduce and conclude the book. The 11 sections are presented in a logical order as they would normally occur in a cardiopulmonary rehabilitation program:

1. Introduction
2. Cardiopulmonary Rehabilitation: Services and Organization
3. Update in the Pharmacological and Non-Pharmacological Treatment of CHF and COPD Patients
4. Integrating New Technologies in Cardiopulmonary Rehabilitation
5. Home Rehabilitation Programs

In this book, no restrictions were put on authors as to which school of thoughts they are part of or are representing. The authors were free to use the format they felt best conveyed their message. Different ideas are presented and the reader must be ready and able to confront contradictory or opposing points of view on how to interpret the body of knowledge at our disposal at the onset of this Millennium. This book is not comprehensive and several topics have been unfortunately left out, without prejudice, mostly because of the limited duration of the Second Symposium during which they were presented.

The reader might be interested to know that abstracts of these papers as well as of the 60 posters presented at the Second Québec International Symposium on Cardiopulmonary Rehabilitation have been published in a supplement of Clinical & Investigative Medicine (19).

# References

1. World Health Organization. Expert Committee. *Rehabilitation of patients with cardiovascular Disease.* Technical report series no 270. Geneva: World Health Organisation, 1964.
2. American Association of CardioVascular and Pulmonary Rehabilitation. Guildelines for Pulmonary Rehabilitation Programs. Champaign, Human Kinetics, 2nd Ed., 1998.
3. American Association of CardioVascular and Pulmonary Rehabilitation. Guildelines for Cardiac Rehabilitation and Secondary Prevention Programs. Champaign, Human Kinetics, 3rd Ed., 1999.
4. Jobin J, Maltais F, Poirier P. La réadaptation cardiorespiratoire: l'intervention sous-utilisée. Le médecin du Québec, 36 (4):97-111, 2001.
5. Denber H.C.B. Cardiac Surgery: Biological and Psychological Implications. Harmonk, Futura publishing, p. 250, 1995.
6. Maltais F., Jobin J., Simard C., LeBlanc P. Cardiopulmonary Rehabilitation in Clinical Practice: The Underused Intervention. In: Jobin J., Maltais F., LeBlanc P., Simard C. Advances in Cardiopulmonary Rehabilitation. Champaign, Human Kinetics, p. 303-306, 2000.
7. Pinsky JL, Jette AM, Branch LG, Kannel WB, Feinleib M. The Framingham Disability Study: relationship of various coronary heart disease manifestations to disability in older persons living in the community. Am J Public Health 80: 1363-7, 1990.
8. Direction de la Santé publique de Québec. Cibles d'action en promotion de la santé et en prévention pour la période 2000-2003. Régie régionale de la santé et des services sociaux de Québec. Bibliothèque nationale du Québec, p. 7, 2000.
9. Dumont S. Cardiovascular Rehabilitation: A Concept in Search of Its Identity. In: Jobin J., Maltais F., LeBlanc P., Simard C. Advances in Cardiopulmonary Rehabilitation. Champaign, Human Kinetics, p. 20-30, 2000.
10. Ades P A. Cardiac Rehabilitation and secondary prevention of Coronary Heart Disease. N Engl J Med, 345(12):892-902, 2001.
11. Jobin J, Doyon J-F. Peripheral Muscle Limitations to Exercise in Patients With Congestive Heart Failure: Implications For Rehabilitation. In: Jobin J., Maltais F., LeBlanc P., Simard C. Advances in Cardiopulmonary Rehabilitation. Champaign, Human Kinetics, p. 90-104, 2000.
12. Maltais F, Jobin J, LeBlanc P. Peripheral Muscle Dysfunction in Patients with Chronic Obstructive Pulmonary Disease. In: Jobin J., LeBlanc P., Simard C. Advances in Cardiopulmonary Rehabilitation. Champaign, Human Kinetics, p. 105-126. 2000.
13. Jobin J., Maltais F., LeBlanc P., Simard C. (eds). Advances in Cardiopulmonary Rehabilitation. Champaign, Human Kinetics, p. 322, 2000.
14. Jobin J., Doyon J.F., Leblanc P., Leblanc M.H., Allaire J., Maltais F., Simard C. Excitabilité des neurones moteurs et stratégies de recrutement d'unités motrices dans les membres inférieurs de patients souffrant d'insuffisance cardiaque chronique : Indices d'anomalie dans les stratégies de recrutement. Le Sport pour Tous et les politiques gouvernementales - Sport for All and Governmental Policies. VIIIe Congrès Mondial du Sport pour Tous – VIII World Sport for All Congress, p. 162, 2000.

15. Dafoe W. Selection of Best Candidates for Cardiac Rehabilitation in the Furture. In : Jobin J., Maltais F., LeBlanc P., Simard C. Advances in Cardiopulmonary Rehabilitation. Champaign, Human Kinetics, p. 54-62, 2000.

16. Bethell H.J.N., Turner S.C., Evans J.A., Rose L. Cardiac Rehabilitation in the United Kingdom. J C R.; 21(2):111-115, 2001.

17. Jobin J., Maltais F., Simard C., LeBlanc P. Current and Future Issues in Cardiopulmonary Rehabilitation. In : Jobin J., Maltais F., LeBlanc P., Simard C. Advances in Cardiopulmonary Rehabilitation. Champaign, Human Kinetics, p. 1-5, 2000.

18. LaMonte M.J., Durstine J.L., Addy C.L., Irwin M.L., Ainsworth B.E. Physical Activity, Physical Fitness, and Framingham 10-Years Risk Score: The Cross-Cultural Activity Participation Study. J C R. 21(2)63-72, 2001.

19. Jobin J, LeBlanc P, Maltais F, Poirier P, Simard C, Eds. Clin. Invest. Med., Suppl. Vol 24, No 3: S1-S64, 2001.

Chapter 2

# Historical Perspective on Integrated Cardiopulmonary Rehabilitation: From Hippocrates to Québec City

Christian Préfaut, MD, France

It is with deep happiness, and emotion that I thank the organizing committee of this congress for giving me the honor of making the opening statement. I have entitled my talk "From Hippocrates to Québec".

I chose Hippocrates because I am from the University of Montpellier where the seal of the Medical School makes reference to Hippocrates. Indeed, the school motto, which may be a bit pretentious, reads as follows "Hippocrates came from Cos and now he is Montpellierain". Montpellier is the oldest existing school of medicine in the Western world and many Arab and Jewish physicians, originally taught by Hippocrates brought his knowledge to Montpellier. Although somewhat embellished, the teaching of Hippocrates was usually presented in its original form. For this reason, Montpellier has always thought of itself as the direct descendent of Hippocrates.

The first question to be asked could be the following: What did Hippocrates think of rehabilitation? I have here portions of a long text written by Hippocrates on respiratory illnesses and more specifically on "the third phthisis". What was this third phthisis? Hippocrates describes phthistic patients as follows: "These patients have a yellowish expectoration and are subject to choking. They may often present with chills and fever and thus likely have secondary infections. The third phthisis generally lasts a little less than ten years, after which the patient dies." We might just wonder if this is not a reference to what is today known as chronic obstructive pulmonary disease. What was Hippocrates' advice with regards to treatment remembering that he was known to be very close to nature and natural solutions? He had a very precise treatment strategy that included the use of astringent white wine, in addition to other medications. When a patient

was under his care, he initially ordered him to walk 20 stades per day, one stade being the equivalent of 180 meters. During the second month, the patient was to walk 10 additional stades, and these distances were to be done before and after dinner. After the fourth month, he asked his patients to walk at least 80 stades each day (14,400 meters). He finally recommended that the distance be increased by five stades per day up to a total of 150 stades each day. At this point, the walking was done in the morning as well as before and after dinner. What is most extraordinary is that Hippocrates concluded that the patient who followed his treatment plan (including physical rehabilitation) was cured after one year of treatment. It therefore seems clear that rehabilitation was already integrated into the treatment of respiratory disorders more than 2500 years ago.

Since I've entitled my talk "From Hippocrates to Quebec", I would like to introduce the topics that will be discussed in Quebec by asking questions that I think can be regrouped into three main categories.

If rehabilitation is to be integrated into the treatment of an illness, the first concern must be the repercussion of rehabilitation on the standard of care of that particular illness and the second the repercussion of treatment on rehabilitation. Will treatment have an effect on how we prescribe rehabilitation in patients receiving beta-blockers, or patients with pacemakers for instance? Will rehabilitation modify traditional treatments? For example, do we need to reduce the amount of hypoglycemic drugs in our diabetic cardiovascular or respiratory patients? Will the oxygen flow in oxygen-dependent patients be reduced by exercise training, or by rehabilitation? Obviously, there are important interrelations between classic treatments and rehabilitation and these must always be taken into account.

I would like for a moment to go back to the issue of oxygen treatment. Can rehabilitation delay the need for oxygen treatment in COPD patients? Considering the overall costs of oxygen therapy as well as individual costs to long-term users, this is an important question which unfortunately is seldom raised and has been overlooked by most investigators. A second important but perhaps more personal question could be the following: What should we do with patients who have exercise-induced desaturation or exercise-induced hypoxia? In a cohort of 200 COPD patients, we found that 60% of individuals desaturated during the walk test while 40% did not. We further divided patients into those who were on long term oxygen therapy and those who were not ($PaO_2 > 60mmHg$). As expected, we found that the majority of oxygen-dependent patients (75%) desaturated. However, 50% of patients with a $PaO_2 > 60$ mmHg, also showed desaturation during a simple walk test. In absolute numbers, this represents 50 individuals to whom we offered oxygen for use during walking. Interestingly, all patients refused and perhaps this is something to think about.

Although rehabilitation can easily be integrated into everyday treatment, questions such as for whom, where, when and how are still unanswered?

In theory, all cardiorespiratory patients could benefit from rehabilitation even if practically, it is not for everyone. Who should be the priority patient? Is it the one with the most severe signs or the one with the worse functional data even if there is discordance between clinical signs and results of testing? Is it the one who has evidence of impaired peripheral muscle function or exercise intolerance or is it for both? What about the patient who has undergone cardiac or pulmonary surgery? These individuals often participate in postoperative rehabilitation programs, but should rehabilitation also be indispensable before surgery? It is even possible that rehabilitation before LVRS might allow some patients to be taken off the operative list. Is it possible that in the future, rehabilitation will be prescribed prophylactically?

Where should rehabilitation be done? Is it best done at the hospital or can it be done on an ambulatory outpatient basis? Can efficient training be done at home? And if we train patients at home, is it safe to do so? These are fundamental questions that I hope will be answered during this symposium.

Should pretreatment evaluation be the same for patients in the hospital versus those who are ambulatory? Do we have indicators as to what are the best tests? For instance, are invasive methods such as cardiac catheterization always indispensable to evaluate the cardiac status? Can we forecast that one day these invasive tests will be replaced by less invasive ones? We also know that there is a need to explore the incapacity, and the handicap. It is better to explore one or the other, or should they always be both evaluated? I do not have an answer for this question.

Up until now, I have been formulating lots of questions for which I unfortunately have very few answers. If you allow me, I would now like to turn to another type of exercise by asking you a multiple-choice question about dyspnea. I have been told that it is absolutely indispensable to quantify dyspnea during an exercise test. Is it also indispensable to evaluate the patient's impairment in order to prescribe the appropriate level of exercise training, and evaluate the efficacy of the exercise program? You have all answered this question, and I agree that all possible answers are correct.

Since dyspnea must be assessed during an exercise test, some physicians think that walking tests will soon supplant the more classical incremental exercise tests. Here again, I would like to show you some data. In 109 consecutive patients with COPD, we studied desaturation during a maximal incremental exercise test on a cycle ergometer and during a 6-minute walking test. During the incremental test, 16.6% of patients experienced desaturation. Two days later the same patients performed the 6-minute walking test and again these same 16.6% showed desaturation. However, 28 % of those who did not desaturate during the ergometer test did so during the walking test. So perhaps the walking test is a better type of examination for diagnosing desaturation. Will it replace the incremental cycling test? I do not know, yet.

What are some of the novel issues in rehabilitation? One question that seems important concerns the usefulness of strength or resistance training. Although we do not have definitive answers, there is increasing evidence indicating that we need to introduce at least a minimum of strength training in rehabilitation programs. What is the best training intensity for endurance training? Should it be high or low intensity? Would ventilatory assistance help to improve the performance results in cardiopulmonary illnesses?

Since integration has now become an important word in our terminology, we have at the very heart of rehabilitation two treatments that are perfectly integrated. These are the symptomatic treatment such as exercise training or physical therapy, and the psychological treatment and social support of the same patient through education, counseling, support groups, and so on. While writing this paper, I also wondered about other questions. Is there anyone in this room who thinks that, if a patient is incapable of stopping smoking we should postpone training programs, or that he or she should not even begin one? Should we withhold rehabilitation when we know that, although the improvements will be less striking, the program will still improve the patient's condition and may even help in the battle to stop smoking?

Since psychological support is so important, how can we bring the patient's significant others—the husband or wife, for example—into the overall program? Lastly, what are the real effects of this approach? The results are indeed difficult to evaluate. Do we even have the elements to determine whether a psychosocial approach can prevent disease progression?

At the end of this brief introduction, I have the firm conviction that we will be hearing presentations of very great interest during the symposium. I thank the organizing committee for their fine work and like most of you, I am convinced that rehabilitation should be a fundamental part of our treatment of patients with chronic respiratory diseases.

PART II

# Cardiopulmonary Rehabilitation: Services & Organization

# Chapter 3

# Distance-Based Technology Applied to Cardiopulmonary Rehabilitation

Michael T. Sharratt, PhD, Canada

## Introduction

Distance-based medicine/telehealth, whether rural or urban, using physicians, nurse practitioners and other health professionals, is going to be the biggest change in health-care that we see in our lifetime.

That prediction is based on the recent explosion of information highway communications along with the escalating growth of electronic technology infrastructure. There have been over one-quarter million "hits" on the word telemedicine with 95% of them coming in the past five years. Telephone companies have laid fibre-optic cable at an unprecedented rate (although much of it is currently sitting unused as "dark fibre") and the race is on to see who will win the financial bonanza of providing affordable wireless capacity in every home. As Robinson points out, the healthcare Internet industry "stands at the end of its beginning" (1).

It's fair to say that Health Informatics is a very hot topic with most governments these days. In the face of potential physician and nurse shortages, there is a concerted effort to explore creative ways of delivering effective service including telehomecare (2). Even before people have need of the health-care system, there is an expanding commitment by governments to provide equal access to correct health information regardless of geographical or other barriers.

To that end, information technology is having a profound impact. Specifically, computers and the Internet have become the technological communication tools which are shrinking the world. Virtually anybody now has access to information, even rehabilitation services which formerly may have been prohibitive in terms of time, effort and expense. However, the seduction of computer engagement may be at the expense of human relationships. Some advocates fail to appreciate that "technology is only a tool, a means to an end, not an end in itself" (3).

At this point in time, there is no guarantee that the health information and/or rehabilitation strategies which are readily available on the Internet... are actually correct (4). In fact, one estimate is that up to two-thirds of the current health information on the Internet is faulty, misleading or downright dangerous.

Therefore, the challenge is substantial for individual consumers and health professionals. Using computers to the information highway, there will be unlimited potential to access credible and verifiable information that can guide prevention. Web-based interactive cardiac disease courses are already available for continuing education or as distance-based courses for academic credit. With on-line education, everybody gets a front-row seat.

In addition to home-based education, there are exciting opportunities for interactive cardiopulmonary rehabilitation that can be tailored to a person's individual circumstances. By bringing the workout into the home or business, there is flexibility to respond to hectic schedules that may involve juggling both career and family.

## Definitions

There are so many electronic terms that it is easy to become bogged down and miss the big picture. It seems reasonable, at least operationally, to consider "informatics" as the broad rubric. In that context, it is reassuring to embrace the statement from Nagendran (5) that "informatics has a key characteristic of a new discipline in a technically transient environment . . . there is no universal definition of it." However, in a broad sense, he goes on to suggest that informatics . . . "is the interface between developing technologies and the decision sciences, in particular, clinical sciences."

Telemedicine does not have a universally accepted definition either even though it began in the 1920's (6). Consequently, for this paper, I will simply use the one that comes from the American Telemedicine Association:

> "Telemedicine is the use of medical information exchanged from one site to another via electronic communications for the health and education of the patient or health care provider and for the purpose of improving patient care".

One has to be cautious with the interpretation of telemedicine to avoid the impression that personal medical interaction with the patient has been abandoned. In fact, the *Advisory Council on Health Infostructure* states that ". . . tools of technology are not intended to replace human contact with medical providers but, rather, to enhance the usefulness of these encounters" (7).

One last definition which is salient to this discussion relates to the word "telehealth" and was presented at an outstanding symposium coordinated by Don Shaw at the 2000 National Meeting of the American Association of Cardiovascular and Pulmonary Rehabilitation in Tampa, Florida.

> "Telehealth includes activities such as health professional's education, community health education, public health, research and administration of health services" (8).

## Why Telehealth . . . Telemedicine?

Now that the context for these terms has been established, the next question is: why should one even be concerned about telehealth and telemedicine?

- It reduces the burden of travel for patients; this has implications for financial and emotional costs.
- It provides 24-hour medical service to remote areas regardless of location, weather conditions or patient mobility.
- It provides transmission of high resolution images from remote areas which can reduce redundant testing, follow-up visits and unnecessary treatment.
- It improves continuity of care.
- It provides support and continuing education for health-care professionals in remote areas.

Clearly, the information highway holds enormous potential for patients and health-care providers who are currently under-served in terms of optimal medical and/or health resources. Fortunately, the infrastructure for this "highway" is being developed at an incredible rate.

## Technology Infrastructure

This aspect of the information highway is rather complex and can be somewhat intimidating to a novice user. Consequently, it is refreshing to come across an article which translates the vagaries of technology infrastructure into meaningful explanations (9). Diener points out that network speed (ie. bandwidth) depends upon both the physical infrastructure/medium (highway) and the communication standard (car).

There are three primary highways or mediums to transport data in the telemedicine system. At the low end of the spectrum is the telephone line, affectionately called POTS (plain old telephone system). Most of the world connects with the Internet through a modem which links a computer with a telephone line at speeds up to 56 kbps (kilobytes per second).

In spite of its lowly status, the telephone line does permit some flexibility in enhancing bandwidth. For example, two individual lines can be linked together or "multiplexed" to double the original modem speed. In addition, there are specialized technologies (Integrated Services Digital Network - ISDN) which can package, compress and transmit data over the public switched network at speeds up to 1.4 megabytes per second (mbps). Staying with telephone lines, Digital Subscriber Lines (DSL) can reach speeds of 8 mbps, at least one way while the return speed may be somewhat slower.

As Diener (9) points out, road speed can be improved if there is no other traffic on it. For example, "dedicated" phone lines which are leased from the distributor, can provide a high quality of data transportation at about 1.5 mbps or 30 times the modem speed. These specialized T-1 and T-3 lines are not widespread.

The next step in the information highway hierarchy involves fibre-optic cable which all telephone companies are laying in urban and some rural areas. Although this network is not well-developed, compared to traditional telephone lines, the potential speed is exceptional at 622 mbps using the asynchronous transfer mode (ATM). This speed is about 11,000 times as fast as the basic telephone modem but there is no guarantee that a potential user may get more than one "strand" in the cable.

While telephone lines are the most widely available communications medium into homes and businesses, cable television is next in popularity. It is possible to split the coaxial cable to a television so that there can be a cable modem attached to a personal computer, with bandwidth capacities up to 10 mbps or 30 times the telephone modem speed. Although one might suspect otherwise, both cable and fibre-optic are not widespread in rural areas.

The final way to speed travel is to leave the road altogether (ie. satellite or wireless). Homes and businesses have been getting information via their television directly from satellite for years. The competition in this arena is for bandwidth. A useful analogy is to consider the size of the pipe used in plumbing. Larger pipes deliver more water per second and similarly, higher bandwidth delivers more data per second. This has direct relevance for cardiopulmonary rehabilitation delivered at a distance because free-flowing physical movements require enhanced bandwidth to transmit high-quality video, free of distortion. For example, a 20 meg dedicated bandwidth would allow video to be shipped without compression, thereby avoiding encoding/decoding delays.

## Issues

There are clearly several issues surrounding the Information Highway which can be looked at as challenges and opportunities for cardiopulmonary applications. If one imagines any remote location, then access springs to mind. From an international perspective, Australia and New Zealand have extensive outlying settlements. Nevertheless, they have collaborated to establish a Telehealth Committee which has a 5-year plan for the integration of telemedicine into mainstream medicine. And Norway, which is cited by Clinica10 as the "most mature of the telemarkets in Europe" has a national program which guarantees equal access to medical services regardless of geographic location.

It's impossible to ignore China with its potentially enormous market and extensive rural population. At present, their national health funding is prioritized to urban areas but they have acknowledged telehealth and telemedicine as cost-effective ways of accessing services to remote rural areas. Closer to home, Canada has a huge rural landscape that would benefit immensely from telehealth and a few experimental programs are showing great success. Indeed, the Canada Health Act (1984) is the cornerstone of the Canadian health system and aims to ensure that all residents of Canada have access to any necessary health-care on a prepaid basis. This legislation can only be truly guaranteed when telemedicine is fully embraced by under-served rural areas. Even in higher density urban cities closer to the United States, "cross-border telemedicine services may inadvertently contribute to a two-tier system" (11).

Recently, a National Broadband Task Force, under the leadership of University of Waterloo president, David Johnston, has presented a compelling challenge for Canada in their report, the New National Dream: Networking the Nation For Broadband Access (available at **http://broadband.gc.ca).** The report calls for high-speed broadband access (ie. 1.5 mbps) by 2004 for all communities in Canada at a cost of between $1.5 billion and $4.5 billion.

Meanwhile, the United States has dealt with this in a proactive way with more than 100 federally funded telemedicine networks and growing support from Medicare. Major applications relate to the prison system and International Space Station. Bashur notes that telemedicine (TM) has "increased access to care for an additional 18 million persons who are now "virtually" located within 40 miles of speciality services"(12).

Cost is definitely a limitation at this time. Regardless of location, if a personal computer is part of the price, one is looking at a minimum of $5,000 for all the connections. Therefore, telemedicine's costs in relation to benefits may account for the slow adoption of TM by mainstream medicine. There is an urgent need for well-guided, scientifically rigorous research. The United Kingdom is onside with this notion, as they have infused $1.45 billion into information technology and the development of telemedicine. Meanwhile, the United States will probably keep its 88% share of the worldwide telemedicine market, followed by Japan and Germany, each with constraints on health-care spending.

Another issue which persists in the face of any communication medium is information quality. Invariably, quality relates to tradeoffs of speed, cost and objectives. Nevertheless, it appears that with today's technology, telemedicine delivers adequate information for a majority of clinical and diagnostic procedures.

The growing complexity of computerized tools and the lack of time to configure them properly have left noticeable security/privacy holes in many physician offices and hospital departments. Patient data made inadvertently accessible to others violates patient confidentiality and opens the door to possible exploitation by insurance companies . . . as well as those who may not have our best interests at heart. Will encryption expertise keep pace? It's too early to tell, but we do have a responsibility to take reasonable safeguards.

## Cardiopulmonary Applications

Although this was not the first application of telemedicine to cardiopulmonary rehabilitation, I would like to acknowledge the sustained contribution of Don Shaw and Ken Sparks to Transtelephonic Exercise Monitoring (TEM) (13). These authors provide an excellent review of TEM, particularly over the past 20 years, following the first report of transtelephonic monitoring by DeBusk et al in 1979 (14). Appropriate acknowledgment is also provided for the outstanding contributions of Phil Wilson who demonstrated, during the 1970's, that cardiac rehabilitation could be done safely at home (15).

A subsequent paper by Shaw (16) presented an interesting snapshot of where telemedicine has been, where it is now, and what the future holds. Notably, 81% of a survey involving five States reported that distance-based physician visits were equal to or better than personal visits. Coincidentally, a paper by Lin et al (17) from Taiwan, reported that over 90% of patients and physicians in their telemedicine project believed that the system was valuable and provided satisfactory services. Shaw further reported that patient satisfaction and outcome scores were "impressive" for home-based cardiac rehabilitation. Nevertheless, as much as this technology "enriches us by removing the boundaries which previously kept us apart" (17) exclusive reliance on contact at a distance could make us "prisoners of our own technology". Stanberry chastens us, in our zeal for speed of contact, not to ignore the intangible comfort and compassion which human beings only truly bring each other when they are face to face (18).

Residents of Northern Alberta in Canada have been the beneficiaries of "Remote Cardiac Rehabilitation" (19) for the past couple years. The actual interaction is via telehealth rather than direct video communications. A more expansive model of web-based delivery of a cardiac program is being conducted by Dr. Joanna Bates out of St. Paul's Hospital in Vancouver (20). The connecting rural site is at Kelowna General Hospital where the participants have access to video clips, live chat sessions, and expert health professionals. Once again, the information is available from a website and this raises two more "issues" that were not noted previously. Each participant had to have his/her own computer and, in many cases, a $2,000 outlay is a significant barrier to "equal" access. Another consideration is literacy, which may be taken for granted in some settings. In more extreme cases, cognitive impairment and substance abuse may be further barriers to opportunities for telehealth.

Distance-based home monitoring is not the sole domain of cardiac patients as noted in a project involving chronic respiratory patients in Spain (21). A spirometer was linked to a local hospital from the patient's home and information could be sent directly via computer by the patient or nurse who visited periodically.

A study by Mulholland et al (22) on neonatal congenital heart defects shows a classic role for specialized telephone lines (ISDN) to transmit clear images from a rural pediatrician to a pediatric cardiologist. In this case, real-time DVD quality was not essential so the cardiologist could still provide rapid feedback as to the need for urgent care, monitoring or simply waiting for the monthly visit of a specialist.

Another example of home-based monitoring (blood pressure in this internet-based system) is reported by Aris et al. (23) from Malaysia. This group was particularly sensitive to minimizing measurement error. This particular model of home-based assessment from remote areas has huge potential for diabetic patients and personal glucose monitoring.

Low bandwidth, Internet-based videoconferencing has been used for several years by Lemaire et al (24) to provide physical rehabilitation consultation services for community hospitals. Remote clinicians rated their satisfaction high with the combination of PC, modem and a separate telephone line for voice. However, it is important to note that while the videoconference capture rate of one frame per second may have been comfortable for physical examinations, the visual interaction would be unacceptable for widespread physical activity in cardiac rehab programs.

Another Ottawa group (25) from the University of Ottawa Heart Institute, also uses low-bandwidth for echo and ECG transport but recognize that at least 4-6 mbps is necessary for a physical examination where video quality is essential.

Finally, I would like to briefly mention our own research (26) where we are investigating the potential of group-based or individual site cardiac rehabilitation in rural settings participating live and interactive with our longstanding community-based program in Kitchener-Waterloo. The instructor of the patient group in K-W would be able to see, and be seen by, the rural patient group. In addition to high quality video, there would be interactive audio. ECG and blood pressure could also be transported by wireless communication. In fact, one company (Health Frontier, Inc.) already has appropriate units on the market which interface with wireless RIM Blackberry transmitters (worn on the belt) that link to a personal computer at a distant location.

It is well-known that at least 80% of cardiac patients do not participate in systematic cardiac rehab programs. Geographical barriers are often part of the problem. If we can take our program to stable patients at a distance, they could receive the benefits that have been documented for participation in systematic cardiac rehabilitation (i.e., a 25% decrease in cardiovascular mortality) (27). Initially, a health professional (e.g., nurse) could be with the distance group to assist with remote monitoring. Preferably, this nurse would be trained in the use of an Automated External Defibrillator (AED), which would also be present. Cardiovascular events, other than a cardiac arrest, are unlikely to be life-threatening. Careful screening and close monitoring should yield the same safe workout results which apply to traditional hospital-based programs.

As part of the initial pilot work, we are simply transmitting video from room to room in the same building. It is easy to produce VHS quality video which is acceptable to the group receiving the instruction at this modest distance. In this controlled setting, we have reduced the bandwidth to simulate distance and determine at what level and quality the transmission becomes annoying to the patients. The next step is to actually transmit from a progressively distant site at a high bandwidth. The ultimate goal is to have a wireless link into the home for this kind of application. At this point in time, several companies are in a frantic race to be the first in the marketplace with an affordable wireless technology. The major difference between traditional videoconferencing and this project is the challenge of transmitting a high-quality image in real time when the activity is free-flowing exercise conducted at a distant site. Without a fibre-optic or cable link, the connection requires a high bandwidth and this is currently expensive.

## Education

As exciting as the research prospects are, it is equally important to educate students who will be knowledgeable and competent in the area of cardiopulmonary rehabilitation. To that end, there are many university courses which provide background material in cardiovascular physiology and a smaller number which focus on coronary heart disease—from pathophysiology to rehabilitation. A course of this nature has existed at the University of Waterloo for 25 years. For 10 years (up to 1999), this course has also been offered via the traditional correspondence route using audio tapes and notes. More recently (2000), this course was converted to an internet-based, interactive mode to provide more flexibility for students near or far. To date, there have been hundreds of students from Canada and the United States taking advantage of getting both the content and a credit out of their own home. In fact, there have been registrants from Europe, Africa and even from jail. The many animations in a web-based course and chat room potential seem to enhance learning and compensate somewhat for the loss of face to face contact. The web-site for further information is **http://webcourses.de.uwaterloo.ca**. Web-based training has been embraced by some medical schools as a new paradigm in computer-assisted instruction (28). This orientation to content and methodology allows the student to exploit increasingly the advantages of the WWW. One variation of this model, in the form of a telerehabilitation system, permits university staff to link with clinicians and students located in remote communities (29). This model, which is most prevalent in a medical setting, could easily be adapted to university programs where health science students rotate between on campus courses and a "co-operative" work term experience (e.g., The University of Waterloo has one of the largest "co-op" programs in the world).

## Conclusion

The information highway has been around for many years but the technology as well as the software has been cumbersome. In the past few years, dramatic advances in both areas have made telehealth and telemedicine less intimidating. Clearly, it is not yet part of mainstream medicine but that situation is about to change in the next few years.

There are still barriers related to access, cost, quality and security. However, they are surmountable and significant progress has been made in both telemedicine and telehealth for under-served areas. This technology will have as much impact, and probably more, in urban areas once optimal use is made of health professionals (e.g., nurses, physiotherapists, kinesiologists) who can enhance both health and health-care at any distance beyond the physician's office. Wireless technology will afford the breakthrough in those areas where fibre-optic cable is not the preferred medium.

Technology has come a long way but still is not as cheap and user-friendly as it should be. However, telemedicine and telehealth are here to stay and for anyone who wants to ride the crest of a wave which will change the face of healthcare as we know it, the timing is perfect.

# References

1.  Robinson JC: Financing the health care internet. *Health Affairs* 2000; 19:72-88.
2.  Chae YM, Lee JH, Ho SH, Kim HJ, Jun KH, Won JU: Patient satisfaction with telemedicine in home health services for the elderly. *Int J Med Informatics* 2001; 61:167-173.
3.  Sinha A: An overview of Telemedicine: The virtual gaze of health care in the next century. *Med Anthropology Quart* 2000; 14:291-309.
4.  Jones R: Developments in consumer health informatics in the next decade. *Health Libraries Review* 2000; 17:26-31.
5.  Nagendran S, Moores D, Spooner R, Triscott J: Is telemedicine a subset of medical informatics? *J Telemedicine and Telecare* 2000; 6 (suppl 2):S2:50-S2:51.
6.  Moore M: The evolution of telemedicine. *Future Generation Computer Systems* 1999; 15:245-254.
7.  Advisory Council on Health Infostructure: Canada Health Infoway: Paths to Better Health. *Health Canada* 1999; Report H21-145/1999F.
8.  Shaw D: Telemedicine: an introduction to the future. *AACVPR Syllabus* 2000.
9.  Diener A, Mueller K, Fletcher J: Assessment of potential uses of and needs for telehealth services in Nebraska. *Nebraska Center for Rural Health Research* 2001; 1-28.
10. Editorial: Telemedicine goes mainstream fuelling high level growth. *Clinica* 2000; 939:8.
11. Bailey M: Legal issues relating to telemedicine in Canada's publicly funded health-care system. *J Telemedicine and Telecare* 2000; 6 (suppl 2):140-142.
12. Bashur RL, Reardon TG, Shannon GW: Telemedicine: a new health care delivery system *Annu Rev Public Health* 2000; 21:613-637.
13. Shaw DK, Sparks KE, Jennings HS: Transtelephonic exercise monitoring: a review. *J Cardiopul Rehab* 1998; 18:263-270.
14. DeBusk RF, Houston N, Haskell W, Fry G, Parker M: Exercise training soon after myocardial infarction. *Am J Cardiol* 1979; 44(7):1223-1229.
15. Wilson PK, Maresh CK, Edgett JW Jr., Gunderson AE: Functional capabilities following coronary bypass surgery. *Med Sci Sports* 1977; 9:77-82.
16. Shaw DK: Telemedicine and cardiopulmonary rehabilitation: where do we stand? *J Cardiopul Rehab* 1999; 19(1):59-61.
17. Lin CC, Chen HS, Chen CY, Hou SM: Implementation and evaluation of a multifunctional telemedicine system in National Taiwan University. *Int J Med Informatics* 2001; 61:175-187.
18. Stanberry B: Telemedicine: barriers and opportunities in the 21st century. *J Intern Med* 2000; 247:615-628.
19. Henderson I, VanLohuizen K, Fenske T: Remote cardiac rehabilitation. *J Telemedicine and Telecare* 2000; 6 (suppl 2):528-529.
20. Bates J: Using the world wide web to deliver a cardiac program to patients at home. *Health Infostructure Support Program of Health Canada* 2000; Project File# 6610-2394-99.
21. de Toledo P, Del Pozo F: A home telecare system for the care of chronic respiratory patients. *Bioengineering and Telemedicine Group*, Technical University of Madrid, Spain 2000.
22. Mulholland HC, Casey F, Brown D et al.: Application of a low cost telemedicine link to the diagnosis of neonatal congenital heart defects by remote consultation. *Heart* 1999; 82:217-221.
23. Aris B, Wagie AAE, Mariun NB, Jammal ABE: An internet-based blood pressure monitoring system for patients. *J Telemedicine and Telecare* 2001; 7:51-53.
24. Lemaire ED, Boudrias Y, Greene G: Low-bandwidth, internet-based videoconferencing for

physical rehabilitation consultants *J Telemedicine and Telecare* 2001; 7:82-89.

25. Cheung ST, Davies RF, Smith K, Marsh R, Sherrard H, Keon WJ: The Ottawa telehealth project. *Telemed J* 1998; 4(3):259-266.

26. Sharratt MT, Carey T: A pilot project to evaluate virtual cardiac rehabilitation using distance-based technology. *Bell University Labs, University of Waterloo*; 2001.

27. Oldridge NB, Guyatt GH, Fischer ME, Rimm AA: Cardiac rehabilitation after myocardial infarction. *JAMA* 1988; 260:945-950.

28. Haag M, Maylein L, Leven FJ, Tonshoff B, Haux R: Web-based training: a new paradigm in computer-assisted instruction in medicine *Int J Med Informatics* 1999; 53:79-90.

29. Liu L, Miyazaki M: Telerehabilitation at the University of Alberta. *J Telemedicine and Telecare* 2000; 6(suppl 2):47-49.

# Chapter 4

# World Wide Cardiopulmonary Rehabilitation . . . Where Are We Now?

Philip K. Wilson, EdD, USA

## Introduction

As we enter the next millennium, we need to determine where cardiopulmonary rehabilitation is in the total service of medicine to both the cardiac and pulmonary patient. Where are we now, compared to a few years ago, and compared to many years ago? Has our professional area of service increased in acceptance, is acceptance the same as a few years ago, or many years ago, or has acceptance decreased? And what is the future of cardiopulmonary rehabilitation? In order for us to make these determinations, we must look at the past, determine the present, and then attempt to predict the future.

## History of Cardiopulmonary Rehabilitation

Historically, cardiopulmonary rehabilitation can be traced to before 1800, however, major events contributing to current cardiopulmonary rehabilitation procedures occurred beginning in 1950. Of major significance in the early 1950s was the work of Hellerstein and Goldston in work classification units, in the assessment of the patient's social and emotional needs, and vocational skills. Their efforts in exercise testing was a continuation of the development in the use of exercise in the determination of a patient's physical capacity (1). In 1952 Millar presented his work of the use of exercise for pulmonary patients (2). In 1953 Morris presented his classic work detailing the relationship between coronary heart disease and physical work capacity (3). The 1960s started with information on exercise as a modality for cardiac patients by Komblueth and Michael

(4), followed by Saltin's report on bed rest and its effect on cardiovascular performance (5), and Cooper's book on Aerobics (6). Highlighting the beginning period of the 1970s was the American Heart Association publication entitled Exercise Testing and Training of Apparently Healthy Individuals: A Handbook for Physicians (7). Wenger in 1973 (8) reported on her inpatient cardiac rehabilitation program, and in 1974 Petty (9) reported on pulmonary rehabilitation. In 1975 the American Heart Association released the document entitled Exercise Testing in Individuals with Heart Disease or at High Risk for its Development (10), and also in 1975 the American College of Sports Medicine released the first edition of Guidelines for Graded Exercise Testing and Exercise Prescription (11). Finally, classic in the use of exercise for cardiac patients was Haskell's 1978 report on the low risk of complications (12). The American Association of Cardiovascular and Pulmonary Rehabilitation was created in 1985. Also in the mid 1980s was the significance of Paffenbargers report on the risk of mortality decreasing with the amount of exercise involvement (13). Finally, the 1990s continued with studies documenting the value of rehabilitation for cardiac and pulmonary patients, and the growth of programs being offered in both North America and throughout the world.

## Where Are we Now?

What is the status of cardiopulmonary rehabilitation today? In fact, what is the status of public attitudes toward the "healthy lifestyle"? Is health and fitness an important part of the lives of people? What do people understand about medical services and procedures? Is there a difference in understandings of people regarding their medical care today, compared to ten years ago?

## The Public

The public of today have a far greater understanding of medical services, and opportunities for their own care, than ever before. Not only do people expect to be fully informed on available medical services, they also have the opportunity to learn about medical services in the lay press. A quick scan of headlines for articles in newspapers indicates the degree to which the public can become informed, far beyond ever before. Examples of newspaper headlines and topics as follows:

- Risk factors:
  "Researchers find a new heart attack risk factor"
  "Obscure cholesterol tied to heart attacks"
- Gene therapy:
  "Trials for gene heart therapy set to go"
  "Cell transplant saves dying heart"
- Surgery:
  "Robot does bypass on beating heart"
  "Heart device tried instead of transplant"
  "Artificial hearts pump ahead"
  "Loss of brainpower after bypass may last"
- Defibrillators:
  "A prescription to save lives"
  "Greater access to defibrillators could save lives"
- Drugs:
  "Heart disease drugs getting major push"

In fact, when you include the Internet, the access of the public to medical information is all the more extensive. A recent report indicated that 52 million Americans go to the Internet for medical information, and that most people who do use the internet for medical information, go on line for that purpose at least once a month. Also emphasized in the report is that as actual time with a physician is decreasing, knowledge by the public is extensively increasing (14).

## Associations

There are many associations, public and professional, in both the area of prevention of cardiovas-

cular disease, and cardiopulmonary rehabilitation. Foremost of public associations is the American Heart Association (AHA), and its related associations throughout the world. Through funded research, and both professional and public information, the American Heart Association and related associations are truly the major organization world wide. However, equally important are professional organizations such as the American Association of Cardiovascular and Pulmonary Rehabilitation (AACVPR), the Canadian Association of Cardiac Rehabilitation (CACR), the Canadian Cardiovascular Society (CCS), the American College of Cardiology (ACC), the American College of Sports Medicine (ACSM) and the companion Canadian organization the Canadian Society of Exercise Physiologists (CSEP). Equally important is the World Council for Cardiovascular and Pulmonary Rehabilitation (WCCPR).

A major impact of these organizations is the development of both independent and joint publications. The Journal of Cardiopulmonary Rehabilitation (JCR) of AACVPR is the number one periodical in the world in the field of cardiopulmonary rehabilitation. Of equal impact is the ACSM's Guidelines for Exercise Testing and Prescription (15).

These two publications are the cornerstone of knowledge, procedures, current practice, and the development of personnel. Of major significance are the joint publications of cooperating organizations. In example, the recent (2000), AHA and AACVPR Scientific Statement on core components of cardiac rehabilitation and secondary prevention programs is a classic example of joint association efforts (16). Discussed in this document is patient assessment, and the program components of nutrition, lipid management, hypertension management, smoking cessation, weight management, diabetes management, psychosocial management, physical activity counseling, and exercise training. Each topic is presented in the format of evaluation, intervention, and expected outcomes.

A second important impact of professional associations is certification, of both cardiac and pulmonary rehabilitation programs and staff. Involved in program certification is the American Association of Cardiovascular and Pulmonary Rehabilitation. Certification programs offered by AACVPR involve the following areas: admissions, assessment, therapeutic plan medical emergencies, personnel outcomes, evaluation, medical records, facilities, equipment, documentation follow up and discharge (17). Since beginning the certification process in 1998, AACVPR has certified 396 cardiac rehabilitation programs and 203 pulmonary rehabilitation programs. The American College of Sports Medicine (ACSM) has offered personnel certification since 1975. The ACSM currently offers certification to personnel involved in preventative programs (health and fitness certification track), and rehabilitation programs (clinical certification track). The health and fitness tract certifies health and fitness directors, fitness instructors, and group exercise leaders. The clinical certification track certifies program directors and exercise specialists (18).

Finally, the ACSM certification process also offers "certificates of enhanced qualification" (CEQs), in the following areas: diabetes, exercise and the older adult, nutrition and exercise, and resistance training (18). In addition to extensive offerings of certification and CEQs in North America, ACSM is currently involved in certification activities in many countries outside of the United States, including the following: Argentina, Belgium, Brazil, Canada, England, Greece, Hong Kong, Ireland, Italy, Japan, Portugal, Singapore, Switzerland, Taiwan, United Arab Emirates. Since beginning the certification of personnel in 1975, over 30,000 professionals have been certified by the American College of Sports Medicine.

## Lifestyle

In North America, are more and more people adopting the healthy lifestyle? Are more and more people practicing the healthy habits of regular exercise, proper diet, non use of tobacco products, limited use of alcohol, and in general, doing everything possible to reduce their risk of the onset of cardiovascular disease? Unfortunately, the answer to this question is no. People are exercising less and eating more. In fact, there is a global epidemic of obesity. The number of people who are obese in the world doubled in most countries in the past 20 years. In the United States since 1960, when 10% of men and 15% of women were obese, the percentages have now increased to 20% men and 25% women (19). The lifestyle one leads, will not only lower the risk for heart disease, but will increase the quality of life. A recent study involving almost 90,000 women and a 14 year follow up, indicated that 82 percent of coronary events (1,128 major coronary events and 296 deaths), could be attributed to a lack of adherence to a low risk lifestyle. A conclusion of the study is that "women who stay active, eat healthful foods and don't smoke, cut their risk of heart disease by 82%" (20). In contrast, the ar-

ticle by Booth and associates identifies that an increase in physical inactivity is directly related to an epidemic of chronic diseases, including heart disease (21). As reported by the Center for Clinical and Lifestyle Research, "there is no longer any serious doubt that daily lifestyle decisions and practices exert a profound impact on both short and long term health and quality of life. Scientific and medical advances over the past 20 years, and particularly over the last five years, have solidified the evidence that positive lifestyle measures are vitally important to good health" (22).

## Length of Life

Though people are exercising less, eating more, and as a rule not giving attention to the healthy lifestyle, we are living longer. However, how soon will the life expectancy be 100 years, 120, 200? In 1900 the life expectancy in the United States was 47, and the life expectancy now is 76 years. The current maximum age is 108. The National Institute of Health in the United States reports that in the past decade the number of centenarians has doubled to 70,000. Also reported is that about 70% of the increase in maximum length of life is due to advances in medical science (23). Many, however, denounce claims of "superlongevity" and that living well past the age of 100 is not possible (24). Those doubters indicate that even if the most common causes of death (cancer and cardiovascular disease) are eliminated, the increase in life expectancy will be no more than 15 years. They site that people will still die from what is commonly termed, the aging process (25).

## Diet and Exercise

Undoubtedly, diet and exercise habits have a major effect upon both quantity and quality of life. Quantity of life is the length of life. Quality of life is the quality of your life today, tomorrow, and the next day. Though it may be argued for years to come the exact and verified length of life, based upon the healthy lifestyle, one cannot argue the effect upon the quality of life. The fit healthy individual, on a daily basis, feels better, has a better attitude, sleeps better, has more stamina, less stress, and basically, is a happier and healthier person. The healthy lifestyle, and the quantity and quality of life, is very significantly affected by diet and exercise. Diet and exercise are certainly two of the major factors in both the prevention of the onset of cardiovascular disease, and survival and rehabilitation from a cardiovascular event (21).

The title of the newspaper article reads "healthier diets boost longevity, 12 year study finds"(26). The article, detailing a release in the Journal of the American Medical Association, quotes, " . . . that people who eat lots of fruit, vegetables and whole grains live significantly longer than those who do not". The study, which involved 42,000 persons, concluded that proper eating habits will dramatically reduce the risk of dying from cancer, heart disease, or stroke (26).

Regarding obesity, is participation in an exercise program enough to show positive effects? According to a report by Ross, Freeman and Janssen, the answer is yes. According to their research and review of existing studies, "exercise with diet restriction is an effective strategy for reducing obesity and related co-morbidity's" (27). Another report by Ades dealing with cardiac rehabilitation patients indicates no. In the review, Ades indicates "exercise only cardiac rehabilitation programs without prescription of a hypocaloric diet, results in little or no weight loss over a 3 month exercise training period" (28, 29, 30).

However, in summary, it would appear logical that a weight loss process involving both exercise and caloric reduction is the best approach. Proper diet will effect weight loss, however the addition of an exercise regime, will not only contribute toward a greater weight loss, but the exercise component will also have positive effect to the patients cardiovascular system. Undoubtedly, we must all be well educated on obesity, with classic references being offered by the Journal of the American Medical Association (31) and Medicine and Science in Sports and Exercise (32). Valuable web sites are **http://www.ajcn.org** (American Journal of Clinical Nutrition); **www.pslgroup.com/OBESITY.HTM** (Doctors guide to Obesity Information and Resources); and **http://www.nlm.nih.gov/** overviews (National Library of Medicine and National Institutes of Health Sources) (33).

It is estimated that 55% of the nearly 100 million Americans are either overweight or obese (34). Ribisl concludes obesity and overweight are associated with increased morbidity and mortality from atherosclerotic diseases, type 2 diabetes, sleep apnea, endometrial and breast cancers, osteoarthritis, and psychological disorders. The three factors that affect obesity are genetics, dietary intake, and physical activity. Those of us in preventative and rehabilitation medicine must address these concerns on a daily basis with our clients and patients (34).

## State of the Art

What is the current state of the art of cardiopulmonary rehabilitation? Where are we now? Certainly, significant advances have been made in our profession in the recent years, but realistically, what is our current status? For certain, we have yet to be totally accepted into the routine everyday treatment of cardiac and pulmonary patients. Granted, the position of cardiac and pulmonary rehabilitation "has come a long way", however we still have a long way to go.

## Pulmonary Rehabilitation

Is pulmonary rehabilitation being offered to all patients? Obviously, no! Is quality of life (QOL), an important factor in the rehabilitation of a pulmonary patient? Obviously yes! Is pulmonary rehabilitation an important service to COPD patients? Again obviously, yes! Pulmonary rehabilitation is an accepted therapy, and has been for a number of years (35, 36, 37, 38, 39, 40). Why then is pulmonary rehabilitation not offered to all patients, other than those with a contraindicated condition? Benzo reports that pulmonary rehabilitation is an accepted therapy for COPD patients, and will improve both exercise capacity and quality of life. Benzo further reports that the use of a Medical Outcomes Survey Short Form 36 item questionnaire will assist in not only determining outcome effect, but the actual use of pulmonary rehabilitation with COPD patients (41). Rehabilitation of the pulmonary patient via exercise therapy, and related services can and should become a routine and required procedure, with definite outcome goals, followed by assessment of those goals that have been attained.

## Cardiac Rehabilitation

Again, is cardiac rehabilitation a routine and always offered and conducted procedure for the qualified cardiac patient? Obvious again, no? Quality of life and favorable changes in coronary risk factors (secondary prevention) for the cardiac patient is effected by the duration of participation of the patient in a cardiac rehabilitation program (42). Other studies further document that the longer a patient participates in a program, the greater the benefits (43, 44). Behavioral lifestyle changes require long tem education (45). Rice recently reported on the effect of designated "education days", separate from "exercise days", upon the goal of offering a meaningful and successful "quality of life" patient education program (46).

Finally, and probably most significant in the success or failure of a program, is the understanding by the involved primary physician of cardiopulmonary rehabilitation, exercise physiology, risk factor reduction, patient education, and all related concepts. We continue to face the dilemma of the ill prepared physician. The state of the art of the primary physician is still not acceptable. Allen recently reported that physicians feel they do not understand adequately the basics of even exercise prescription, and they admit they know little about motivating patients toward the practice of healthy habits (47).

Physiologically, cardiopulmonary rehabilitation is proven to benefit involved patients. Our task continues to be how to educate medical specialists (physicians, nurses, etc.), of the need for cardiopulmonary rehabilitation. A related task, and a shared responsibility with the primary physician, is then the motivation of the patient to both enter the rehabilitation process, and to continue in the practice of healthy habits throughout life.

## Future

What is the future of cardiopulmonary rehabilitation? Obviously, the future is determined by current problems and challenges. Are the problems consistent throughout the world? Obviously, no! The problems in developing countries varies significantly from the problems in developed countries. And of the developed countries, do problems differ from region to region? Are the problems in Europe different than the Orient, or North America? What is the status of the problems world wide?

## Developed Countries

The status of cardiopulmonary rehabilitation in developed countries varies significantly from region to region. For example, in an effort to determine the

current problems and challenges in the United States, a small number of "authorities" were surveyed on their opinions. The following is a summary of their opinions, listed in order of most important, to next most important, etc.:

1. Reimbursement/financial—in the United States we are continually facing a decrease in the amount of funds provided for cardiopulmonary rehabilitation. This problem, is by far the most significant to our profession. The availability of funds, either via third party reimbursement, or by any other manner, is critical to the future of cardiopulmonary rehabilitation.
2. Personnel—the availability of qualified personnel is a very significant problem. Qualified personnel must have the availability of training sites, with skilled and knowledgeable staff.
3. Referrals—as discussed, cardiopulmonary rehabilitation is yet to be totally accepted by both medical personnel, and the lay public.
4. Compliance—motivation to the participant and adherence is still a major problem.

Referrals and compliance are significant problems in the United States. In the article entitled "Exercise rehabilitation for cardiac patients . . . A beneficial but underused therapy", Thompson states as follows:

"Exercise based cardiac rehabilitation is currently underused, even though exercise is one of the few nonsurgical interventions that can make heart disease patients feel better physically and medically. Benefits include increased muscle strength, lower heart rate, increased stroke volume, and increased submaximal and maximal working capacity. Patients in cardiac rehabilitation programs, however, often do not exercise enough to obtain maximal benefit. Programs should ideally be initiated under supervision to provide the correct regimen and requisite vigorous activity. Subsequent moderate exercise regimens can be done at home. All patients should engage in lifelong maintenance programs (48)."

In contrast, and in examination of programs in Europe, review of The Carinex Study reveals that a number of programs do not even offer pulmonary rehabilitation (49). In Europe and many other developed countries, a major effort must be extended to education of the public in the effects of smoking.

In addition, in these regions there must be a parallel action in legislation against tobacco companies.

## Developing Countries

Finally, a major concern world wide must be the lack of significant efforts on cardiopulmonary rehabilitation in developing countries. Poverty in many of these countries and environmental pollution contributes to major health concerns. Concern must be given to not only the general lack of significant rehabilitation programs, but a similar lack of efforts on risk factor identification, evaluation, and education. An overall concern must be given to the related lack of public education in healthy habits, and the need for the healthy lifestyle.

A possible answer to developing countries would be to adopt model programs which currently exist in developed countries. This process would provide an expedited mechanism for needed services. Model programs exist, and would be eager to provide assistance. An example would be the Toronto Cardiac Rehabilitation and Secondary Prevention Program. Developed in 1968 by Dr. Terrance Kavanagh, this program continues to be one of the most successful in the world. The program continues to maintain "state of the art" policies and procedures. Annually over 1,800 new patients are referred to the program, from over 400 referring physicians (50).

## World Wide

Many problems are world wide, though certainly to a greater degree in some regions more than others. Lack of funding for necessary education and intervention in cardiovascular disease is world wide. A similar lack of funding for both primary and secondary prevention (rehabilitation) is world wide. Additional funding for research is also universal. Finally, a lack of equality in both the availability of programs to minorities, and the interest in programs by minorities, is universal.

## Conclusion

What then is the status of cardiopulmonary rehabilitation world wide? In summary, in some regions of the world, the profession exists and is functioning. However, in these areas (e.g., United States),

the problems of reimbursement, personnel, and referrals must be solved. If not solved, the eventual result may be diminishing existence of programs as we know now, and even the possibility of the overall elimination of all programs. In other countries, the scope of programs must be expanded to address all aspects of cardiovascular concerns, and specifically, pulmonary rehabilitation. Finally, developing regions must begin to address the actual need for cardiopulmonary rehabilitation, and establish programs which address not only rehabilitation, but equally important, preventative programs.

Cardiopulmonary disease is a leading cause of morbidity and mortality in the United States, North America, and throughout developed countries. Cardiopulmonary disease will increase significantly in the developing countries in the next decade. The long term existence of cardiopulmonary rehabilitation is dependent upon program review, and then appropriate program expansion. Expansion must be realistic to program needs, and available financial resources.

## References

1. Hellerstein HK, Goldston E. Rehabilitation of patients with heart disease. *Postgrad Med* 1954:1 5:265-278.
2. Millar WF. Physical therapeutic measures in the treatment of chronic brochopulmonary disorders. *Am J Med* 1958:24:929.
3. Morris JN, Heady JA, Raffle PA, Roberts CG, Parks JW. Coronary heart disease and physical activity of work. *Lancet* 1953:2:1053-1057.
4. Komblueh IH, Micheal E. Outline of exercise program for patients with myocardial infarction. *Pa Med* 1961:60:1575-1578.
5. Saltin BG, Blomquist JH, Mitchell R. Response to exercise after bed rest and training. *Circulation* 1968:7:71-78.
6. Cooper KH. Aerobics 1968; New York, Bantam Books.
7. American Heart Association. Exercise testing and training of apparently healthy individuals: A handbook for physicians. 1972:New York, American Heart Association.
8. Wenger NK, Hellerstein HK, Blackburn H, Castranova SV. Uncomplicated myocardial infarction. Current physician practice in patient management. *JAMA* 1973:224:511-514.
9. Petty TL. Pulmonary rehabilitation. Basics of RD. 1975; New York, American Thoracic Society.

10. American Heart Association. Exercise testing and training of individuals with heart disease or at high risk for its development. 1975:Dallas, American Heart Association.

11. American College of Sports Medicine. Guidelines for graded exercise testing and prescription. 1975:Philadelphia: Lea and Febiger.

12. Haskell W. Cardiovascular complications during exercise training of cardiac patients. *Circulation* 1978:57:920-924.

13. Paffenbarger RS, Hyde RT, Wing AL, Hsieh CC. Physical activity, all cause mortality, and longevity of college alumni. *N Eng J Med* 1986: 314:605-613.

14. Chicago Tribune: Many surfing internet for health advice report finds. 11/20/01, p.1.

15. ACSM's guidelines for exercise testing and prescription. 2000: 6th edition, Baltimore: Lippincott, Williams and Wilkins.

16. AHA/AACVPR. Scientific statement, core components of cardiac rehabilitation and secondary prevention programs. *J Cardiopulm Rehab* 2000:20:310-316.

17. AACVPR: Program certification: Evolution of the process. National convention presentation, 1999:9/16/99, 2:30-4:30 p.m.

18. ACSM certification resource center catalog, 2001. Baltimore: Lippincott, Williams and Wilkins.

19. USA Today: Weight of world on our shoulders. 10/30/00, p.8d.

20. Lifestyle can lower heart disease risks. *Fitness Management* 2000:9:8.

21. Booth FW, Gordon SE, Carlson CJ, Hamilton MT. Waging war on modern chronic diseases: primary prevention through exercise biology. *J Appl Physiol* 2000:774-787.

22. Lynch DJ. Eye on the future: ACSM's Health and Fitness Journal 2000:Jan-Feb:4/1,p.40.

23. USA Today. Forget 100: try living past 120. 10/2/00.

24. Chicago Tribune. 100 year life expectancy may be 500 years off. 2/19/01, p1/1.

25. USA Today. Long life has limits, experts on aging say. 2/20/01, p.6d.

26. Chicago Tribune. Healthier diets boost longevity, 12 year study finds. 4/26/00,p.6.s 1.

27. Ross R, Freeman JA, Janssen I. Exercise alone is an effective strategy for reducing obesity and related comorbidities. *ACSM Exercise and Sports Science Reviews* 2000:28:4:165-170.

28. Ades PA. Obesity and CAD: Science and practice. AACVPR national convention presentation, 2000:9/21/00, 2:30-4:30 p.m.

29. Lavie CJ, Milani RV. Effects of cardiac rehabilitation, exercise training, and weight reduction on exercise capacity, coronary risk factors, behavioral characteristics and quality of life in obese coronary patients. *Am J Cardio* 1997:79:397-401.

30. Brochu M, Poehlman ET, Savage P, Ross S, Ades PA: Coronary risk profiles in male coronary patients: Effects of body composition, fat distribution, age and fitness. *Coronary Artery Disease* 2000:11:137-144.

31. Special Obesity Issue. *JAMA* 1999:vol 282, No.16, 10/27.

32. Special Physical Activity and Obesity Supplement. Medicine and Science in Sports and Exercise 1999: 31 (#11 supplement): 663-667, November.

33. NIH clinical guidelines on the identification, evaluation, and treatment of overweight and obesity in adults. *American Journal of Clinical Nutrition* 1998: (Oct), 68 (4):899-917.

34. Ribisl PM. The new Y2k problem: Obesity, genes, gluttony, or sloth. AACVPR national convention presentation. 2000:9/23/00, 9:00-10:00 a.m

35. Ries AL. Position paper of the AACVPR: scientific basis of pulmonary rehabilitation. *J Cardiopulm Rehab* 1990:10:418-441.

36. Hodgkin JE, Connors GL, Bell CW. Pulmonary rehabilitation: Guidelines to success. 1993: Philadelphia, J.B. Lippincott.

37. Casaburi R. Principles and practice of pulmonary rehabilitation. 1993: Philadelphia, W.B. Saunders.

38. Ries AL, Kaplan RM, Limberg TM, Prewitt LM. Effects of pulmonary rehabilitation on physiologic and psychosocial outcomes in patients with chronic obstructive pulmonary disease. *Ann Intern Med* 1995: 122:823-832.

39. Foster S, Thomas HM. Pulmonary rehabilitation in lung disease other than chronic obstructive pulmonary disease. *Am Rev Respir Dis* 1990:141:601-604.

40. Crouch R, MacIntyre NR Pulmonary rehabilitation of the patient with nonobstructive lung disease. *Respir Care Clin N Am* 1998:4:59-67.

41. Benzo R, Flune PA, Turner D, Tempest M. Effect of pulmonary rehabilitation on quality of life in patients with COPD: The use of SF-36 summary scores as outcomes measures. *J Cardiopulm Rehab* 2000:20:231-234.

42. Morrin L, Black S, Reid R. Impact of duration in a cardiac rehabilitation program on coronary risk profile and health related quality of life

outcomes. *J Cardiopulm Rehab* 2000:200: 115-121.

43. Rogers MA, Yamomoto C, Hagberg JM, Holloszy JO, Ehsari AA. The effect of 7 years of intense exercise training on patients with coronary artery disease. *J Am Coll Cardial* 1987:10:321-326.

44. Oldridge N, Gottieb M, Guyatt G, Jones N, Streiner D, Feeny D. Predictions of health related quality of life with cardiac rehabilitation after myocardial infarction. *J Cardiopulm Rehab* 1990:10:130-140.

45. Steele JM, Ruzicki D. An evaluation of the effectiveness of cardiac teaching during hospitalization. *Heart Lung* 1987:16:306-311.

46. Rice CR, Berkuzsen MA, Nauright L, Sperling LS. Phase II cardiac rehabilitation: meeting the time challenge. *J Cardiopulm Rehab* 1999:19:347-351.

47. Allen M, Mann K, Putnam W, Richard J. Prescribing exercise for cardiac patients: knowledge, practices and needs of family physicians and specialists. *J Cardiopulm Rehab* 2000:20:333-339.

48. Thompson PD. Exercise rehabilitation for cardiac patients. *The Physician and Sports Medicine* 2001:29(1), 69-75.

49. Vanhees L, Dugmore IV, Pentilla JV. The Carinex Survey. Vitgeverij Acco 1999: Belgium.

50. Hamm LF, Kavanagh T. The Toronto cardiac rehabilitation and secondary prevention program: 1968 into the new millennium. *J Cardiopulm Rehab* 2000:20:16-22.

Chapter 5

# The Inclusive Chronic Disease Model: Reaching Beyond Cardiopulmonary Patients

Paul M. Ribisl, PhD, USA

The populations in most developed nations are aging and according to the U.S. Census Bureau, since 1900 the percentage of Americans aged 65 and older has tripled. In 2000 the number of Americans aged 85 and older, representing 4.0 million individuals, was 43 times larger than in 1900 (1). Each year in the United States, chronic diseases claim the lives of more than 1.7 million Americans, or 7 of every 10 deaths. The medical care costs for individuals with chronic diseases exceeds $400 billion annually, accounting for more than 60% of total medical care expenditures (2). Thus, with the economic burden of chronic disease growing exponentially, appropriate care for everyone cannot be provided without posing a significant threat to the health care system. The application of high cost technology is responsible for most of this cost and yet it has been ineffective in reversing this trend. Since much of the chronic disease burden is preventable, effective preventive and rehabilitative efforts must be implemented to a greater degree if this trend is to be reversed.

In spite of widely published guidelines for physicians (3,4) and the much heralded Surgeon General's report (5), the majority of physicians still fail to prescribe exercise to their patients (6-9). Successful physical activity programs have been developed for promotion in clinical settings, (10) but this is not the norm. There is ample evidence that those physicians who have been trained in counseling and who maintain healthful personal lifestyles, counsel their patients more effectively than those who do not practice these personal behaviors and/or feel inadequate in patient counseling (11). There is recent evidence that patients who are most likely to change behavior have been counseled on health-related behaviors by a physician (12); additionally, Pronk and others (13) found that never-smokers with a BMI of 25 kg/m² and who participated in physical activity 3 days per week had mean annual health care charges that were approximately 49% lower than physically inactive smokers with a BMI of 27.5 kg/m². Given the body of evidence that prevention is effective and that Americans are becoming increasingly sedentary, this message must continue to be promoted within the medical community – much like the messages in the past that have been proven to be effective in reducing smoking, cholesterol, and hypertension in Americans.

It is common knowledge that the typical patients entering most cardiopulmonary rehabilitation programs today have multiple sub-clinical and clinical diseases (14) and yet many programs do not get enough referrals to ensure financial stability. This is true in spite of evidence that not only are they cost effective (15-17), but they have also been shown to reduce morbidity (18,19) and mortality (20). Given the knowledge of the cost effectiveness and efficacy of cardiopulmonary rehabilitation programs, Hall (21,22) has recommended that these programs be redesigned to include patients with additional chronic disease diagnoses because this approach is cost-effective and reduces personnel, program, and facility redundancy. It is becoming increasingly clear that programs must be redesigned to attract and manage this new and expanding group of patients, using a new approach while adhering to current clinical guidelines (23-29).

## Statement of Purpose

The purpose of this paper is to outline a new model of care that will address the challenge of managing an aging population with multiple chronic diseases using an inclusive, multi-dimensional model.

## Physical Activity and Chronic Disease

The literature is replete with research that demonstrates the health benefits of implementing behavioral modifications for diet, smoking cessation, stress management, as well as appropriate medication in the prevention and rehabilitation treatment plan for patients with the major chronic diseases. Stampfer and colleagues (30) found that women in the Nurses' Health Study who were in the low risk group had a relative risk of only 0.17 (95% CI 0.07-0.41) for coronary events compared to all other women. Low risk behavior was defined as not smoking, maintaining BMI <25 kg/m², consuming alcohol moderately, engaging in moderate-vigorous activity for 30min/day on average, and scoring high on a healthy diet scale. At this point it should be made clear that a comprehensive program of prevention and rehabilitation must include interventions for several behaviors, including nutrition, physical activity, smoking cessation, stress management, etc; however, for simplicity, this paper will focus primarily on studies that incorporate *physical activity* as the primary treatment modality for only the following chronic diseases: cardiovascular disease, pulmonary disease, obesity, diabetes, osteoarthritis, and osteoporosis.

## Cardiovascular Disease

There is increasing recent evidence that supports the benefits of physical activity in the prevention of cardiovascular disease in both men and women. Drygas and others (31) followed adult males for 5 years to study the effects of differing levels of energy expenditure upon coronary heart disease risk factors and found that in comparison to being sedentary, long-term stabilization of risk factors was achieved with physical activity expenditure above 1,000 kcal/wk and that >2,000 kcal/wk was associated with additional benefits. Rockhill and others (32) examined the recreational activity of middle-aged and older women in the Nurses' Health Study and found that levels of physical activity were inversely related with mortality risk from cardiovascular as well as other disease. Manson and others (33) compared walking with vigorous exercise and found a strong, graded inverse association between physical activity and the risk of coronary events. As compared with those who were most sedentary, those women in the highest quintile group for en-

ergy expenditure had approximately half the risk of coronary events. Lakka and others (34) have demonstrated that higher levels of cardiorespiratory fitness are associated with a slower progression of early atherosclerosis in middle aged men who were followed for 4 years using carotid atherosclerosis assessed by B-mode ultrasonography. These data and others on the benefits of exercise in halting, slowing, and reversing cardiovascular disease are convincing and continue to justify the inclusion of exercise as one of the core components in cardiac rehabilitation programs (23); the remaining sections will focus on other chronic diseases.

## Pulmonary Disease

The incidence, morbidity and mortality of chronic obstructive pulmonary disease (COPD) is rising throughout the world and the total economic cost of COPD in the US in 1993 was estimated to be over $15.5 billion, with $6.1 billion for hospitalization, $4.4 billion for physician and other fees, $2.5 billion for drugs, $1.5 billion for nursing home care and $1.0 billion for home care (35). Exercise has significant benefits for individuals with COPD and extensive guidelines are available for the development of multidisciplinary programs of pulmonary rehabilitation (25,36,37). While exercise training does not reverse the damage associated with pulmonary disease, there are important changes in the upper and lower extremities that allow improved functional capabilities for ambulation, Activities of Daily Living (38-40), and Quality of Life (41).

## Obesity

It is estimated that 55% of the population or nearly 100 million Americans are either overweight or obese and the increase is approximately 10-20% since 1980s (42). The total costs attributable to obesity-related disease approaches $100 billion annually and Americans spend in excess of $50 billion/year on diet related products. With the advent of the automobile, elevators, computers, television, and energy saving devices at home and in the workplace, Americans no longer expend the energy to offset their intake. Recent reviews support the role of physical activity in weight management (28,43,44). A recent study from Finland (45) demonstrates that regular physical activity is effective in preventing weight gain in adults. This was a prospective 10-year follow-up study using a regionally representative cohort of over 5,000 men and women. The main outcome measures were average body mass change during the 10 years of follow-up and clinically significant body mass gain; the latter is defined as a body mass gain of >5kg and/or a body mass index (BMI) of >26 at the end of the follow-up. The results of this study revealed that men and women who had reduced their weekly activity or became sedentary at the end of the follow-up were at 1.6 to 2.0 times greater risk for clinically significant body mass gain, respectively, in comparison with the most active group. The dose-response relationship between physical activity and weight gain in these and other studies supports the causal nature of this association. These findings are consistent with the hypothesis that regular physical activity prevents body mass gain and that physical inactivity is a powerful risk factor for obesity among adults. It also points out the fact that primary care physicians (46) should encourage regular physical activity throughout life if the typical trends of the past 20 years are to be reversed in older Americans.

## Diabetes

Diabetes is a chronic disease that affects nearly 16 million Americans, with over 10 million cases diagnosed, and is characterized by serious, costly, and potentially fatal complications. The total cost of diagnosed cases of diabetes in the U.S. in 1992 was estimated to be $92 billion (47). Several large-scale preventive trials are currently underway in the U.S. (48) and Finland (49). In addition, the American Diabetes Association has developed a recent position statement (27) on diabetes and exercise that supports the need for exercise in a comprehensive treatment plan for diabetics. Diabetes is associated with an increased risk of cardiovascular disease (50) and recent studies reveal improvements in cardiovascular risk factors, fitness, and glucose tolerance with an exercise program for both men (51) and women (52,53).

## Osteoarthritis

Osteoarthritis (OA), the most common form of arthritis, increases in prevalence with age and places older adults at risk for significant disability since it is the most common reason for total hip and knee replacements (54). There are numerous risk factors for OA (i.e., genetics, gender, nutrition, etc.) but local biomechanical factors are also very important, including joint injury, joint deformity, sports participation, and obesity. While traumatic injury from sport is a common cause of OA, there is no evidence that running increases the risk of OA (55). Knee extensor strength is negatively associated with risk of osteoarthritis (56) while obesity shows a positive relationship (57). A recent retrospective study (58) compared men and women with either a low or high number of cumulative hours in recreational activity and found a significant reduction in risk of knee osteoarthritis requiring arthroplasty (45% lower in women and 65% lower in men) as individuals increased their hours of recreational physical exercise. In a study of older individuals with diagnosed OA, an 18-month program of aerobic and resistance exercise significantly reduced knee pain and physical disability as well as improved strength, endurance, and physical function (59), suggesting that exercise should be prescribed as part of the treatment for knee osteoarthritis. These studies make a clear case for the need to remain active and maintain normal body weight in order to prevent or decrease the risk of developing OA in aging adults.

## Osteoporosis

Osteoporosis poses a major health threat in the Unites States and while 10 million persons already have osteoporosis, another 18 million have low bone mass that places them at high risk for this disorder. The conclusion of an NIH Consensus Panel is that osteoporosis is largely preventable and that optimization of bone health is a process that must occur throughout life in both men and women (26). A comprehensive approach requires an assessment of risk factors as well as early intervention, depending upon the cause(s) of osteoporosis. While age, gender, gonadal steroids, and genetics play an important role, the modifiable risk factors include diet and physical activity as a means of preventing and/or treating individuals with osteoporosis. The panel recommends regular exercise, especially in the form of resistance and high-impact activities, as a means of developing peak bone mass in adults and children in addition to reducing the risk of falls in older persons. Fuchs and others (60) have demonstrated an increase in bone mass of the spine and femoral neck of prepubertal children as a result of a 7-month high-intensity jumping program and strongly recommend that vigorous weight bearing activity be incorporated into school programs for youth. In a 15 year longitudinal study, Welton and others (61) followed a group of 84 males and 98 females longitudinally from age 13 until age 28 and concluded that regular weight-bearing exercise and at least a normal age-related body weight in adolescence and young adulthood are of key importance in reaching the highest lumbar peak bone mass at the age of 27 years. High impact activity has also been demonstrated to increase bone mineral density in the weight-bearing site (femoral neck) but not in the non-weight bearing site (distal radius) of premenopausal women. (62) Gregg and others (63) have shown that higher levels of leisure time, sport activity, and household chores and fewer hours of sitting daily were associated with significantly reduced relative risk for hip fracture in elderly women (>65 yrs). Similar results were found in men, where there was an inverse relationship between physical activity and osteoporotic hip fracture (64). However, as Winters and Snow have demonstrated, detraining will reverse these positive effects (65) and therefore, lifelong high-impact weight bearing activity (66) and resistance training (67) are essential for optimal bone health.

## Discussion

It is apparent that convincing evidence continues to mount regarding the influence of lifestyle behaviors upon health and well-being, making it imperative that in addition to other preventive and rehabilitative strategies, nutrition and physical activity should be incorporated into the disease management plans for patients with each of these chronic diseases. The most effective way to do this would be to develop *Disease Management Centers* that are dedicated to providing the medical care that meets the current standards of practice. The model shown in figure 5.1 demonstrates a theoretical approach that is based upon independent studies that have proven to be successful in changing health-related behaviors. In this model, patients with one or more chronic diseases that are amenable to lifestyle modification are referred to their Primary Care Physician through several sources: a worksite physician or nurse, a medical specialist, or even through self-referral. The Primary Care Physician is key to the success of this model as s/he would then refer this patient to the Preventive/Rehabilitative Center for an initial contact and evaluation. At this initial evaluation, the clinical staff would assess the readiness of the patient to participate in one of the interventions (68), identify the needs of the patient, and develop an individualized program of intervention that is tailored to meet those needs. These programs will be described in more detail later in this chapter.

## Application to Practice

The challenge is to first develop these programs and then encourage the referral base that allows these programs to remain solvent while still providing the standard of care dictated by the health care industry. While clinical guidelines should dictate physician practice, it is common knowledge that preventive care is not effectively implemented due to competing demands and other important

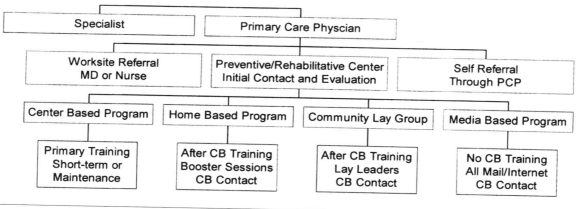

**Figure 5.1**  Flow chart for disease management program

primary care responsibilities of Primary Care Physicians. Goodwin and others (69) addressed this issue and demonstrated significant increases in screening services, health habit counseling, and global preventive service delivery rates as a result of a comprehensive training program delivered to community family practices. Their approach has potential for being incorporated into the model proposed in this paper.

It is important that Primary Care Physicians be encouraged to think of lifestyle intervention as the first step in the management of their patients who have one or more of these chronic diseases. This is not the common trend in medicine today although considerable work has been expended in an effort to help physicians put prevention into practice (70,71). Next, physicians must make referrals to appropriate health care professionals who can then apply proven techniques of behavioral intervention (72-74) in concert with the medical management provided by the referral physician (75). The multidisciplinary team that would manage such an endeavor is presented in figure 5.2.

To the knowledge of this writer, the model proposed in this paper has never been implemented as a comprehensive, integrated approach to preventive care within a managed care organization. However, each of the four essential programmatic components has been successfully implemented separately in: Center-Based Programs (76,23); Home-Based Programs (77-79); Lay Community Groups (80,81), and Mail/Internet Self-Management Programs (82,83).

This proposed model requires significant coordination between the Primary Care Physicians in a community and the staff at the Preventive/Rehabilitative Center. This model is initiated upon referral from a Primary Care Physician, where the patient is evaluated through a comprehensive screening process that incorporates existing test results plus data from the patient history to provide a basis for establishing patient goals. Next, the appropriate health care professionals, including case managers (79) and behavioral therapists (7,74), will set short and long term goals, in concert with the patient, that are based upon current clinical guidelines. An intervention strategy is then developed using proven behavioral techniques (84) that can be implemented through one or more of the four programmatic options: the Center-Based Program, the Home-Based Program, the Lay Community Groups, or the Mail/ Internet Based Self-Management Programs. At the same time, specific outcomes must be established that are based upon knowledge, function, quality of life, and disease progression (22).

The **Center-Based Program** is the traditional cardiopulmonary rehabilitation model that has been the standard in most communities for the past 25 years (23,24,85). While it is also the most time/staff-intensive and expensive, it can be modified to include at least three options: 1) a short 3-session plan, 2) an intermediate 36 session plan, or 3) a long (> 1 year) plan, depending upon patient preference, time/distance barriers, or and/or finances. In this new inclusive model, it is recommended at a minimum that all patients report initially to the Center-Based Program for at least the short 3-session plan to prepare them for one of the next program levels.

Next, the **Home-Based Program**, which is a more recent development (77,86), can be implemented at the time the patient transitions out of the Center-Based Program. The Home-Based model allows the patient the freedom to exercise at home at times that are most convenient and does not involve the barriers of time, travel, and expense that are associated with the Center-Based Program The Home-Based Program is an attractive alternative to the Center-Based Model because it can be maintained indefinitely and patients

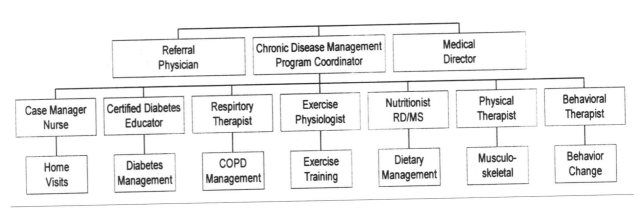

**Figure 5.2**   Chronic disease management team.

can then be followed and monitored using the standard case-manager approach (79).

For those patients who are not inclined to adopt a Home-Based Program but would prefer a group support approach outside of the Preventive/ Rehabilitative Center, the **Lay Community-Based Program** (80,81) is a logical option as it provides the patient with expertise in disease management along with social support—but at a low cost in terms of time, travel, and financial expense. In this approach, patients with multiple chronic diseases are trained by medical specialists to serve as lay leaders and conduct self-management programs in the community for other patients with multiple chronic diseases.

For those patients who for one reason or another cannot participate in any of the previously described programs, the final options are the **Mail-Based** or **Internet-Based Programs.** These programs will appeal to those who prefer to take more responsibility for their health behaviors but still need guidance and expertise that can be accessed at their convenience. The Mail-Based Program designed by Fries (87) has been used effectively in multiple studies (82) with improved health outcomes and significant cost savings. Internet-Based Programs, while relatively new, show promise as a supplemental means of promoting physical activity (88); a recent study (83) demonstrated that is can be used successfully in a weight loss program.

## Summary

The time is overdue for the development of a comprehensive disease management plan that can be universally adopted by health care professionals and endorsed by HMOs, Medicare, and other insurers. The essential components of a comprehensive program have already been developed and it remains to be seen if these components can be fully integrated into preventive medicine in a timely manner. The benefits will reduce the chronic disease burden on society by promoting cost savings, reducing morbidity/mortality, and improving quality of life.

## References

1. U.S.Department of Health and Human Services. Programs and initiatives for an aging America. 5-3-2001. HHS Press Office.

2. National Center for Chronic Disease Prevention and Health Promotion and Chronic Disease Prevention. Chronic diseases and their risk factors: the nation's leading causes of death. 1999.

3. Weingarten S. Using practice guideline compendiums to provide better preventive care. *Ann Intern Med* 1999; 130(5):454-458.

4. U.S.Department of Health and Human Services. Clinician's Handbook of Preventive Services. Put Prevention into Practice. 1998.

5. U.S.Department of Health and Human Services. Physical activity and health: a report of the Surgeon General. 1996. Atlanta: Department of Health and Human Services, Centers for Disease Control and Prevention, National Center for Chronic Disease Prevention and Health Promotion.

6. Wee CC, McCarthy EP, Davis RB, Phillips RS. Physician counseling about exercise. *JAMA* 1999; 282(16):1583-1588.

7. Sherman SE, Hershman WY. Exercise counseling: how do general internists do? *J Gen Intern Med* 1993; 8(5):243-248.

8. Damush TM, Stewart AL, Mills KM, King AC, Ritter PL. Prevalence and correlates of physician recommendations to exercise among older adults. *J Gerontol A Biol Sci Med Sci* 1999; 54(8):M423-M427.

9. Ribisl PM. Exercise: the unfilled prescription. *Am J Med Sports* 3, 13-21. 2001.

10. Prochaska JJ, Zabinski MF, Calfas KJ, Sallis JF, Patrick K. PACE+: interactive communication technology for behavior change in clinical settings. *Am J Prev Med* 2000; 19(2):127-131.

11. Thompson SC, Schwankovsky L, Pitts J. Counselling patients to make lifestyle changes: the role of physician self-efficacy, training and beliefs about causes. *Fam Pract* 1993; 10(1):70-75.

12. O'Connor PJ, Rush WA, Prochaska JO, Pronk NP, Boyle RG. Professional advice and readiness to change behavioral risk factors among members of a managed care organization. *Am J Manag Care* 2001; 7(2):125-130.

13. Pronk NP, Goodman MJ, O'Connor PJ, Martinson BC. Relationship between modifiable health risks and short-term health care charges. *JAMA* 1999; 282(23):2235-2239.

14. Richardson LA, Buckenmeyer PJ, Bauman BD, Rosneck JS, Newman I, Josephson RA. Contemporary cardiac rehabilitation: patient characteristics and temporal trends over the past decade. *J Cardiopulm Rehabil* 2000; 20(1):57-64.

15. Ades PA, Pashkow FJ, Nestor JR. Cost-effectiveness of cardiac rehabilitation after myocardial infarction. *J Cardiopulm Rehabil* 1997; 17(4):222-231.

16. Levin LA, Perk J, Hedback B. Cardiac rehabilitation—a cost analysis. *J Intern Med* 1991; 230(5):427-434.

17. Oldridge NB. Comprehensive cardiac rehabilitation: is it cost-effective? *Eur Heart J* 1998; 19 Suppl O:O42-O50.

18. Hedback B, Perk J, Wodlin P. Long-term reduction of cardiac mortality after myocardial infarction: 10-year results of a comprehensive rehabilitation programme. *Eur Heart J* 1993; 14(6):831-835.

19. Hamalainen H, Luurila OJ, Kallio V, Knuts LR. Reduction in sudden deaths and coronary mortality in myocardial infarction patients after rehabilitation. 15 year follow-up study. *Eur Heart J* 1995; 16(12):1839-1844.

20. Jolliffe JA, Rees K, Taylor RS, Thompson D, Oldridge N, Ebrahim S. Exercise-based rehabilitation for coronary heart disease (Cochrane Review). Cochrane Database Syst Rev 2001; 1:CD001800.

21. Hall LK. Health and disease management: expandingt the cardiac and pulmonary rehabilitation model. Clinical Exercise Physiology 1[1], 42-46. 199.

22. Hall L. Management models: disease management algorithms stratify risks and interventions. *The Journal for Respiratory Care Practitioners* June/July, 71-72. 97.

23. Balady GJ, Ades PA, Comoss P, Limacher M, Pina IL, Southard D et al. Core components of cardiac rehabilitation/secondary prevention programs: A statement for healthcare professionals from the American Heart Association and the American Association of Cardiovascular and Pulmonary Rehabilitation Writing Group. *Circulation* 2000; 102(9):1069-1073.

24. Wenger NK, Froelicher ES, Smith LK, Ades PA, Berra K, Blumenthal JA et al. Cardiac rehabilitation as secondary prevention. Agency for Health Care Policy and Research and National Heart, Lung, and Blood Institute. *Clin Pract Guidel Quick Ref Guide Clin* 1995;(17):1-23.

25. Guidelines for Pulmonary Rehabilitation Programs. Connors G, Hilling L, editors. 2nd. 2001. Champaign, Illinois, Human Kinetics. 1998.

26. Osteoporosis prevention, diagnosis, and therapy. *JAMA* 2001; 285(6):785-795.

27. American Diabetes Association. Diabetes Mellitus and Exercise. *Diabetes Care* 1999;49s.

28. Clinical Guidelines on the Identification, Evaluation, and Treatment of Overweight and Obesity in Adults—The Evidence Report. National Institutes of Health [published erratum appears in *Obes Res* 1998 Nov;6(6):464] [see comments]. *Obes Res* 1998; 6 Suppl 2:51S-209S.

29. Felson DT, Lawrence RC, Hochberg MC, McAlindon T, Dieppe PA, Minor MA et al. Osteoarthritis: new insights. Part 2: treatment approaches. *Ann Intern Med* 2000; 133(9):726-737.

30. Stampfer MJ, Hu FB, Manson JE, Rimm EB, Willett WC. Primary prevention of coronary heart disease in women through diet and lifestyle. *N Engl J Med* 2000; 343(1):16-22.

31. Drygas W, Kostka T, Jegier A, Kunski H. Long-term effects of different physical activity levels on coronary heart disease risk factors in middle-aged men. *Int J Sports Med* 2000; 21(4):235-241.

32. Rockhill B, Willett WC, Hunter DJ, Manson JE, Hankinson SE, Colditz GA. A prospective study of recreational physical activity and breast cancer risk. *Arch Intern Med* 1999; 159(19):2290-2296.

33. Manson JE, Hu FB, Rich-Edwards JW, Colditz GA, Stampfer MJ, Willett WC et al. A prospective study of walking as compared with vigorous exercise in the prevention of coronary heart disease in women. *N Engl J Med* 1999; 341(9): 650-658.

34. Lakka TA, Laukkanen JA, Rauramaa R, Salonen R, Lakka HM, Kaplan GA et al. Cardiorespiratory fitness and the progression of carotid atherosclerosis in middle-aged men. *Ann Intern Med* 2001; 134(1):12-20.

35. Friedman M, Hilleman DE. Economic burden of chronic obstructive pulmonary disease. Impact of new treatment options. *Pharmacoeconomics* 2001; 19(3):245-254.

36. ACCP, AACVPR. Pulmonary rehabilitation: joint ACCP/AACVPR evidence-based guidelines. ACCP/AACVPR Pulmonary Rehabilitation Guidelines Panel. American College of Chest Physicians. American Association of Cardiovascular and Pulmonary Rehabilitation. *Chest* 1997; 112(5):1363-1396.

37. Advances in Cardiopulmonary Rehabilitation. Champaign, IL: Human Kinetics, 2001.

38. Resnikoff PM, Ries AL. Maximizing functional capacity. Pulmonary rehabilitation and adjunctive measures. *Respir Care Clin N Am* 1998; 4(3):475-492.

39. Resnikoff PM, Ries AL. Pulmonary rehabilitation for chronic lung disease. *J Heart Lung Transplant* 1998; 17(7):643-650.

40. Ries AL, Kaplan RM, Limberg TM, Prewitt LM.

ologic and psychosocial outcomes in patients with chronic obstructive pulmonary disease. *Ann Intern Med* 1995; 122(11):823-832.

41. Shafazand S, Canfield J, Kuschner WG. Improved quality of life among patients completing a pulmonary rehabilitation program: one center's early experience. *Respir Care* 2001; 46(6):595-600.

42. National Task Force on the Prevention and Treatment of Obesity. Overweight, obesity, and health risk. *Arch Intern Med* 2000; 160(7):898-904.

43. Wing RR, Hill JO. Successful weight loss maintenance. *Annu Rev Nutr* 2001; 21:323-341.

44. Ribisl P, McInnis KMJRJ. The next y2k problem—obesity: genes, gluttony, or sloth? *Am J Med Sports* 3, 171-179. 2001.

45. Haapanen N, Miilunpalo S, Pasanen M, Oja P, Vuori I. Association between leisure time physical activity and 10-year body mass change among working-aged men and women. *Int J Obes Relat Metab Disord* 1997; 21(4):288-296.

46. Nawaz H, Adams ML, Katz DL. Physician-patient interactions regarding diet, exercise, and smoking. *Prev Med* 2000; 31(6):652-657.

47. Diabetes Statistics. NIDDK. 6-6-2001. Internet Communication

48. The Diabetes Prevention Program. Design and methods for a clinical trial in the prevention of type 2 diabetes. *Diabetes Care* 1999; 22(4):623-634.

49. Eriksson J, Lindstrom J, Valle T, Aunola S, Hamalainen H, Ilanne-Parikka P et al. Prevention of Type II diabetes in subjects with impaired glucose tolerance: the Diabetes Prevention Study (DPS) in Finland. Study design and 1-year interim report on the feasibility of the lifestyle intervention programme. *Diabetologia* 1999; 42(7):793-801.

50. Lotufo PA, Gaziano JM, Chae CU, Ajani UA, Moreno-John G, Buring JE et al. Diabetes and All-Cause and Coronary Heart Disease Mortality Among US Male Physicians. *Arch Intern Med* 2001; 161(2):242-247.

51. Laukkanen JA, Lakka TA, Rauramaa R, Kuhanen R, Venalainen JM, Salonen R et al. Cardiovascular fitness as a predictor of mortality in men. *Arch Intern Med* 2001; 161(6):825-831.

52. Hu FB, Stampfer MJ, Solomon C, Liu S, Colditz GA, Speizer FE et al. Physical Activity and Risk for Cardiovascular Events in Diabetic Women. *Ann Intern Med* 2001; 134(2):96-105.

53. Walker KZ, Piers LS, Putt RS, Jones JA, O'Dea K. Effects of regular walking on cardiovascular risk factors and body composition in normo-glycemic women and women with type 2 diabetes. *Diabetes Care* 1999; 22(4):555-561.

54. Felson DT, Lawrence RC, Dieppe PA, Hirsch R, Helmick CG, Jordan JM et al. Osteoarthritis: new insights. Part 1: the disease and its risk factors. *Ann Intern Med* 2000; 133(8):635-646.

55. Lane NE, Oehlert JW, Bloch DA, Fries JF. The relationship of running to osteoarthritis of the knee and hip and bone mineral density of the lumbar spine: a 9 year longitudinal study. *J Rheumatol* 1998; 25(2):334-341.

56. Slemenda C, Brandt KD, Heilman DK, Mazzuca S, Braunstein EM, Katz BP et al. Quadriceps weakness and osteoarthritis of the knee. *Ann Intern Med* 1997; 127(2):97-104.

57. Felson DT, Zhang Y, Hannan MT, Naimark A, Weissman B, Aliabadi P et al. Risk factors for incident radiographic knee osteoarthritis in the elderly: the Framingham Study. *Arthritis Rheum* 1997; 40(4):728-733.

58. Manninen P, Riihimaki H, Heliovaara M, Suomalainen O. Physical exercise and risk of severe knee osteoarthritis requiring arthroplasty. *Rheumatology* (Oxford) 2001; 40(4):432-437.

59. Ettinger WH, Jr., Burns R, Messier SP, Applegate W, Rejeski WJ, Morgan T et al. A randomized trial comparing aerobic exercise and resistance exercise with a health education program in older adults with knee osteoarthritis. The Fitness Arthritis and Seniors Trial (FAST). *JAMA* 1997; 277(1):25-31.

60. Fuchs RK, Bauer JJ, Snow CM. Jumping improves hip and lumbar spine bone mass in prepubescent children: a randomized controlled trial. *J Bone Miner Res* 2001; 16(1):148-156.

61. Welten DC, Kemper HC, Post GB, Van Mechelen W, Twisk J, Lips P et al. Weight-bearing activity during youth is a more important factor for peak bone mass than calcium intake. *J Bone Miner Res* 1994; 9(7):1089-1096.

62. Heinonen A, Kannus P, Sievanen H, Oja P, Pasanen M, Rinne M et al. Randomised controlled trial of effect of high-impact exercise on selected risk factors for osteoporotic fractures. *Lancet* 1996; 348(9038):1343-1347.

63. Gregg EW, Cauley JA, Seeley DG, Ensrud KE, Bauer DC. Physical activity and osteoporotic fracture risk in older women. Study of Osteoporotic Fractures Research Group. *Ann Intern Med* 1998; 129(2):81-88.

64. Kujala UM, Kaprio J, Kannus P, Sarna S, Koskenvuo M. Physical activity and osteoporotic hip fracture risk in men. *Arch Intern Med* 2000; 160(5):705-708.

65. Winters KM, Snow CM. Detraining reverses positive effects of exercise on the musculoskeletal system in premenopausal women. *J Bone Miner Res* 2000; 15(12):2495-2503.

66. Andreoli A, Monteleone M, Van Loan M, Promenzio L, Tarantino U, De Lorenzo A. Effects of different sports on bone density and muscle mass in highly trained athletes. *Med Sci Sports Exerc* 2001; 33(4):507-511.

67. Kerr D, Ackland T, Maslen B, Morton A, Prince R. Resistance training over 2 years increases bone mass in calcium-replete postmenopausal women. *J Bone Miner Res* 2001; 16(1):175-181.

68. Counseling: intervention effects on mediators of motivational readiness for physical activity. *Ann Behav Med* 2001; 23(1):2-10.

69. Goodwin MA, Zyzanski SJ, Zronek S, Ruhe M, Weyer SM, Konrad N et al. A clinical trial of tailored office systems for preventive service delivery. The Study to Enhance Prevention by Understanding Practice (STEP-UP). *Am J Prev Med* 2001; 21(1):20-28.

70. Dickey LL, Gemson DH. Put prevention into practice: shifting the curve toward success? *Am J Prev Med* 1997; 13(5):343-344.

71. McBride P, Underbakke G, Plane MB, Massoth K, Brown RL, Solberg LI et al. Improving prevention systems in primary care practices: the Health Education and Research Trial (HEART). *J Fam Pract* 2000; 49(2):115-125.

72. Marcus BH, Dubbert PM, Forsyth LH, McKenzie TL, Stone EJ, Dunn AL et al. Physical activity behavior change: issues in adoption and maintenance. *Health Psychol* 2000; 19(1 Suppl):32-41.

73. Bock BC, Marcus BH, Pinto BM, Forsyth LH. Maintenance of physical activity following an individualized motivationally tailored intervention. *Ann Behav Med* 2001; 23(2):79-87.

74. Wetter AC, Goldberg JP, King AC, Sigman-Grant M, Baer R, Crayton E et al. How and why do individuals make food and physical activity choices? *Nutr Rev* 2001; 59(3 Pt 2):S11-S20.

75. DeBusk RF, West JA, Miller NH, Taylor CB. Chronic disease management: treating the patient with disease(s) vs. treating disease(s) in the patient. *Arch Intern Med* 1999; 159(22):2739-2742.

76. Maines TY, Lavie CJ, Milani RV, Cassidy MM, Gilliland YE, Murgo JP. Effects of cardiac rehabilitation and exercise programs on exercise capacity, coronary risk factors, behavior, and quality of life in patients with coronary artery disease. *South Med J* 1997; 90(1):43-49.

77. Brubaker PH, Rejeski WJ, Smith MJ, Sevensky KH, Lamb KA, Sotile WM et al. A home-based maintenance exercise program after center-based cardiac rehabilitation: effects on blood lipids, body composition, and functional capacity. *J Cardiopulm Rehabil* 2000; 20(1):50-56.

78. Oka RK, De Marco T, Haskell WL, Botvinick E, Dae MW, Bolen K et al. Impact of a home-based walking and resistance training program on quality of life in patients with heart failure. *Am J Cardiol* 2000; 85(3):365-369.

79. DeBusk RF, Miller NH, Superko HR, Dennis CA, Thomas RJ, Lew HT et al. A case-management system for coronary risk factor modification after acute myocardial infarction. *Ann Intern Med* 1994; 120(9):721-729.

80. Lorig KR, Sobel DS, Stewart AL, Brown BW, Jr., Bandura A, Ritter P et al. Evidence suggesting that a chronic disease self-management program can improve health status while reducing hospitalization: a randomized trial. *Med Care* 1999; 37(1):5-14.

81. Lorig K, Gonzalez VM, Laurent DD, Morgan L, Laris BA. Arthritis self-management program variations: three studies. *Arthritis Care Res* 1998; 11(6):448-454.

82. Fries JF, Harrington H, Edwards R, Kent LA, Richardson N. Randomized controlled trial of cost reductions from a health education program: the California Public Employees' Retirement System (PERS) study. *Am J Health Promot* 1994; 8(3):216-223.

83. Tate DF, Wing RR, Winett RA. Using Internet technology to deliver a behavioral weight loss program. *JAMA* 2001; 285(9):1172-1177.

84. Zimmerman GL, Olsen CG, Bosworth MF. A 'stages of change' approach to helping patients change behavior. *Am Fam Physician* 2000; 61(5):1409-1416.

85. Carlson JJ, Johnson JA, Franklin BA, VanderLaan RL. Program participation, exercise adherence, cardiovascular outcomes, and program cost of traditional versus modified cardiac rehabilitation. *Am J Cardiol* 2000; 86(1):17-23.

86. King AC, Haskell WL, Taylor CB, Kraemer HC, DeBusk RF. Group- vs home-based exercise training in healthy older men and women. A community-based clinical trial. *JAMA* 1991; 266(11):1535-1542.

87. Fries JF, McShane D. Reducing need and demand for medical services in high-risk persons. A health education approach. *West J Med* 1998; 169(4):201-207.

88. Marcus BH, Nigg CR, Riebe D, Forsyth LH. Interactive communication strategies: implications for population-based physical-activity promotion. *Am J Prev Med* 2000; 19(2):121-126.

Chapter 6

# Close Follow-Up for the Congestive Heart Failure Patient Using Outpatient, Home and Palliative Care

Susan E. Qualietti RN, MSN, ANP, USA

## Introduction

Congestive heart failure (CHF) is a major chronic illness through out the world with an enormous impact on health care costs. It is estimated that over 4 million persons in the United States (US) have CHF and is present in almost 10% of persons over 70 years old. It is the only cardiovascular disease that is increasing in incidence and prevalence (1). Various disorders of the pericardium, myocardium and endocardium can lead to heart failure but 80% of CHF is due to left ventricular systolic dysfunction. Coronary artery disease is the leading cause of heart failure, occurring in approximately two thirds of CHF patients. Non-ischemic cardiomyopathy can be caused by hypertension, alcohol abuse, thyroid disease, myocarditis and idiopathic reasons (idiopathic dilated cardiomyopathy). Heart failure is the most common diagnosis in hospitalized patients over 65 years. One third of the patients hospitalized for CHF are re-admitted within 90 days of discharge (1). Prognosis with CHF is poor, with one in five patients dying within 1 year of diagnosis and half within 5 years (1). Survival estimates are worse for men than women; fewer than 20% of patients regardless of age or gender survive longer than 10 years and CHF prognosis is worse in elderly subjects of both sexes. Annual direct health care expenditures for CHF in the US have been estimated at $20-40 billion, with $8-15 billion spent on hospitalization alone (1).

Over the last two decades, new therapeutic options have improved the mortality associated with left ventricular systolic dysfunction. Because CHF patients have improved survival expectancy, their health cares needs vary depending upon their stage of illness, age, socio-economic status, social support and other disabling diseases. Cardiac rehabilitation has traditionally provided care for the coronary artery disease patient, but now these programs welcome the CHF patient even though they are considered "high risk" (2). Alternative approaches to the delivery of cardiac rehabilitation services using home monitoring and telephone contact have been supported by the Agency for Health Care Policy and Research (AHCPR) clinical practice guidelines on cardiac rehabilitation. These types of approaches for managing heart failure have been reported in the literature in the last ten years, with the goal of reducing hospitalizations and improving implementation of guideline recommendations. Other approaches such as disease management models offer chronic care coverage across the continuum, aiming to provide continuity.

In general, many of the newer CHF models of care use a multidisciplinary approach and most assume the basic principles of cardiac rehabilitation: provide close follow up, patient oriented goals, behavioral management for diet, guidance for exercise and medication adherence, risk assessment for risk modification counseling, symptom management, and improvement in quality of life. Unfortunately, models aimed at care for the advanced heart failure patient are only beginning to emerge. This paper reviews the clinical and research issues associated with integrated care for the CHF patient in the clinic, the home and when palliation is the major issue.

## Health Care Utilization and Outcomes With CHF

Despite the research that has led to improved survival with medical therapy, CHF is still associated with poor outcomes, high health care utilization and requires further investigation to help improve outcomes. Patient characteristics such as socio-economic status, race, gender and social support can influence delivery of care and recurrence of hospitalization (3,4). Table 6.1 lists the factors associated with increased health care services for the CHF patient. (5).

Poor quality of life (QOL) can result from decreasing functional status and poor symptom control. Burns and colleagues (1997) described the impact of CHF on patients following hospitalization and reported that of the 519 CHF patients reviewed, 35% were short of breath walking less than 1 block, 62% had fair or poor perceived health, 32% received

**Table 6.1   Factors Contributing to Health Care Utilization in Congestive Heart Failure Patients**

1. Demographic and socioeconomic factors
   age (older, greater than 65)
   sex (female)
   race and ethnicity (African-American)
   lower socioeconomic status
   type of health insurance (Medicare)

2. Clinical factors
   additional comorbid illnesses (diabetes, COPD, arthritis, stroke)
   poorer functional status
   depressed left ventricular function
   depression

3. Patient non-compliance with treatment
   lack of knowledge concerning medication use
   difficulty adhering to diet recommendations
   delay with seeking follow-up care

4. Health-care system factors
   type of provider (cardiologist vs. non-cardiologist)
   premature hospital discharge

5. Follow-up care
   inadequate diagnosis
   inadequate treatment according to CHF guidelines
   adverse drug reactions
   inadequate patient education
   lack of follow-up care (no referral for rehabilitation or home care)
   poor continuity of care (case management not utilized)

some formal care and 46% were re-hospitalized within 1 year of discharge (6). The relation of daily activity levels in patients with CHF and long term prognosis were analyzed in 84 patients with Class II-III heart failure, all with ejection fraction (EF) less than 35% for over one year (7). Reduced measures of daily activity by pedometer score were a stronger predictor of death (p<0.001) than laboratory-based exercise tests. The SUPPORT investigators found that survival among 1390 adult CHF patients with median age of 68 years was only 61.5% at one year (8). At six months, 40% of patients were dependent in one or more activity of daily living (ADL) even though 59% of patients reported quality of life between good and excellent. Many studies list high rates of comorbid problems such as coronary artery disease (CAD), chronic obstructive pulmonary disease (COPD) and diabetes mellitus (DM) which ultimately compound functional decline.

Hospitalization rates for CHF doubled between 1973 and 1986, with the steepest increase among those over 74 years (9). Croft et al. reviewed Medicare hospital claims of 631,306 patients from 1986 and 803,506 patients from 1993 who had initial hospitalizations for CHF (10). Age-standardized hospitalization rates for any diagnosis of CHF was higher during 1993, discharge to home health services doubled (6% to 12%) and over 25% of all admissions regardless of race or sex were in patients 85 years or older. Hospitalization rates may even be higher, depending on which reporting measures are used. Goff and colleagues report that reliance on ICD codes during hospitalization resulted in missing 1/3 of the patients with clinical evidence of acute CHF (11).

Sixty five percent of patients admitted for heart failure exacerbation were due to lack of compliance with either drugs, dietary indiscretions or both (12). Ni and associates reported that of 113 patients, 86% said they knew "little or nothing" or "some" about CHF (13). Forty percent did not recognize the importance of daily weights and only one third always avoided salty foods. Poor adherence to self-care was associated with unmarried status; lower perceived self-efficacy, lack of knowledge about self-care and no prior hospitalization.

Edep and colleagues report that there are significant differences between internists, general/family practitioners, and cardiologists for implementing the AHCPR guidelines for CHF (14). Only 60-70% of non-cardiologists used angiotensin converting enzyme (ACE) inhibitor therapy. In addition to underutilization of medications (possibly due to unfamiliarity with doses and side effects), over-burdened primary care providers also feel time constraints during clinic visits that limit their ability to provide education on diet, exercise and medication. Senni and colleagues also report that advances with CHF diagnosis and therapy management have not been incorporated into community settings over the last 10 years (15).

Patient preferences for CHF therapy outcomes have not been extensively studies though this should impact CHF care. Stanek and colleagues conclude after analyzing survival vs. symptom preferences in 50 patients, symptom control was of greater importance than longer survival (16).

## Methods of Follow-Up

There is general agreement between the various heart failure guidelines that counseling concerning diet (fluid and salt restriction), exercise, symptom management, risk factor management, medication use (dosing, polypharmacy, effect on survival), prognosis (life expectancy, advanced directives) should be included in the management of the CHF patient. In a recent consensus on the recommendations for the management of chronic heart failure, it is stated that "Of the general measures that are recommended in patients with heart failure, possibly the most effective (yet least utilized) is close attention and follow-up" (1). Currently, no guidelines mention models other than standard clinic visits on implementing these aspects. Lack of systematic monitoring of patients after hospital discharge can impact the effectiveness of CHF management. General suggestions such as utilizing interdisciplinary health care providers, involving family members, scheduling group educational meetings and providing nursing interventions have been discussed. Due to limited research, there is no consensus on the "best" method on how or where to provide these services. Despite the prevalence of CHF in the elderly and the eventual debilitating progression this disease, research trials have also not been conducted evaluating palliative care for the advanced CHF patient. As a result, specific recommendations for this group of CHF patients are not available.

Various home-based and clinic programs utilizing a disease management approach for CHF have begun to surface. Problems such as disease severity causing homebound status, lack of transportation to access the out patient clinic and insurance limitations on home care benefits can impact which patients are referred for home or clinic management. Identifying whether patient outcomes differ with primary care providers, cardiology practices or joint management is being investigated. Despite these various clinical problems, there is a growing body of information supporting either telephone, clinic based or home care for the CHF patient. Each of these will be reviewed below.

## Out Patient Based Care-Telephone Follow-Up

Several studies support a nurse monitored telephone program that closely follows symptoms and medical compliance (see table 6.2). In addition to telephone contact, patient education, diet counseling, symptom management, medication recommendations, automated reminders and assistive devices for blood pressure and weight have been included as interventions. Care was usually coordinated through a physician, a cardiologist, primary care provider or both.

Of the studies reviewed, 3 out of 4 report significant reductions in hospitalizations and readmissions (17,18,19,20). It is difficult to generalize outcome benefits from these studies since most were not controlled trials, patients varied in age and existing support structures were not defined to determine clinic accessibility.

## Out Patient Care-Clinic Follow-Up

### Nurse Directed Out Patient Clinics

Clinic management for the CHF patient can be provided by various health personnel and can include many aspects of care (see table 6.2). Nurse directed clinics have shown significant results in implementing and managing secondary prevention in patients with coronary heart disease as well as with heart failure management (21,22,23,24). Recently, nurse managed CHF clinics have been associated with reduced hospitalizations and decreased LOS. The registered nurse (RN) usually has experience with heart failure management, is able to provide education on heart failure and self- management and can be accessible for unscheduled clinic appointments. Collaboration with a physician, dietician and social worker can be particularly effective in improving outcomes (23).

Patients enrolled in heart failure programs are typically managed by physicians with an expertise

**Table 6.2 Management of the Congestive Heart Failure Patient Using Phone, Clinic and Home Care**

| Author | Enrolled patients | Study design | Follow-up | Intervention | Reduced hospitalization | Decreased LOS | Decreased cost | Improved medicine therapy | Improved functional status/QOL |
|---|---|---|---|---|---|---|---|---|---|
| West, 1997 | 51 | Observ | 4.5 m | Phone/nurse | X | | | X | X |
| Shah, 1998 | 27 | Observ | 8.5 m | Phone/nurse | X | X | | | |
| Heidenreich, 1999 | 68 | Observ | 12 m | Phone/nurse | X | X | X | | |
| Fulmer, 1999 | 50 | Rand | 2.5 m | Phone/nurse | | | | X | X |
| Cintron, 1983 | 15 | Observ | 24 m | Clinic/nurse | X | X | X | | |
| Lasater, 1996 | 80 | Observ | 6 m | Clinic/nurse/team | X | X | X | | |
| Cline, 1998 | 190 | Rand | 12 m | Clinic/nurse | | X | X | X | |
| Gattis, 1999 | 181 | Rand | 6 m | Clinic/phone | | | | X | |
| Kostis, 1994 | 20 | Rand | 3 m | Clinic | X | | | | X |
| Hanumanthu, 1997 | 187 | Observ | 12 m | Clinic | X | | | X | X |
| Fonarow, 1997 | 214 | Observ | 6 m | Clinic/phone | X | | X | X | X |
| Lazarre, 1997 | 34 | Observ | 7 m | Home/nurse/team | X | | | | |
| Kornowski, 1995 | 42 | Observ | 12 m | Home/team | X | X | | X | X |
| Rich, 1995 | 282 | Rand | 3 m | Home/nurse/team/phone | X | | X | | X |
| Rich, 1996 | 156 | Rand | 1 m | Home/team | | | | X | |
| Stewart, 1999 | 200 | Rand | 6 m | Home/nurse/team | X | X | | | |
| Stewart, 1999, 1998 | 97 | Rand | 18 m | Home/team | X | X | X | | |

Observ= observational; Rand= randomized; m= month; QOL=quality of life; Team= staff other than cardiologist, nurse or other physician; Nurse= primary manager of care using a registered nurse (RN) or advanced practice RN; Home= community based or hospital based home care; Phone= telephone contact with / or without assistive devices; Clinic= primary follow up in out patient setting.

in heart failure, receive specialized testing such as echocardiograms or exercise testing with hemodynamic monitoring and education regarding non-pharmacological therapy. Nurse practitioners (NP) functioning as providers in CHF clinics can assist with interval exams, patient education and telephone care. Typically, the NP is available to see deteriorating patients between scheduled visits, thus avoiding unnecessary emergency room visits. Improved patient satisfaction, decreased hospitalizations and reduced patient costs have been reported using a NP in CHF clinics (22).

## Out Patient Heart Failure Programs

Heart failure programs or multidisciplinary programs have also been used in clinic practice (see table 6.2). These programs managed patients with chronic heart failure though some programs accepted patients waiting for heart transplantation (25,26,27). Many programs have education groups and individual sessions lead by a heart failure clinical nurse specialist who reviews dietary guidelines, exercise prescription, diuretic therapy and prognosis. Telephone follow-up was incorporated into some of the programs. Telephone calls were made after medication change and at routine intervals. Vigilant follow up with regular personal contact from the heart failure team improved medical compliance and functional status, decreased hospitalizations and CHF costs (26,27).

Gattis and colleagues randomized 181 CHF patients attending a Cardiology clinic to usual care vs. clinical pharmacist evaluation during clinic care (28). For the intervention group, the pharmacist consulted with the cardiologist, provided patient education on medication use and contacted patients by phone at 2, 12 and 24 weeks after initial evaluation. After 6 months of follow up, the intervention group had lower all- cause mortality events and higher ACE inhibitor use (p<.001).

For clinic evaluation, patients must be cognitively intact and have regular transportation available. If these patient conditions change, the effectiveness of out patient management can be altered. Most of the patients listed in the out patient studies were less than 75 years and were NYHA class II or III. No studies listed social variables or concomitant medical problems that could also impact clinic attendance. If patients have visual or hearing deficits, phone follow up alone without social support may not be effective. Consistent contact, whether by phone or clinic, with a specified team member knowledge-able with CHF management has been associated with hospital reduction, better medication compliance and improved life-style modification.

## Home Care in the CHF Patient

Kane and associates reviewed patterns of post-hospital care in 2248 Medicare patients (29). Of the total 490 CHF patients, mean age was 78 years, 44% lived alone and 67% required prior help before hospitalization. Thirty four percent required home care services.

Home care appears a necessary component for heart failure treatment because of increasing numbers of elderly patients diagnosed with CHF, the associated functional decline and the significant amount of caregiver stress with patients managed at home. Patients referred to a community home care agency must meet home care guidelines for acceptance. These CHF patients must have a skilled nursing need and will receive time-limited follow-up determined upon entry into the agency program.

Home care agencies have begun to feature specialty programs for patients with heart failure (30,31). Programs offer a variety of services such as inotropic therapy, intravenous diuretic administration, pulse oximetry as well as case management using a multidisciplinary team. Customized cardiac home rehabilitation programs educate patients with new onset or exacerbation of heart disease on nutrition, exercise, medication use and risk factors (31). Outcome-based critical pathways are being used by home care agencies to document and track standards of practice while monitoring costs (32).

## Clinical Trials Using Home Care for CHF Patients

Home care programs providing interdisciplinary approaches for patients with chronic illness have been reported in the literature since the early 1990s (33). Multiple studies using home care follow up for CHF patients have been associated with reduced hospital admissions, improved functional status and decreased heath care costs (30,34,35,36,37,38). Patients have been evaluated through traditional home care coverage or using a multidisciplinary approach (see table 6.2)

In contrast, Wilson et al. reported higher frequency of hospitalization with the implementation of a home health care in 35 patients referred to from a university heart failure program (39). After referral to home care, patients were hospitalized 0.66 per month as compared to 0.45 per month before referral (p<0.05). These patients had a high mortality and most patients were referred for intensive, aggressive medical therapy (inotropic or intravenous diuretic therapy) unlike the older patients enrolled in other home care studies for post hospitalization medical and symptom management.

In general, multidisciplinary home care for elderly patients with CHF is associated with decreased hospital admissions and health care costs. Home care ranged from routine assessment with patient education to intravenous therapy. Patients generally appear to benefit from close follow up that provides symptom management, patient education and medication review. Patients eventually return to out treatment with home care primarily reinforcing discharge instructions and thus preventing readmission from CHF exacerbation. Coordinating cardiology care with primary care providers during home care also seems to encourage adherence to guideline.

## Patients With Advanced Heart Failure

There has been some controversy defining advanced heart failure in the literature. Current literature suggests that the definition should include the persistence of severe clinical symptoms despite treatment, marked left ventricular dysfunction (resting ejection fraction of less than 30%) and poor exercise capacity (less than 14ml/kg/min on symptom-limited exercise test). Levels of advanced heart failure can be categorized according to response to therapy: level 1 are patients who will probably benefit from aggressive recommended therapy, level 2 are patients who may improve with advanced specialty treatment and level 3 are patients who continue to have refractory symptoms despite aggressive specialty care (40). Levels of additional treatment that are not yet evidence based are recommended according to the level of advanced heart failure. Level 1 includes promising strategies such as multidisciplinary management and anticoagulation therapy. Level 2 and level 3 are either research strategies that may provide benefit for patients in whom traditional therapy has failed. More traditional approaches such as cardiac transplantation are only available to a small, highly selected group of patients, usually not the elderly. Other surgical procedures such as partial left vetriculectomy and

cardiomyoplasty are still under investigation. Additional problems with classification can occur when patients have reversible ventricular dysfunction or they functional improve with medical therapy.

High mortality rates, unplanned hospital admissions and medical therapies contribute to the high costs associated with CHF, especially those with advanced disease. The direct cost of hospitalization exceeds $7.5 billion per year while the total cost of evaluation and long-term care management may exceed $10 billion (41). The staggering costs demand a hard analysis of cost of care vs. benefit to patient regarding survival as well as QOL, especially as new, expensive, selective treatments become available.

Due to the progressive, marked physical decline in the advanced CHF patient, symptom management is a hallmark of treatment. Continued, repetitive efforts to manage reversible or precipitating factors that exacerbate CHF are crucial components of care. Pharmacological therapy includes maximal doses of ACE inhibitors, digoxin, diuretics and other combinations of afterload therapy if ACE drugs are not tolerated (42). Use of other inotropic therapy, antiarrhythmic agents and anticoagulants are being studied to allow for better risk stratification with use. Other newer pharmacological agents such as neurohormonal modulators are being investigated (40). Invasive procedures such as implantable defibrillators and permanent pacemakers can be difficult to ascertain the risk/benefit ratio to the patient without large clinical trials documenting efficacy.

Ultimately, the complex patient will become refractory to standard therapy recommendations and continue to experience severe symptoms. The patient and care provider must discuss when care may become too aggressive. Advanced planning is more likely to occur with continued patient-provider relationships, thus health care models that support continuity of care for the CHF patient using constant providers should improve treatment planning and discussion about end of life care (43). Preferences for either QOL or survival become more crucial when discussing treatment preferences in the advanced CHF patient. Decisions regarding therapy recommendations can be difficult. Recommended drugs such as beta-blockers and invasive procedures such as automatic implantable cardiac defibrillators (AICD) can improve survival but do not necessarily improve quality of life (QOL). There have been no large clinical trials of outpatients receiving home inotropic infusion therapy that demonstrate improved QOL or survival. Long-term dobutamine therapy has been associated with higher mortality rates (42). Lewis and colleagues report that over 70% of patients (n=75) interviewed would trade all or none of 2 years to feel better (44). Recently, algorithms have been proposed for managing complex or refractory heart failure that include home therapy and hospice choices (45).

Coping with advanced heart failure can be difficult since the patient eventually must deal with depression, uncertainty regarding prognosis, loss due to decline in physical status, hostility and anger. Dracup and colleagues evaluated psychosocial adjustment in 134 advanced heart failure patients waiting for transplant (46). Depression, hostility and functional status accounted for 43% of the variance for psychosocial adjustment to heart failure. In a prospective study of 391 CHF patients, Vaccarino et al. report that the higher the level of depressive symptoms, the higher the rate of death or functional decline (47). Patterns of uncertainty can arise when new or changing symptoms occur, misinformation regarding disease, inability to distinguish disease symptoms from aging and general loss of control over illness (48).

There are no studies in the literature that address long-term home care for the NYHA class III-IV patient. Reimbursement through Medicare and private health insurance has not been traditionally covered. Since US legislation now allows nurse practitioners to receive direct reimbursement for patients billed under Medicare B, frail elderly CHF patients who have difficulty accessing clinics are now eligible for long-term home care. Management of advanced heart failure requires an interdisciplinary team to address medical, psychological, social and spiritual needs. New home care models such as the Medicaring Collaborative Project emphasize coordinated care consistent with patient wishes, symptom management to prevent exacerbations, maintaining function and QOL using good medical care, patient education with concentration on treatment preferences and family support especially time near death (49). Some problems such as adequate 24 hour coverage must be incorporated into these advanced CHF treatment models.

## Palliative and End of Life Care

None of the CHF guidelines published address end of life care for the CHF patient and currently there are no well-defined models of care for this group of patients (1,50,51,52,53). A 6-month prognosis must

be determined to enroll the patient in a hospice program and the patient must agree to non-aggressive care. In contrast to cancer, predictions of timing of death can be difficult for CHF. Deaths can result from strokes, myocardial infarction, arrhythmias or infection. Most patients will continue to functionally decline and become resistant to increasing doses of medical therapy with their cause of death resulting from progressive hemodynamic decline. Ultimately, it is difficult for the physician to predict terminal heart failure from advanced heart failure. Fox and colleagues were unable to predict a survival prognosis of 6 months or less in CHF patients using various criteria based on national hospice guidelines (54). Of the CHF patients who died, almost 80% were predicted to live 6 more months just 3 days before death.

Inability to predict actual time to death leads to continued hope making the transition from gravely ill to terminally ill difficult (55). In the last six months of life, various problems such as poor symptom control of pain and dyspnea, poor prediction of death, poor utilization of hospice services, poor adherence to patient's treatment preferences, patient indecision regarding code status and uncertainty regarding the course of disease become barriers to care during end of life. To date, the SUPPORT trial is the largest trial analyzing patient preferences, prognosis, treatment and outcomes (56). In this trial, only 23% of 936 NYHA class IV CHF patients refused resuscitation. Of the 600 who responded 2 months later, 19% changed their preferences. The SUPPORT investigators also characterized the dying experience of older and seriously ill patients in 4124 patients through family report (57). Even though 59% of the patients desired comfort care during the last days of life, symptoms such as pain, dyspnea and fatigue were very prevalent and care was at odds with preference in 10% of cases. Of the 263 CHF patients, over 65% suffered severe dyspnea three days before death. Over 40% of the CHF group received at least one of three life-sustaining treatments (feeding tube, ventilator, CPR) during the last 3 days before death. Unfortunately, this emphasizes most patients, regardless of preference, were treated aggressively.

To receive hospice care, the patient must agree to palliative care. This terminal care is generally mutually exclusive and separate from treatments that cure the underlying disease or treat the underlying pathophysiology. Symptomatic care whether offered in the home or with in-patient hospice can include diuresis, morphine or supplemental oxygen without hospitalization. Many patients are not ready to accept this course of treatment unless impending death is foreseeable. It is not surprising that the average terminally ill patient enters hospice 1 month before death and 16% enter only 1 week before death (58). Of the 263 CHF patients in the SUPPORT trial, 58% died in the hospital, 27% at home and only 3% in hospice (57).

In a recent study where patients, families and providers were interviewed regarding the components of a good death, six important themes were noted (60). These included pain and symptom management, clear decision-making, preparation for death, completion, contributing to others and affirmation of the whole person were six important themes during end of life care. These results highlight the importance of discussing treatment preferences during the advanced and terminal phases of heart failure.

Due to Medicare restrictions, hospice is utilized late in life and other options for end of life care should be available before such severe decline. Hospice care can save costs if used in the last 2 months of life. It does this by reducing hospitalizations but becomes more costly if provided for a full year before death (43). Cost savings to the health care industry from advanced planning for end of life thus far have been minimal. Patients seem to prefer home treatment of an acute illness as an alternative if the outcomes are equivalent to those of hospitalization (59). Overall, patients preferred treatment at the site associated with the greatest chance of survival. These types of site preferences need to be analyzed during various phases of CHF. Services included in the MEDICARING model are: constant primary care provider regardless of setting, case management of home, personal and emergency care, access to 24 hour urgent care advice, and in-patient respite care. These type of model allow, for home care that is not time-limited or restricted by hospice criteria.

## Conclusions

Preliminary research suggests disease management programs providing close follow up for the CHF patient appear to be effective in reducing hospital admissions. In addition, they lowered cost and improved quality of life, functional capacity, compliance with medication and diet recommendations and patient satisfaction. Poor prognosis and increasing prevalence of CHF among the elderly underscore the importance of documenting the long-term

effects of these models of care. Components of successful programs included multidisciplinary care, phone follow up and coordination of care with primary care providers. Utilizing medical staff experienced in heart failure management contributed to adherence with guideline recommendations.

## Areas for Further Research

Previous research trials have mainly been observational using small sample sizes and diverse interventions. Other interventions such as exercise and psychosocial intervention have not been adequately studied. The effect of close follow-up on survival as well as end of life is unknown. Further research needs to be conducted despite the initial positive outcomes. Realistic programs need to be developed that can be incorporated in academic and rural settings with sufficient reimbursement.

Even though the multidisciplinary approach to heart failure seems advisable, there is not an "optimal" method that adjusts for NYHA class and functional status, type of intervention, site of care and recommended health care provider. What are the benefits of home care if patients are able to access the clinic setting? When can phone follow-up adequately provide patient care in conjunction with limited clinic follow-up? How can registered and advanced practice nurses complement physician care? CHF management programs must tailor services, considering frailty, sensory deficits, transportation access and family/social support as well as costs associated with service utilization. New research suggests using advanced practice nurses for comprehensive discharge planning and 6 month home care follow-up in the frail elderly reduced admissions, lengthened time between discharge and readmission and decreased health care costs (61). With the estimated $20.2 billion costs associated with CHF, cost effectiveness of multidisciplinary care is desperately needed along with the cost analysis of drug therapy alone (62).

The importance of quality of life and psychosocial factors as part of CHF outcomes has not been adequately investigated. Unfortunately, the prevalence of depression in the elderly CHF patient is not known and is probably under reported (63). Vaccarino and group recently reported that increasing depressive symptoms is a negative prognostic factor for patients with CHF (47). As patients progress to advanced heart failure, symptom management rather than mortality may be the goal of treatment (64). Relief of symptoms, psychological well-being, social interaction, minimal assistance with self-care, good cognitive function can all be markers associated with positive quality of life. Of the 292 CHF patients reviewed who were hospitalized and aged greater than 65 years, absence of emotional support was associated as an independent predictor of fatal and nonfatal cardiovascular events in the year after admission (65). New health status measures for CHF that are easily distributed and obtain clinically meaningful outcomes are being developed (66). QOL vs. survival decisions are unique for each patient and therefore emphasize the importance of implementing patient negotiated goals involving treatment preferences throughout all phases of heart failure.

Guidelines for advanced heart failure are necessary due to the eventual, progressive functional decline and unpredictable prediction of death. Programs such a MEDICARING can offer comprehensive care with creative combinations of aggressive and supportive care instead of traditional rescue care (49). In-patient hospice units can also provide palliative care while also providing 24-hour medical care and easing caregiver burden. Management of terminal CHF patients by palliative care services and not independently by cardiologists is slowly being reported in the literature (67).

Suggested goals for treatment are listed in table 6.3. Frequency and type of intervention could be stratified according to the patient's clinical status, risk of readmission and adherence to therapeutic regimens (5). Since adherence to diet and medication recommendations can be less than 50% and up to 50% of patients miss follow-up appointments, strategies aimed at behavior modification are important to support (68). Jaarsma and colleagues report that intensive, systematic, tailored and planned education supported by routine contact from a nurse increased patient self-care behavior (69). CHF disease management using a multidisciplinary heart failure team and repeated patient education sessions in an indigent population helped improve functional status, reduced hospitalizations and lowered net costs (70). National organizations such as the American Heart Association (AHA) continue to support team management for the CHF patient (71).

**Table 6.3   Goals of Treatment for CHF Patient**

1. Reduce hospital admissions and readmissions as well as emergency room visits.
2. Provide patient-centered, goal-directed care.
3. Utilize evidence-based practice guidelines to direct care.
4. Coordinate care with multidisciplinary team members and primary care providers.
5. Provide a continuum of care from initial diagnosis through end of life.
6. Stratify care approaches according to patient need using telemonitoring, out patient care, home care or combination of approaches.
7. Emphasize quality of life by controlling symptoms, delaying functional decline and discussion treatment preference.

# References

1. Packer M, Cohn JN. Consensus recommendations for the management of chronic heart failure. *Am J Cardiol* 1999;83:1A-79A.
2. Wenger N, Froelicher E et.al. Clinical Practice Guidelines, Number 17 Cardiac Rehabilitation. AHCPR Publication No. 96-0672, October 1995.
3. Philbin E, DiSalvo T. Influence of race and gender on care process, resource use, and hospital-based outcomes in congestive heart failure. *Am J Cardiol* 1998;82:76-81.
4. Philbin E, Dec GW, Jenkins P, DiSalvo T. Socioeconomic status as an independent risk factor for hospital readmission for heart failure. *Am J Cardiol* 2001;87:1367-1371.
5. Stewart S, Blue L. Improving outcomes in chronic heart failure: a practical guide to specialist nurse intervention. 2000 BMJ Books.
6. Burns RB, McCarthy EP, Moskowitz MA, Ash A, Kane RL, Finch M. Outcome for older men and women with congestive heart failure. *J Am Geriatr Soc* 1997;45:276-280.
7. Walsh JT, Charlesworth A, Andrews R, Hawkins M, Cowley AJ. Relation of daily

activity levels in patients with chronic heart failure to long-term prognosis. *Am J Cardiol* 1997;79:1364-1369

8. Jaagosild P, Dawson NV, Thomas C, Wenger NS, Tsevat J, Knaus WA, Califf RM, Goldman L, Vidaillet A, Connors AF; for the SUPPORT Investigators. Outcomes of acute exacerbation of severe congestive heart failure. *Arch Intern Med* 1998;158:1081-1089.

9. Ghali JK, Cooper R, Ford E. Trends in hospitalization rates for heart failure in the United States, 1973-1986: Evidence for increasing population prevalence. *Arch Intern Med* 1990;150:769-773.

10. Croft JB, Giles WH, Pollard RA, Casper ML, Anda RF, Livengood JR. National trends in the initial hospitalization for heart failure. *J Am Geriatr Soc* 1997;45:270-275.

11. Goff D, Pandey D, Chan F, Ortiz C, Nichaman M. Congestive heart failure in the United States: Is there more than meets the I(CD Code)? The Corpus Christi Heart Project. *Arch Intern Med* 2000;160:197-202.

12. Ghali JK, Kadakia S, Cooper R, Ferlinz J. Precipitating factors leading to decompensation of heart failure. *Arch Intern Med* 1988;148:2013-2016.

13. Ni H, Nauman D, Burgess D, Wise K, Crispell K, Hershberger RE. Factors influencing knowledge of and adherence to self-care among patients with heart failure. *Arch Intern. Med.* 1999 Jul 26;159(14):1613-9.

14. Edep ME, Shah NB, Tateo IM, Massie BM. Differences between primary care physicians and cardiologists in management of congestive heart failure: Relation to practice guidelines. *J Am Coll Cardiol* 1997;30:518-526.

15. Senni M, Tribouilloy C, Rodeheffer R, Jacobsen S, Evans J, Bailey K, Redfield M. Congestive heart failure in the community: trends in incidence and survival in a 10-year period. *Arch Intern Med* 1999;159:29-34.

16. Stanek EJ, Oates MB, McGhan WF, Denofrio D, Loh E. Preferences for treatment outcomes in patients with heart failure: symptoms vs. survival. *J Card Fail.* 2000 Sep;6(3):225-32.

17. West JA, Miller NH, Parker KM, Senneca D, Ghandour G, Clark M, Greenwald G, Heller RS, Fowler MB, DeBusk RF. A comprehensive management system for heart failure improves clinical outcomes and reduces medical resource utilization. *Am J Cardiol* 1997;79:58-63.

18. Shah NB, Der E, Ruggerio C, Heidenreich PA, Massie BM. Prevention of hospitalizations for heart failure with an interactive home monitoring program. *Am Heart J* 1998;135:373-378.

19. Heidenreich P, Ruggerio C, Massie B. Effect of a home monitoring system on hospitalization and resource use for patients with heart failure. *Am Heart J* 1999;138:633-640.

20. Fulmer T, Feldman P, Kim TS, Carty B, Beers M, Molina M, Putman M. An intervention study to enhance medication compliance in community-dwelling elderly individuals. *Journal of Gerontological Nursing* 1999;25(8):6-14.

21. Campbell NC, Ritchie LD, Thain J, Deans HG, Rawles JM, Squair JL. Secondary prevention in coronary heart disease: a randomized trail of nurse led clinics in primary care. *Heart* 1998;80:447-452.

22. Cintron G. Bigas C, Linares E, Aranda JM, Hernandez E. Nurse practitioner role in a chronic congestive heart failure clinic: In-hospital time, costs, and patient satisfaction. *Heart & Lung* 1983;12(3):237-240.

23. Lasater M. The effect of a nurse-managed CHF clinic on patient readmission and length of stay. *Home Heathcare Nurse* 1996;14(5):351-356.

24. Cline CMJ, Israelsson BYA, Willenheimer RB, Broms K, Erhardt LR. Cost effective management program for heart failure reduces hospitalization. *Heart* 1998;80:442-446.

25. Kostis JB, Rosen RC, Cosgrove NM, Shindler DM, Wilson AC. Norpharmacologic therapy improves functional and emotional status in congestive heart failure. *Chest* 1994;106:996-1001.

26. Hanumanthu S, Butler J, Chomsky D, Davis S, Wilson JR. Effect of a heart failure program on hospitalization frequency and exercise tolerance. *Circulation* 1997;96:2842-2848.

27. Fonarow GC, Stevenson LW, Walden JA, Livingston NA, Steimle AE, Hamilton MA, Moriguchi J, Tillisch JH, Woo MA. Impact of a comprehensive heart failure management program on hospital readmission and functional status of patients with advanced heart failure. *J Am Coll Cardiol* 1997;30:725-732.

28. Gattis W, Hasselblad V, Whellan D, O'Connor C. Reduction in heart failure events by the addition of a clinical pharmacist to the heart failure management team. *Arch Intern Med* 1999;159:1939-1945.

29. Kane RL, Finch M, Blewitt L, Chen Q, Burns, Moskowitz M. Use of post-hospital care by Medicare patients. *J Am Geriatr Soc* 1996;44:242-250.

30. Lazarre M, Ax S. Patients, chronic heart failure, and home care. *CARING Magazine* 1997; June:20-24.

31. Green K, Lydon S. Home health cardiac rehabilitation. *Home healthcare Nurse* 1995;13(2):29-39.

32. Maturen V, Van Dyck L. Using outcome-based critical pathways to improve documentation. *Home Health Care Manage Prac* 1996;8(2):48-58.

33. Cummings JE, Hughes SL, Weaver FM, Manheim LM, Conrad KJ, Nash K, Braun B, Adelman J. Cost-effectiveness of Veterans Administration hospital based home care. *Arch Intern Med* 1990;150:1274-1280.

34. Kornowski R, Zeeli D, Averbuch M, Finkelstein A, Schwartz D, Moshkovitz M, Weinreb B, Hershkovitz R, Eyal D, Miller M, Levo Y, Pines A. Intensive home-care surveillance prevents hospitalization and improves morbidity rates among elderly patients with severe congestive heart failure. *Am Heart J* 1995;129:762-766.

35. Rich MW, Beckham V, Wittenberg C, Leven CL, Freedland KE, Carney RM. A multidisciplinary intervention to prevent the readmission of elderly patients with congestive heart failure. *N Engl J Med* 1995;333:1190-1195.

36. Rich MW, Baldus D, Beckham V, Wittenburg C, Luther P. Effect of a multidisciplinary intervention on medication compliance in elderly patients with congestive heart failure. *Am J Med* 1996;101:270-276.

37. Stewart S, Marley JE, Horowitz JD. Effects of a multidisciplinary, home-based intervention on unplanned readmissions and survival among patients with chronic congestive heart failure: A randomized controlled study. *Lancet* 1999; 354:1077-1083.

38. Stewart S, Vandenbroek AJ, Pearson S, Horowitz JD. Prolonged beneficial effects of a home-based intervention on unplanned readmissions and mortality among patients with congestive heart failure. *Arch Intern Med* 1999;159:257-261.

39. Wilson JR, Smith JS, Dahle KL, Ingersoll GL. Impact of home health care on health care costs and hospitalization frequency in patients with heart failure. *Am J Cardiol* 1999;83:615-616.

40. O'Connor C, Gattis W, Swedberg K. Current and novel pharmacological approaches in advanced heart failure. *Am Heart J* 1998; 135:S249-S263.

41. Schulman K, Mark D, Califf R. Outcomes and costs within a disease management program for advanced congestive heart failure. *Am Heart J* 1998; 135:S285-S292.

42. Gheorghiade M, Cody R, Francis G, McKenna W, Young J, Bonow R. Current medical therapy for advanced heart failure. *Am Heart J* 1998:135:S231-S248.

43. Miles SH, Koepp RM, Weber EP. Advance end-of-life treatment planning. *Arch Intern Med* 1996;156:1062-1068.

44. Lewis EF, Johnson PA, Johnson W, Collins CM, Flavell CM, Griffin LM, Stevenson LW. Heart failure patients express strong polarity of preferences for either quality of life or survival. *Circulation* 1998: 98 Supp I:I-866.

45. Stevenson L, Massie B, Francis G. Optimizing therapy for complex or refractory heart failure: a management algorithm. *Am Heart L* 1998; 135:S293-S309.

46. Dracup K, Walden J, Stevensen L, Brecht ML. Quality of life in patients with advanced heart failure. J Heart Lung Transplant 1992;11:273-9.

47. Vaccarino V, Kasl S, Abramson J, Krumholz H. Depressive symptoms and risk of functional decline and death in patients with heart failure. *J Am Coll Cardiol* 2001;38:199-205.

48. Winters C. Heart failure: living with uncertainty. *Prog Cardiovasc Nurs* 1999;14:85-91.

49. Lynn J, Wilkinson A, Cohn F, Jones SB. Capitated risk-bearing managed care systems could improve end-of-life care. *J Am Geriatr Soc* 1998; 46(3):322-330.

50. Potter JF, Galindo D, Aronow WS. Heart failure: Evaluation and treatment of patient's with left ventricular systolic dysfunction. *JAGS* 1998;46:525-529.

51. Remme, WJ. The treatment of heart failure: The task force of the working group on heart failure on the European Society of Cardiology. *European Heart Journal* 1997;18:736-753.

52. Williams JF, Bristow MR, Fowler MB, Francis GS, Garson A, Gersh BJ, Hammer DF, Hlatky MA, Leier CV, Packer M, Pitt B, Ullyot DJ, Wesler LF, Winters WL. Guidelines for the evaluation and management of heart failure: Report of the ACC/AHA Task Force on Practice Guidelines (Committee on Evaluation and Management of Heart Failure). *Circulation* 1995;92:2764-2784.

53. Konstam M, Dracup K, Baker D, et al. Heart Failure: Evaluation and Care of Patients With Left Ventricular Systolic Dysfunction: Clinical Practice Guideline No. 11. Rockville, Md: Agency for Health Care Policy and Research; 1994. Publication AH-CPR 94-0612.

54. Fox E, Landrum-McNiff K, Zhong Z, Dawson N, Wu A, Lynn J. Evaluation of prognostic criteria for determining hospice eligibility in patients with advanced lung, heart, or liver disease. *JAMA* 1999; 282:1638-1645.

55. Finucane T. How gravely ill becomes dying: A key to end-of-life care. *JAMA* 1999; 282(17):1670-1672.

56. Krumholz HM, Phillips RS, Hamel MB, Teno JM, Bellamy P, Broste SK, Califf RM, Vidaillet H, Davis RB, Muhlbaier LH, Connors AF, Lynn J, Goldman L: for the SUPPORT Investigators. Resuscitation preferences among patients with severe congestive heart failure. *Circulation* 1998;98:648-655.

57. Lynn J, Teno J, Phillips R, Wu A, Desbiens N, Harrold J, Claessens M, Wenger N, Kreling B, Connors A. Perceptions by family members of the dying experience of older and seriously ill patients. *Ann Intern Med* 1997; 126:97-106.

58. Lo B. Care at the end of life: Guiding practice where there are no easy answers. *Annals of Internal medicine* 1999; 130(9):772-773.

59. Fried TR, van Doorn C, Tinetti ME, Drickamer MA. Older persons' preferences for site of treatment in acute illness. *J Gen Intern Med* 1998;13:522-527.

60. Steinhauser KE, Clipp EC, McNeilly M, Christakis NA, McIntyre LM, Tulsky JA. In search of a good death: Observations of patients, families and providers. *Ann Intern Med.* 2000; 132:825-832.

61. Naylor MD, Brooten D, Campbell R, Jacobsen BS, Mezey MD, Pauly MV, Schwartz JS. Comprehensive discharge planning and home follow-up of hospitalized elders. *JAMA* 1999; 281:613-620.

62. Rich M, Nease R. Cost-effectiveness anaylsis in clinical practice- the case of heart failure. *Arch Intern Med* 1999;159:1690-1700

63. Freedland K, carney RM, Rich MW, Carracciolo A, Krotenberg JA, Smith LJ, Sperry J. Depression in elderly patients with congestive heart failure. *Journal of Geriatric Psychiatry* 1991: 24(2):59-71.

64. Cleland J. Are symptoms the most important target for therapy in chronic heart failure? *Progress in Cardiovascular Diseases* 1998; 41(1):59-64.

65. Krumholz H, Butler J, Miller J, Vaccarino V, Williams C, Menedes de Leon C, Seeman T, Kasl S, Berkman L. Prognostic importance of emotional support for elderly patients hospitalized with heart failure. *Circulation* 1998;97:958-964.

66. Green CP, Porter CB, Bresnahan DR, Spertus JA. Development and evaluation of the Kansas City Cardiomyopathy Questionnaire: A new health status measure for heart failure. *J Am Coll Cardiol* 2000; 35:1245-1255.

67. Thorns A, Gibbs L, Gibbs JS. Management of severe heart failure by specialist palliative care. *Heart* 2001;Jan:85(1):93.

68. Evangelista L, Dracup K. A closer look at compliance research in heart failure patients in the last decade. *Progress in Cardiovasc Nursing* 2000;15:97-103.

69. Jaarsma T, Halfens R, Abu-Saad H, Dracup K, Gorgeis T, van Ree J, Stappers J. Effects of education and support on self care and resource utilization in patients with heart failure. *Eur Heart J* 1999;20:673-682.

70. O'Connell A, Crawford M, Abrams J. Heart failure disease management in an indigent population. *Am Heart J* 2001;141:254-8.

71. Grady K, Dracup K, Kennedy G, Moser D, Piano M, Stevensen L, Young J. Team management of patients with heart failure: a statement for healthcare professionals from the cardiovascular nursing council of the American Heart Association. *Circulation* 2000; 102:2443-2456.

PART III

# Update On the Pharmacological and Non-Pharmacological Treatment of CHF and COPD Patients

# Chapter 7

# The Pharmacological Treatment of Heart Failure

Marie-Hélène LeBlanc, MD, Canada

## Introduction

Among the causes of death and major morbidities related to cardiovascular diseases, heart failure is probably the most important one. Its incidence and prevalence continue to increase, reflecting the longer lifespan and more effective treatment of acute cardiovascular events (1). Despite recent therapeutic advances that have improved survival and exercise tolerance, the overall prognosis of heart failure is still poor. Indeed in mild cases, the annual mortality rate is 5-10% while it goes up to 50-60% in patients with advanced symptomatology (2). It is the most common hospital discharge diagnosis in patients older than 65 years and together coronary artery disease and high blood pressure are responsible for 60-70% of all episodes of congestive heart failure.

In recent years, considerable progress has been made with our understanding of the pathophysiology of heart failure. The clinical manifestations of heart failure are, however, heterogeneous and they reflect not only the primary hemodynamic abnormalities caused by cardiac dysfunction but also the multiple secondary compensatory mechanisms such as vasoconstriction, neurohormonal activation and metabolic imbalance (3,4,5). Because vascular resistance is increased, one of the most important clinical features of the disease is exercise intolerance due to impaired functional capacity of peripheral blood vessels to dilate in response to increased flow. This reduced peripheral vasodilatation capacity is due to the inability of the endothelium to release nitric oxide, resulting in vascular endothelial dysfunction (6,7).

## Non-Pharmacological Approach to Management of Heart Failure

Patient's education about signs and symptoms of heart failure, purpose of medication and need for compliance should be done and reinforced frequently. Advices on how to maintain fluid and salt restriction as well as need of weighing themselves every morning should also be given. Emphasis should be placed on body weight. Smoking cessation is important in all patients and must be encouraged. Vaccination against influenza and pneumococcal disease should be provided to all patients (8). Control of arrhythmias, especially atrial fibrillation, as well as avoidance of nonsteroidal anti-inflammatory drugs and of most calcium channel blockers is mandatory.

Although its effect on survival is unknown, low level exercise, such as walking should be encouraged as there is some evidence that appropriate physical conditioning leads to improvement in quality of life and exercise capacity (8,9).

Sleep disorders are present in up to 50% of patients with heart failure and these include central sleep apnea known as Cheynes-Stokes respiration in 36% of cases, obstructive sleep apnea in 12% of cases and a combination of both patterns in 52% of cases. Cheynes-Stokes respiration is more common in men than in women and it may lead to sleep fragmentation and fatigue. In these individuals, sympathetic overactivation is present and higher norepinephrine levels are associated with poorer prognosis. Nocturnal hypoxia increases the likelihood of ventricular ectopy (10,11).

The correction of Cheynes-Stokes respiration may improve the mechanical efficiency of the failing heart. Continuous positive airway pressure (CPAP) applied via a nasal mask during the night is a promising approach as it provides an increase in intrathoracic pressure thus augmenting stoke volume and cardiac output. It also reduces mitral regurgitation and improves cardiac function especially in patients who have central sleep apnea (12,13).

# Pharmacologic Approach to Management of Heart Failure

## Diuretics

Diuretics are essential for symptomatic treatment of volume overload. Loop diuretics, thiazides, and metolazone are all used at different stages in the treatment of congestive heart failure, sometimes in combination. It is suggested to use the lowest possible dose permitting weight stabilization and control of symptoms.

## Aldosterone Antagonist

By promoting myocardial fibrosis, magnesium wasting and arrhythmias, aldosterone has a significant role in the pathophysiology of heart failure. In the "RALES" study, patients suffering from severe heart failure and who had a left ventricular ejection fraction of less than 35% were assigned to receive 25 mg of spironolactone daily or placebo in addition to their regular medication. This study was discontinued early because in the spironolactone treated group there was a 30% risk reduction of death and a 35% reduction of hospitalization for worsening heart failure. There was also a significant improvement in the functional class of these patients (14). Spironolactone should be considered for patients with more severe heart failure. In these patients, careful monitoring of potassium levels should be carried out especially if the patient has concomitant diabetic renal disease or other renal dysfunction.

## Digitalis

The use of digitalis in the treatment of congestive heart failure remains controversial despite the results of the "DIG" trial which showed reduced hospitalization and symptom improvement in patients

with severe heart failure (class III-IV, NYHA). It should be used in conjunction with an angiotensin converting enzyme inhibitor and a betablocker and care should be taken to closely monitor older patients with diminished renal function as toxicities are more likely to occur in these individuals (15).

## Angiotensin Converting Enzyme (ACE) Inhibitors

Evidence concerning the beneficial effects of ACE inhibition has accumulated over the last 15 years. Large trials conducted in patients with mild as well as severe forms of congestive heart failure have all shown reductions in mortality and in number of hospitalizations (16). On average, the clinical improvement associated with ACE inhibitor treatment results in a reduction of 0.5-1.0 level in the NYHA classification, a 15% decrease in hospitalization for heart failure and a reduction in 1 year mortality of 16% in moderate cases of heart failure and of 31% in severe cases (17). In patients with left ventricular dysfunction and asymptomatic heart failure, ACE inhibitions leads to a 37% reduction in the risk of developing symptomatic heart failure (18,19). There is a 2% average increase of the left ventricular ejection fraction with the use of an ACE inhibitor. The Consensus Recommendations are that all patients with heart failure due to left ventricular systolic dysfunction should receive an ACE-inhibitor unless they are intolerant or there is a specific contraindication. All patients with asymptomatic left ventricular dysfunction should also receive an ACE-inhibitor. In general, one should aim for target doses recommended in the large-scaled studies (1).

## Hydralazine/Nitrate Combination

The combination of hydralazine and isosorbide dinitrate can be used in patients who cannot tolerate an ACE-inhibitor because of renal insufficiency. Two major studies (V-HEFT I and V-HEFT II) have shown the benefits of this combination to reduce mortality and increase ejection fraction and exercise tolerance. In those two studies, there were, however, no effect on the number of hospitalizations (20,21). The improved survival figures may be due to the direct effect of nitrate on myocardial remodeling while although not supported by hard data, this regimen may have additive effect if the patient is already on an ACE-inhibitor.

## Angiotensin-Receptor Blockers (ARB's)

According to some investigators, ARB's may be more effective than ACE inhibitors in blocking the effects of angiotensin II. ARB's selectively antagonize the angiotensin II type I (AT1) receptor, thereby blocking the effects of angiotensin II (AT2) that contribute to hypertension and cardiovascular remodeling. In addition, by blocking AT1 receptors, more AT2 becomes available to activate AT2 receptors, which mediate potentially beneficial antiproliferative and vasodilatory actions. Currently, the role of ARB's as therapy for heart failure is still a matter of debate because many large scale studies have failed to show superior effects of ARB's over ACE-inhibitors. The *"Elite II trial"* was designed to address the question of whether losartan was superior to captopril to lower mortality rates from all causes. The secondary endpoint of this trial was the reduction of sudden deaths and/or resuscitated cardiac arrests while other endpoints included combined outcomes of mortality and hospitalization from all causes, safety, and tolerability. There was no significant difference in mortality over a median follow-up time of 1.5 years, although trends were consistently in favor of captopril. Losartan was better tolerated than captopril with 14.5% of patients withdrawing from captopril compared with to 9.4% withdrawing from losartan (p< 0.001) (22). The addition of losartan to an ACE inhibitor has been found to improve exercise capacity when compared with ACE inhibitors alone. Data from the *"RESOLVD trial"* suggest that the combination of both medications may be better to reduce neurohormonal activation and ventricular dilatation (23). Trials are now underway to determine the safety and benefit of a more complete blockade of the renin-angiotensin-aldosterone system.

Currently, ACE inhibitors remain the therapy of choice in patients with left ventricular dysfunction while ARB's should only be used in patients unable to tolerate ACE-inhibitors because of cough or angioedema.

## Beta-Blockers

Over the past few years, the most extensively studied drug class used to manage heart failure has been that of β-adrenergic antagonists. Overall, there is strong evidence that these agents can improve symptoms, morbidity and survival in all classes of heart failure patients. The benefits however are not in terms of short-term relief of symptoms but rather in terms of improvement in LV function and long-term survival. A meta-analysis looking at the results of 18 published double-blind, placebo-controlled parallel-group trials of β-blockers in mostly moderate heart failure patients concluded that β-blockers could produce a wide range of favorable effects when added to conventional therapy. Indeed, there was a significant impact on morbidity and mortality with a 32% reduction in the risk of death, 41% risk reduction of hospitalization for heart failure and 37% reduction in the combined risk of morbidity and mortality. There was also a 29% increase in left ventricular ejection fraction and 32% increase in functional improvement (24).

Both selective and non-selective β-blockers have been used in large scale trials. Metoprolol and bisoprolol do not block myocardial $\beta_2$-receptors and have no effect on the $\beta_2$-receptor-mediated peripheral vasodilatation. Carvedilol does not upregulate $\beta_1$-receptor but blocks $\beta_2$-receptors as well as $\alpha_1$-adrenergic receptors. Carvedilol also has anti-oxidant, anti-proliferative and anti-endothelin effects. Although carvedilol may have favorable effects on heart function because of its peripheral vasodilating actions, it is not known if such activity remains during long term therapy or if tolerance develops to the $\alpha_1$-blocker.

The *"Carvedilol or Metoprolol European Trial (COMET)"* is an ongoing large-scale trial evaluating the pharmacologic differences of these drugs on mortality in patients with moderate to severe heart failure. More than 3,000 patients will be randomized on a 1:1 basis (25). Experience with β-blockers in patients with moderate to severe systolic heart failure is considerable and recent recommendations suggests that all patients with stable NYHA class II or III heart failure should receive a β-blocker unless contraindicated. The recent *"COPERNICUS Trial"* evaluated severely disabled heart failure patients (class III-IV) with LVEF< 25%. Patients were randomized to receive carvedilol up to 25 mg twice a day, for up to 29 months (mean 10.4 months). Because of the unexpected efficacy of the drug, the trial was stopped prematurely with a 35% reduction in mortality, and 29% reduction in the combined risk of death or hospitalization (26). Taking into account the results of many large scale trials, the use of β-blockade in patients with heart failure of varying severity is mandatory unless there is a specific contraindication. The medication should be started at a low dose and then slowly increased especially in patients with more advanced heart failure. β-blockers with an intrinsic sympathomimetic activity such as bucindolol, do not appear to have a beneficial effect in the treatment of heart failure.

## Anticoagulants and Antiplatelets Agents

Because of left ventricular dilatation, stasis in the cardiac chambers and low cardiac output, patients with advanced heart failure are more at risk for thromboembolic complications. Anticoagulation is therefore recommended if there is clinical evidence of embolic disease and for patients in atrial fibrillation where the value of anticoagulation for stroke prevention is well established. Antiplatelet agents are recommended in the treatment of coronary artery disease, as they reduce post-infarction mortality and risk of subsequent myocardial infarction. Unfortunately, no definitive clinical studies have been done in patients with heart failure and left ventricular dysfunction.

## Antiarrythmic Agents

Most heart failure patients die suddenly rather than through progression of the disease. In this context, complex ventricular arrhythmias should be treated with class III agents such as amiodarone. Patients should also be monitored closely for evidence of thyroid, pulmonary and hepatic toxicities.

# Conclusion

The management of congestive heart failure has changed considerably over the last few years and currently optimal pharmacologic treatment is both recommended or required if one is to improve survival and quality of life of patients suffering from this multifaceted disease. With the development of more multidisciplinary heart failure clinics, it will soon become possible to manage heart failure management more aggressively and therefore potentially decrease the economic burden of this disease.

# References

1. Consensus recommendations of the management of chronic heart failure. *Am J Cardiol* 1999; 83: 1A-38A.

2. Zannad F, Briancon S, Juillère Y et al and the EPICAL Investigators. Incidence, clinical and etiologic features and outcomes of advanced chronic heart failure: The EPICAL Study. *J Am Coll Cardiol* 1999; 33: 734-42.

3. Floras J. Clinical aspects of sympathetic activation and parasympathetic withdrawal in heart failure. *J Am Coll Cardiol* 1993; 22: 72A-84A.

4. Hirsch AT, Pinto YM, Schunkert D et al. Potential role of the tissue renin-angiotensin system in the pathophysiology of congestive heart failure. *Am J Cardiol* 1990; 66: 22D-32D.

5. Hirsch AT, Creager MA. The peripheral circulation in heart failure. In Congestive Heart Failure. Edited by Hosenpred JD, Greenberg BH. Heidelberg: Springer-Verlag; 1994: 145-160.

6. Harrington D, Coats AJ. Mechanism of exercise intorelance in congestive heart failure. *Curr Opin Cardiol* 1997; 12: 224-32.

7. Kubo SH, Rector TS, Bank AJ, Williams RE, Heifetz SM. Endothelium-dependant vasodilatation is attenuated in patients with heart failure. *Circulation* 1991; 84: 1589-96.

8. Packer M, Cohn JN. Consensus Recommendations for the management of Chronic Heart Failure. *J Am Coll Cardiol* 1999; 83 (2A): 1A-38A.

9. Coats AJS, Adamopoulos S, Meyer TE, Conway J, Sleight P. Effects of physical training in chronic heart failure. *Lancet* 1990; 335:j 63-6.

10. Lipkin DP. Sleep-disordered breathing in chronic stable heart failure. *Lancet* 1999; 354: 531-532.

11. Lanfranchi PA, Braghiroli A, Bosimini E et al. Pronostic value of nocturnal Cheynes-Stokes respiration in Chronic Heart Failure. *Circulation* 1999; 99: 1435-1440.

12. Tkacova R, Liu PP, Naughton M.T, Bernard DC et al. Effects of continuous positive airway pressure on atrial natriuretic peptide and mitral regurgitation fraction in patients with heart failure and central sleep apnea. *J Am Coll Cardiol* 1997; 30: 739-45.

13. Sin DD, Logan AG, Fitzgerald FS, Liu PP, Bradley TD. Effects of continuous positive airway pressure on cardiovascular outcomes in heart failure patients with and without Cheynes-Stokes respiration. *Circulation* 2000; 102: 61-66.

14. Pitt B, Zannad F, Remme WJ et al. The effects of spironolactone on morbidity and mortality in patients with severe heart failure. Randomized Aldactone Evaluation Study Investigators. *N Engl J Med* 1999; 341: 709-717.

15. The Digitalis Investigation Group. The effects of digoxin on mortality and morbidity in patients

with heart failure. *N Engl J Med*, 1997; 336: 525-33.

16. CONSENSUS Trial Study Group. Effects of Enalapril on mortality in severe congestive heart failure. Results of the North Scandinavian Enalapril Survival Study. *N Engl J Med* 1987; 316: 1429-35.

17. The SOLVD Investigators. Effects of enalapril on survival in patients with reduced left ventricular ejection fractions and congestive heart failure. *N Engl J Med*, 1991; 325: 293-302.

18. The SOLVD Investigators. Effects of enalapril on mortality and the development of heart failure in asymptomatic patients with reduced left ventricular ejection fraction. *N Engl J Med* 1992; 327: 685-91.

19. Pfeffer MA, Braunwald E, Moye LA et al for the SAVE Investigators. Effetcs of Captopril on mortality and morbidity in patients with left ventricular dysfunciton and myocardial infarction. Results of the Survival And Ventricular Enlargement Trial. *N Engl J Med*, 1992; 327: 669-77.

20. Cohn JN, Johnson G, Ziesche S, Cobb F, Francis G et al. A comparison of enalapril with hydralazine-isosorbide dinitrate in the treatment of chronic congestive heart failure. *N Engl J Med*, 1991; 325: 303-310.

21. Cohn JN, Archibald DG, Ziesche S, Franciosa JA et al. Effect of vasodilator therapy on mortality in chronic congestive heart failure: results of the Veterans Administration Cooperative Study. *New Engl J Med*, 1986; 314: 1547-52.

22. Pitt B, Poole-Wilson PA, Segal R et al. Effect of Losartan compared with Captopril on mortality in patients with symptomatic heart failure; randomized trial the Losartan Heart Failure Survival Study Elite II. *Lancet*, 2000; 355: 1582-87.

23. McElvie RS, Yusuf S, Pericak D et al. Comparison of Candesartan, Enalapril and their combination in congestive heart failure: randomized evaluation of strategies for left ventricular dysfunction (RESOLVD) pilot study. The RESOLVD Pilot Study Investigators. *Circulation* 1999; 100: 1056-1064.

24. Lechat P, Packer M, Cholon S, Cucherat M, Arab T, Boissel JP. Clinical effects of β-adrenergic blockade in chronic heart failure. A meta-analysis of double-blind, placebo-controlled, randomized trials. *Circulation* 1998; 98: 1184-91.

25. Metra M, Nodari S, D'Aloia A, Bontempi L, Boldi E, Dei Cas L. A rationale for the use of β-blockers as standard treatment for heart failure. *Am Heart J*, 2000; 139 (3): 511-521.

26. Packer M, Coats AJS, Fowler MB et al. Effects of Carvedilol on survival in severe chronic heart failure. *N Engl J Med* 2001; 344: 1651-8.

## Chapter 8

# Pharmacological Treatment of Patients With Chronic Obstructive Pulmonary Disease: Update and Future Directions

Pierre LeBlanc, MD, Canada

An effective management plan for patients with chronic obstructive pulmonary disease (COPD) must include four components: 1) Assessment and monitoring of the disease; 2) Reduction of risk factors; 3) Management of stable disease and; 4) Management of exacerbations (GOLD). The main goals of treatment are to prevent disease progression, relieve symptoms, improve exercise tolerance, improve health status, prevent and treat complications, and ultimately reduce mortality. Patients should be identified before they reach the end stage of their illness where disability is substantial. Once symptom control has been achieved, reduction in therapy is not usually possible but appropriate measures to prevent exacerbations should be implemented as quickly as possible. By optimizing the pharmacological treatment of COPD, it may be possible to prevent exacerbations of the disease as well as to reduce symptoms and allow the patient to increase its level of activity. This will contribute significantly to improve quality of life, which is the most important goal of this type of intervention. In order to adjust therapy with progression, each follow-up visit must include a discussion of the current therapeutic regimen. Dosages of various medications, adherence to the regimen, inhaler techniques, effectiveness of the current regime at controlling symptoms, and side effects of treatment should also be monitored.

## Prevention of Deterioration of Airway Obstruction

### Smoking Cessation

Smoking cessation impacts positively on progression of COPD. Fletcher and Peto (1) showed that 15-20% of smokers had an increased susceptibility to tobacco smoke and that smoking cessation could modify the rate of decline in $FEV_1$. These findings were confirmed more recently by the Lung Health Study (2) which showed that smoking cessation was of major benefit for all participants regardless of their age, lung function and gender. Early detection of COPD followed by smoking cessation resulted in the best clinical outcome.

In tobacco, nicotine is the primary agent which leads to addiction and over the past few years, advances have been made in the treatment of this addiction (3). Nicotine gums with increased dosage and transdermal patches are now available and lead to higher success rates. The ideal duration of nicotine replacement is not yet established but usually it is suggested to treat for a period of a 6 to 8 weeks. Nicotine replacement therapy allows the smoker to give up smoking without going through a full syndrome of nicotine withdrawal (4). More recently, a sustained release form of the antidepressant, bupropion, has been shown to improve cigarette abstinence (5,6). Bupropion was more effective than nicotine transdermal patches or placebo in helping patients to maintain abstinence at 12 months. When bupropion was combined with transdermal patches, a higher rate of continuous abstinence was obtained.

### Vaccination

Patients with COPD are at higher risk for developing pneumonia specially pneumococcal infections. In 1997, Koivula et al. (7) showed the value of pneumococcal immunization in patients with chronic diseases, such as COPD to reduce the incidence of pneumococcal pneumonia. Recommendations for vaccination have recently been updated and it is now recommended for all COPD patients (8). Another new recommendation is to administer a booster vaccination 5 years after initial vaccination in all patients who are less than 65 years of age at the time of their original vaccination.

Influenza and its complications are responsible for increased mortality and morbidity in elderly patients including those with chronic lung disease. In 1999, Nichols et al. (9) showed the efficacy and cost effectiveness of influenza vaccination when they reported a 70% reduction in the risk for death from any cause (odd ratio = 0.3).

## Protease Inhibitors

Hereditary deficiencies in $\alpha_1$-antitrypsine are characterized by the development of severe emphysema at an early age and smoking is considered to be a significant contributing factor. Even though $\alpha_1$-antitrypsine replacements have been shown to be biologically active, there has never been a randomized study to document their clinical efficacy. A recently published German-Danish study suggest however that weekly infusions of human $\alpha_1$-antitrypsine may slow the annual decline of $FEV_1$ in patient with an initial $FEV_1$ between 30% and 65% of predicted value (10).

## Pharmacological Therapy to Optimize Lung Function, Symptomatology, and Health Status

### Short Acting Bronchodilators

Some bronchodilators have been shown to be beneficial in stable COPD patients. These include anticholinergic drugs (ipartropium bromide), short-acting $\beta_2$-agonist or a combination of both drugs.

Anticholinergic drugs given to patients with COPD produce the same or significantly greater bronchodilation than $\beta_2$-agonists (11). Even when anticholinergics produce levels of bronchodilation equivalent to $\beta_2$-agonists, they can generate greater improvements in symptoms and quality of life. Side effects are minimal even when the drug is administered at doses much higher than recommended. Based on these informations, ipratropium bromide is now considered the preferred and first-line agent when standard treatment for COPD is required (12-15). Long-term anticholinergic usage provides sus-

tainable and beneficial effects, without tachyphylaxis or receptor downregulation. Long term usage does not, however, influence COPD disease progression as determined by the rate of annual decline in $FEV_1$.

Short-acting $\beta_2$-agonists provide a rapid response which makes them useful for symptom relief and protection from exercise-induced dyspnea. Although there is virtually no sympathetic innervation of airway smooth muscles, membrane-associated $\beta_2$-receptors located in smooth muscles are activated through circulating cathecolamines, which antagonize muscle contraction and lead to bronchodilation. As a membrane-associated receptor, $\beta_2$-receptors can downregulate by internalisation of receptor (16). This down regulation is dependent on the intensity and duration of $\beta_2$-agonist exposure and it accounts for the tachyphylaxis observed with prolonged $\beta_2$-agonist use. In one study (17), regular treatment with $\beta_2$-agonist was associated with minimal changes in baseline function and decline in acute response to bronchodilator therapy after 90-day administration. By contrast, regular treatment with ipratropium bromide was associated with improvement both in baseline lung function and acute response to bronchodilator therapy. Treatment with corticosteroids upregulates mRNA production and partially reverse $\beta_2$-agonist-induced tachyphylaxis (18).

### Theophylline

The use of theophylline has decreased significantly over the past 10 years although it may still have several potentially useful effects. Unfortunately, randomized clinical trials have not shown consistent improvements in respiratory symptoms, exercise capacity and health status. In three trials (19-21) in which a validated instrument was used, theophylline improved health status. It also improved exercise capacity in two of these three studies (20-21). Based on these results, there is still a rationale for the use of theophylline in COPD patients who are symptomatic despite inhaled bronchodilators. Combinations of $\beta_2$-agonists, anticholinergics and/or theophylline may produce additional improvements in lung function and health status although increasing the number of drugs is likely to increase costs. In some cases, an equivalent benefit can be obtained by increasing the dose of one bronchodilator specially when side effects are not a limiting factor. (GOLD)

## Long Acting Bronchodilators

Although long-acting bronchodilators have been developed in the form of $\beta_2$-agonists and anticholinergics, only $\beta_2$-agonists (salmeterol and formoterol) are currently available for clinical use. Long acting $\beta_2$-agonists have a prolonged effect on smooth muscles of the airway and they also have non bronchodilator properties. One of their main advantages is their long duration of action. Both salmeterol and formoterol increase lung function for at least 12 hours compared to 4-6 hours for salbutamol (22-23). Formoterol is highly efficient at the $\beta_2$-receptor while salmeterol is a partial agonist. These pharmacological properties do not, however affect either clinical efficacy or responsiveness to short acting $\beta_2$-agonist during exacerbations of the disease (24). In a study where salmetrol was given at doses of 50 or 100µg twice a day, both groups of patients showed a significant increase in $FEV_1$, while only those receiving 50 µg had clinically significant improvement in health-related quality of life. In a recent review by the Cochrane Airways Group (25) of the use of long acting $\beta_2$-agonists in COPD, it was concluded that improvements in quality of life and reduction of breathlessness could occur with only small changes in lung function.

## Newer Inhaled Bronchodilators

Only one compound, tiotropium (Spiriva), has been developed as a long-acting-anticholinergic bronchodilator. This new generation compound has been shown to have unique pharmacologic activities, one of the most important being its prolonged binding to muscarinic receptors. In clinical trials carried out in COPD patients, this property has translated into effective bronchodilation when the drug was administered only once a day. Tiotropium, like ipratropium is a competitive antagonist of acetylcholine at muscarinic receptors of the M1 to M5 subtypes and this activity results in smooth muscle relaxation and inhibition of mucus secretion.

The first clinical evidence of reduction of cholinergic tone with tiotropium was reported by Maesen et al. (26) who observed long-lasting increases in airflow following a single dose. These observations set the stage for the development of the first once-daily-inhaled bronchodilator for the treatment of COPD. The first clinical trial involving various doses of this drug was reported by Littner et al. (27) who observed significant bronchodilation over doses ranging from 4.5 to 36 µg. After 4 weeks of once-daily inhalation of 18 µg tiotropium, $FEV_1$ was 0.13 litre above the baseline whereas it was at 0.15 litre immediately after the first inhalation. From these clinical observations, the 18 µg dose was selected as being optimal for long-term clinical trials. More recently, Van Noord et al. (28) showed that tiotropium at a dose of 18 µg inhaled once daily using the Handi-Haler was significantly more effective than 40 µg ipratropium given four times a day in improving trough, average, and peak lung function over a 13-week period. In that study, the safety profile of tiotropium was similar to that of ipratropium. One year data from a clinical trial comparing tiotropium to placebo showed improvements in $FEV_1$, transitional dyspnea index, and health status as measured by the St. George's Respiratory Questionaire (SGRQ) (29). Tiotropium is therefore a safe and effective once-daily anticholinergic bronchodilator drug which should prove useful as first-line maintenance therapy in COPD.

Viozan is a new drug in the same class as dual D2 dopamine receptors and $\beta_2$-adrenoceptor agonists. All symptoms of COPD can potentially be mediated by neuronal mechanisms and sensory afferent nerves activated by endogenous and exogenous irritants can generate reflexes iliciting cough, mucus production, bronchoconstriction, and changes in the depth of breathing. In general, peripheral D2-receptors have an inhibitory role and activation of these receptors on the presynaptic terminals of postganglionic sympathetic nerves inhibits the release of noradrenaline thereby modulating vascular tone. It was therefore postulated that stimulation of dopamine D2-receptors on sensory nerves may suppress reflex mediated cough, sputum production and dyspnea in COPD. Viozan is a potent full agonist at D2-receptor sites, a potent partial agonist at $\beta_2$-adrenoreceptor sites and it has no significant activity at $\alpha_2$-, $\beta_1$- and $\beta_3$-adrenoceptors sites. In addition, it has low potency at $\alpha_1$-receptors sites. The efficacy and safety of Viozan have been assessed in phase II trials carried out in symptomatic COPD patients. In a 6-week dose-ranging study, where Viozan was compared to a placebo (30), Viozan dose dependently (1) improved individual symptom scores for cough, sputum production, breathlessness and total symptom scores, (2) improved morning and evening peak flows, (3) reduced requirements for rescue medications, (4) improved health status and quality of life as measured by SGRQ by total scores and individual three quality of life domains, and

(5) was positively thought to be efficient by both patient and investigator. In a placebo-controlled study of 4-week duration (31), Viozan was compared to salbutamol and ipratropium bromide. Viozan was showed to be significantly better than the other two drugs at improving total symptom score of cough, sputum production and breathlessness. In these studies, Viozan was well tolerated and side effects were attributable to the $\beta_2$-properties of the compound. The combination of D2-receptor agonist activity to modulate sensory nerve reflexes with $\beta_2$-adrenoceptor agonist activity to provide bronchodilatation is a novel approach in the management of COPD.

## Corticosteroids

Historically, physicians tended to apply established therapies used in asthma to COPD patients, mostly because of the diagnostic confusion that frequently exists between these two conditions. Pathophysiologic studies done in patients with COPD have shown that there is a low-grade inflammatory reaction in the airways which may lead to occlusive, fibrotic changes over many years. This chronic inflammation has also been implicated in the pathogenesis of emphysema (32). Suppression of these inflammatory responses provides the rationale for using corticosteroids. The question of efficacy is important because corticosteroids may have major adverse effects, particularly when given systematically over a long period of time.

## Oral Corticosteroids

Before concluding that a patient may benefit from oral corticosteroids, the patient's disease and pulmonary function must be stable and the potential benefits documented objectively. A meta-analysis estimated that the percentage of patients with stable COPD, who improved their $FEV_1$ at least by 20% with 20 mg of prednisone or more given during at least 7 days, was only 10% more (95% confidence interval, 2-18%) than in a placebo group. The percentage of patients who may benefit from oral corticosteroid therefore appears to be marginal while the potential for adverse effects is a significant problem. (33) Only one randomized prospective trial looked at long-term effects of corticosteroids in COPD patients. In that study (34), 58 patients were randomized to receive 1600 µg per day of budesonide, 1600 µg per day of budesonide plus 5 mg per day of oral prednisolone, or placebo. Treatment with corticosteroids significantly reduced pulmonary symptoms but changes in $FEV_1$ over two years did not reach statistical significance.

## Inhaled Corticosteroids

The pathophysiologic features of COPD are distinct from those observed in asthma. In COPD, there is an increase in CD8-lymphocytes, neutrophils and squamous metaplasia but there is no thickening of the basal membrane or disruption of the airway epithelium. In theory, inhaled corticosteroids may suppress these inflammatory reactions therefore slowing down the decline in lung function. In the few short-term studies in which small number of patients were identified according to their response to oral steroids, the proportion of patients and the size of the effect have been consistently less in patients receiving inhaled corticosteroids than those receiving oral corticosteroids (35). In the large population of patients who do not improve significantly with oral corticosteroids, inhaled corticosteroids, even at high doses, fail to show beneficial physiological and functional effects (36).

Five major trials have assessed the long-term efficacy of inhaled corticosteroids in patients with COPD. The international COPD Study group (37) was the first to compare the effects of inhaled corticosteroids versus placebo in a large multicenter trial opened to patients with moderately severe COPD (mean $FEV_1$ = 1.56L). Two hundred and eighty one patients were randomized to either treatment with inhaled fluticasone propionate (500 µg twice a day for 6 months) or with placebo. Over the duration of the study, 37% of patients in the placebo group and 32% in the treatment group experienced one exacerbation of their disease, a non statistically significant difference (primary outcome). However, there were more exacerbations (111 vs 76) and severe exacerbations in the placebo group. At 6 months the average $FEV_1$ improved by about 150 mL more in patients receiving fluticasone than in patients receiving placebo fluticasone diproprionate caused a measurable reduction in serum cortisol levels although the clinical significance of this finding is uncertain.

In the EUROSCOP trial (38), the investigators compared budesonide (400 µg twice daily) to placebo in actively smoking subjects with mild COPD (mean $FEV_1$ of 2.54L) over a 3-year period. The primary outcome was the rate of decline in post-bronchodilator $FEV_1$. During the first 6 months of study, $FEV_1$ improved by about 10 mL in the budesonide group whereas it declined by 40 mL in the placebo group. After 9 to 36 months, however, the rate of $FEV_1$ decline did not differ significantly between both groups. The clinical significance of these results remains uncertain.

In the ISOLDE trial (39) the rate of post bronchodilator $FEV_1$ was also the primary outcome of the study. In that trial, the authors compared fluticasone diproprionate, (500 μg twice a day) to placebo in 751 subjects with moderately severe COPD (mean $FEV_1$ of 1.41). The $FEV_1$ was significantly higher by 100-150 mL in the fluticasone diproprionate group throughout the study but no effect on the rate of decline in $FEV_1$ (50 ml/year in the fluticasone diproprionate group and 57 ml/year in the placebo group, P = 0.16) was observed. There were 25% less disease exacerbations (P = 0.03) and fewer withdrawals for respiratory causes (P = 0.02) in the fluticasone diproprionate group.

In the Copenhagen City Heart Study epidemiology survey (40) 290 patients with mild COPD (mean $FEV_1$ of 2.37) were enrolled in a randomized, double-blind, placebo-controlled trial. They received either 1200 μg of budesonide daily for 6 months followed by 400 μg twice daily for 30 months or placebo. Again, the mean outcome was the rate of decline in $FEV_1$. There was no significant difference in this outcome between the two groups nor was there an effect on COPD exacerbations (155 in the budesonide group versus 161 in the placebo group).

Finally the results of the Lung Health Study II (41) were recently published. In that trial, 1116 patients with mild to moderate COPD (mean $FEV_1$ of 2.13) were randomized to receive either inhaled triamcinilone acetonide (1200 μg daily) or placebo for a period of 3-3.5 years. Inhaled triamcinolone had no effect on the slope of $FEV_1$ over time but caused a modest improvement in selected respiratory symptoms as well as some decrease in health resource use.

Based on these results the GOLD (42) statement is that inhaled corticosteroids do not modify the long-term decline in $FEV_1$ in patients with COPD. Consequently, regular treatment with inhaled corticosteroids is only appropriate for symptomatic patients with documented spirometric responses to inhaled corticosteroids, or for those with a $FEV_1$ <50% of predicted and repeated exacerbations requiring treatment with antibiotics or oral corticosteroids. This last recommendation is an extrapolation from the results of the previously mentioned 5 large multicenter studies in which this question was not specifically addressed. It is finally worth noting that the dose-response relationship to inhaled corticosteroids in COPD is still not known.

It therefore appears important that future investigations looking at the efficacy of corticosteroids in the treatment of COPD carefully consider the exact clinical and histopathlogical profile of the patients included in the study. Conclusions pertaining to one group (e.g., those with relatively pure emphysema and sparse inflammation) may differ markedly from those applicable to another group such as the one which include patients with chronic bronchitis and neutrophil or eosinophil airway inflammation.

## Pharmacological Therapy for COPD Exacerbations

### Systemic Corticosteroids

There are five large randomized, controlled trials that looked at the use of systemic corticosteroids for COPD exacerbation. In 1980, Albert et al. (43) randomized 44 hospitalized patients ($FEV_1$ < 0.64 L) to receive either intravenous methylprednisolone 0.5 mg/kg every 6 hours or placebo for 3 days. $FEV_1$ improved at a significantly faster rate in those who received methlyprednisolone but unfortunately, the observations ended after 3 days and no other clinically important endpoints were evaluated.

In 1989, Emerman et al. (44) randomized 96 patients presenting to an emergency departement for COPD exacerbations ($FEV_1$ < 30% of predicted value). They compared a single 100 mg dose of intravenous methylprednisolone to placebo. They observed no significant changes in spirometric values and no significant difference in the hospitalization rate between both groups but as noted by the authors, the duration of therapy was probably too brief to show beneficial effects.

Thompson et al. (45) randomized 27 COPD patients (mean $FEV_1$ = 1.3L) with an exacerbation of their disease. These were treated as out-patients, with a 9-day, tapering dose of oral prednisone or with placebo. Prednisone improved arterial blood gases and $FEV_1$ at 3 and 10 days and treated patients experienced fewer treatment failures.

In 1999, the US Department of Veterans Affairs Cooperative Studies Program sponsored a study (46) in which 1840 patients hospitalized for COPD exacerbation were registered and 271 were randomized to one of three treatment arms ($FEV_1$ <0.8L). There were two active treatment groups where patients received 125 mg of intravenous methylprednisolone four times a day for three days followed by 60 mg of oral prednisone. These individuals were then randomized to a tapering dose of prednisone over 2 or 8 weeks. The third group received placebo. Systemic corticosteroids were found to reduce treatment failures defined as death from any cause, intubation and mechanical ventilation, readmission for COPD exacerbation, or the need to intensify pharmacological treament at the earlier time points. The absolute rates of treatment failure were also reduced by corticosteroids at 30 days (33% to 23%, p=0.04) and at 90 days (48% to 37%, p=0.04). The two most common treatment failures were hospital readmission for COPD exacerbation and need to intensify administration of corticosteroids. Eight weeks of treatment were no more effective than two weeks. The maximum improvement of $FEV_1$ was 100 mL and it was obtained after only 24 hours of treatment. There was finally no significant difference in mortality at six months between treatment and placebo group.

Davies et al. (47) studied 56 patients who were randomized to receive either 30 mg once daily of oral prednisolone or placebo. All patients received otherwise standard therapy. At day 5, post-bronchodilator $FEV_1$ increased by 90 mL/day in the treatment group and only by 30 mL/day in the placebo group (p=0.039). The hospital length of stay was also shorter in the treatment group than in the placebo group. The benefits of treatment did not extend beyond hospital discharge.

Based on these observations, patients with COPD exacerbations should be treated with systemic corticosteroids. The dose should be minimal (30 mg daily) and the duration of treatment should not extend beyond 2 weeks. Benefits and risks of the repetitive use of systemic corticosteroids are still largely unknown.

In an attempt to find an alternative to systemic corticosteroids in acute exacerbations of COPD, a double blind, double dummy, parallel group comparison study was designed to investigate the efficacy of nebulized budesonide and prednisolone in comparison to placebo in hospitalized patients (48). At 72 hours, mean changes of postbronchodilatation $FEV_1$ were substantially greater with active treatments than with placebo (95% confidence interval): inhaled steroids versus placebo 0.11 L (0.02-0.19); prednisolone versus placebo 0.16 L (0.08-0.25). Although higher incidences of hyperglycemia and minor psychiatric disorders can be observed with prednisolone, nebulized budesonide may be an alternative to oral prednisolone.

## Antibiotics

The prescription of antibiotics to facilitate early recovery of acute exacerbations of COPD has become routine despite unanswered questions concerning their true benefits. In 1987, Anthonisen et al. (49) reported the results of the highest quality clinical study to date and concluded that antibiotics improved outcomes. They randomized 173 outpatients to receive either placebo or broad-spectrum antibiotics during 362 COPD exacerbations. These exacerbations were classified according to their severity from type 1 (the most severe with increases in dyspnea, sputum volume, and sputum purulence) to type 3 (the least severe with only one symptom plus one other finding among sore throat, rhinorrhea, fever, increased wheezing or increased cough. Compared with placebo, antibiotics shortened the duration of exacerbations by about 2 days (P<0.02) and accelerated recovery of peak expiratory flow rates (P<0.02). Treatment success, defined as resolution of symptoms within 21 days, occurred in 55% of the placebo group and 68.1% of patients receiving antibiotics (P<0.05). Among the patients with type 1 exacerbations, clinical deterioration occurred more than twice as often with placebo than with antibiotics. A clinician would therefore need to treat roughly 8 exacerbations to avoid a single deterioration. The authors concluded that the strongest reason to give antibiotics to patients with acute exacerbations of COPD is to avoid a deleterious outcome. They also stated that antibiotics are clearly indicated in type 1 exacerbations, of no benefits in type 3 exacerbations, and probably useful in patients with type 2 exacerbations. A recent meta-analysis (50) identified only nine randomized, placebo-controlled trials of at least 5 days of antibiotics treatment. An effect of antibiotic treatment was noted to be positive in 7 of these trials and negative in 2. Overall, a small benefit in favor of antibiotic treatment was demonstrated. More recently Grossman et al. (51) suggested that acute exacerbations should be classified in four categories based on clinical status, risk factors, and probable pathogens and they proposed choices of antibiotics. This rationale is likely to reduce treatment failures as well as decrease costs of treatment (51-52). Nowadays, exacerbations of COPD are routinely treated with antibiotics. Unfortunately these drugs are becoming more and more expensive even if their superiority over older antibiotics is not documented (53).

## Bronchodilator treatment

During acute exacerbations of COPD, the apparent advantages of ipratropium bromide are not as clear as they are in stable disease and in emergency settings, the addition of nebulized ipratropium bromide to nebulized $\beta_2$-agonist seems to produce a similar degree of bronchodilation. It would therefore, seem that there is no difference in effect and no advantage in combining these two drugs in acute exacerbation (54).

## Conclusions

There has recently been renewed interest in the management of COPD and the publication of the GOLD guidelines, the development of new molecules such as tiotropium and viozan and the exciting research on airway inflammation are good examples of this. Smoking cessation remains however the only proven intervention that may change the evolution of the disease while all other therapeutic modalities are aimed at reducing symptoms. A better understanding of the physiopathology of the disease may improve future pharmacotherapy. For instance, focusing on reversal of damages is not a realistic goal in COPD patients because the structural changes that have occurred are mostly irreversible. We should therefore aim at developing new drugs effective in halting the progression of the disease. Finally, the evaluation of new pharmacological treatments should not only be based on measurements of physiopathological markers but also on evaluation of functional and health status.

## References

1. Fletcher C., Peto R. 1977. The natural history of chronic airflow obstruction. *Br Med J* 1:1645-1648.
2. Anthonisen N., Cornett J, Kiley J et al. The Lung Health Study: effects of smoking cessation and the use of an inhaled anticholinergic bronchodilator on the rate of decline of $FEV_1$. The Lung Health Study. *JAMA* 272:1497-1505.
3. Henningfield JE. Nicotine medications for smoking cessation. *N Engl J Med* 1995, 333:1196-1203.
4. Fiore M, Smith S, Jorenby D, Baker T. The effectiveness of the nicotine patch for smoking cessation. *JAMA* 1994; 271:1940-1949.
5. Hurt RD, Sachs DPL, Glover ED et al. A comparison of sustained-released bupropion and placebo for smoking cessation. *N Engl J Med* 1997; 337:1195-1202
6. Jorenby DE, Leischow SJ, Nides MA et al. Bupropion, nicotin patch or both for smoking cessation. *N Engl J Med* 1999:340:685-691.
7. Koivula I, Sten M, Leinonen M, et al. Clinical efficacy of pneumococcal vaccine in the elderly: A randomised, single-blind population-based trial. *Am J Med* 1997; 103:281-290.
8. Center for Disease Control: Prevention of pneumococcal and influenza: Recommendations of the Advisory Committee on Immunization Practices (ACIP). *MMWR Morb Mort Wkly Rep* 1999 48:1-28.
9. Nichols KL, Baken L, Nelson A. Relation between influenza vaccination and outpatient visits, hospitalisation and mortality in elderly persons with chronic lung disease. *Ann Int Med* 1999; 130:397-403.
10. Seersholm N, Wencker M, Banik N, et al. Does Alpha 1-antitrypsine augmentation therapy slow the annual decline in $FEV_1$, in patients with severe hereditary Alph 1-antitrypsin deficiency? *Eur Respir J* 1997;10:2260-2263.
11. Combivent Inhalation Aerosol Group: In chronic obstructive pulmonary disease, a combinaison of ipratropium and albuterol is more effective than either agent alone: An 85-day multicenter trial. *Chest* 1994; 105:1411-1419.
12. Ferguson GT, Cherniack RM. Management of chronic obstructive pulmonary disease. *N Engl J Med* 1993; 328:1017-1022.
13. American Thoracic Society: Statement: Standards for the diagnosis and care of patients with chronic obstructive pulmonary disease. *Am J Respir Crit Care Med* 1995 152(suppl):77-121.
14. British Thoracic Society: BRS guidelines for the management of chronic obstructive pulmonary disease: COPD guidelines group of the standards care committee of the BTS. *Thorax* 1997; 52 (suppl):1-28.
15. Siafakas NM, Vermeire P Pride NB, et al. European Respiratory Society-consensus statement: Optimal assessment and mangement of chronic obstructive pulmonary disease (COPD) *Eur Respir J* 1995; 8:1398-1420.
16. Barnes PJ. State of the art: B-Adrenergic receptors and their regulation. *Am J Respir Crit Care Med* 1995;152:838-860
17. Rennard S, Serby C, Ghabouri M et al. Extended therapy with ipratropium is associated with improved lung function in COPD: a retrospective

analysis of data from seven clinical trials. *Chest* 1997; 112:336-340.

18. Giannin D, Bacci E, Dente FL et al. Inhaled beclomethasone diproprionate reverts tolerance to protective effect of salmeterol on allergen challenge. *Chest* 1999; 115:629-634.

19. Mahler DA, Matthat RA, Snyder DK, et al. Sustained-release theophylline reduces dyspnea in nonreversible obstructive airway disease. *Am Rev Respir Dis* 1985;131:22-25.

20. Guyatt GH, Berman LB, Townsend M et al. A measure of quality of life for clinical trials in chronic lung disease. *Thorax* 1987; 42:773-778.

21. Kirsten D, Wegner R, Jorres R, et al. Effects of theophylline withdrawal in severe chronic obstructive pulmonary disease. *Chest* 1993;104:1101-1107.

22. Matera MG, Cazzola M, Vinciguerra A et al. A comparison of the bronchodilating effects of sameterol, salbutamol and ipratropium bromide in patients with chronic obstructive pulmonary disease. *Pulm Pharmacol* 1995; 8:267-271.

23. Maesen BLP, Wertermann CJJ, Duurkens VAM et al. Effects of formoterol in apprently poorly reversible chronic obstructive pulmonary disease. *Eur Respir J* 1999; 13:1103-1108.

24. Johnson M, Coleman RA. Mechanism of action of B2-adrenoceptor agonists. In Busse WW, Holgate ST (eds). Asthma and Rhinitis. Cambridge, Blackwell, 1995, pp1278-1295.

25. Appleton S, Smith B, Veale A, Bara A. Long-acting β2-agonists for chronic obstructive airways disease. Cochrane Database Syst Rev 2000;2:CD001104.

26. Maesen FPV, Smeets JJ, Costongs MAL et al. BA 679 BR, a new long-acting antimuscarinic bronchodilator: A pilot dose-escalation study. *Eur Respir J* 1993;6:1031-1036.

27. Littner MR, Ilowite JS, Tashkin DP et al. Long-acting bronchodilation with once daily dosing of tiotropium (Spiriva) in stable COPD. *Am J Respir Crit Care Med* 2000; 161;1136-1142.

28. Van Noord JA, Bantje ThA, Eland ME, Korducki L, Cornelissen PJG, on behalf of the Dutch Tiotropium Study Group. A randomized controlled comparison of tiotropium and ipratropium it the treatment of chronic obstructive pulmonary disease. *Thorax* 2000;55:289-294.

29. Mahler DA, Montner P, Brazinski SA et al. Tiotropium (Spiriva), a new long-acting anticholinergic bronchodilator, improves dyspnea in patients with COPD. *Am J Respir Crit Care Med* 2000;161:A892.

30. Wenzel S, Ind PW, Laursen LC, D et al. Viozan (AR-C68397AA) reduces breathlessness cough and sputum production in COPD patients. *Am J Respir Crit Care Med* 2000;161:A490.

31. Laitinen LA, Laursen LC, Wouters E et al. Viozan (AR-C 68397AA) versus salbutamol and iprotropium bromide in the management of COPD. *Am J Respir Crit Care* 2000;161:A490.

32. Niewoehner DE. Cigarette smoking, lung inflammation, and the development of emphysema. *J Lab Clin Med* 1988;111:15-27.

33. Callaghan CM, Dittus RS, Katz BP. Oral corticosteroid therapy for patients with stable chronic obstructive pulmonary disease. *Ann Intern Med* 1991;114:216-223.

34. Renkema TEJ, Schouten JP, Koeter GH, et al. Effects of long-term treatment with corticosteroids in COPD. *Chest* 1996;109:1156-1162.

35. Shim CS, Williams, Jr MH, Aerosol beclomethasone in patients with steroid-responsive chronic obstructive pulmonary disease. *Am J Med* 1985;78:655-658.

36. Bourbeau J, Rouleau M, Boucher S. A randomized controlled trial of inhaled corticosteroids in patients with advanced obstructive pulmonary disease. *Thorax* 1998;53:477-482.

37. Paggiaro PL. Dahle R, Bakran I, et al. Multicentre randomised placebo-controlled trial of inhaled fluticasone propionate in patients with chronic obstructive pulmonary disease. *Lancet* 1998;351:773-780.

38. Pauwels RA, Lofdahl CG, Laitinen LA et al. Long term with inhaled budesonide in persons with mild chronic obstructive pulmonary disease who continue smoking. *N Engl J Med* 1999;340:1948-1953.

39. Burge PS, Calverly PMA, Jones PW et al. Randomised, double blind, placebo controlled study of fluticasone proprinate in patients with moderate to sever chronic obstructive pulmonary disease. The ISOLDE trial. *BMJ* 2000;320:1297-1303.

40. Vestbo J, Sorensen T, Lange P, et al. Long-term effect of inhaled budesonide in mild and moderate chronic obstructive pulmonary disease: a randomised controlled trial. *Lancet* 1999;353:1819-1823.

41. The Lung Health Study Research Group. Effect of inhaled trimcinolone on the decline in pulmonary function in chronic obstructive pulmonary disease. *N Engl J Med* 2000;343:1902-1909.

42. Pauwles RA, Buist AS, Calverly PMA, Jenkins CR, Hurd SS on behalf of the GOLD scientific Committee. Global strategy for the diagnosis, management, and prevention of chronic obstructive pulmonary disease. NHLBI/WHO Global initiative for chronic obstructive lung disease (GOLD) workshop summary. *Am J Respir Crit Care Med* 2001;163:1256-1276.

43. Albert RK, Martin TR, Lewis SW. Controlled clinical trial of methylprednisolone in patients with chronic bronchitis and acute respiratory insufficiency. *Ann Int Med* 1980;92:753-758.

44. Emerman CI, Connors AF, Lukens TW et al. A randomized controlled trial of methylprednisolone in the emergency treatment of acute exacerbations of COPD. *Chest* 1989;95:563-567.

45. Thompson WH, Wielson CP, Carvalho P et al. Controlled trial of oral prednisone in outpatients with acute COPD exacerbations. *Am J Respir Crit Care Med* 1996;154:407-412.

46. Niewoehner DE, Erbland ML, Deupree RH et al. Effects of systemic glucocorticoids on exacerbations of chronic obstructive pulmonary disease. Departement of Veteran Affairs Cooperative Study Group. *N Engl J Med* 1999;340:1941-1947.

47. Davies L, Angus RM, Calverley PM. Oral corticosteroids in patients admitted to hospital with exacerbations of chronic obstructive pulmonary disease: a prospective randomized controlled trial. *Lancet* 1999;354:456-460.

48. Maltais F, Bourbeau J, Tonnel A et al. Comparison of nebulized budesonide and oral prednisolone with placebo in the treatment of acute exacerbations of COPD. *Eur Repir J* 1999;14(Suppl 30)2815.

49. Anthonisen NR, Manfreda J, Warred CP et al. Antibiotic therapy in exacerbations of chronic obstructive pulmonary disease. *Ann Intern Med* 1987;106:196-204.

50. Saint S, Bent S, Vittinghoff E, Grady D. Antibiotics in chronic obstructive pulmonary disease exacerbations: a meta-analysis. *JAMA* 1995;273:957-960.

51. Grossman RF, Mukerjee J, Vaughan D et al. A 1-year community-based health economic study of ciprofloxacin vs usual antibiotic treatment in acute exacerbations of chronic bronchitis. *Chest* 1998;113:131-141.

52. Destaches CJ, Dewan N, O'Donohue WJ, et al. Clinical and economic considerations in the treatment of acute exacerbations of chronic bronchitis. *J Antimicrob Chemother* 1999;43 (Suppl A) 107-113.

53. Cazzola M, Vinciguerra A, Beghi G, et al. Comparative evaluation of the clinical and microbiological efficacy of co-amoxiclav vs cefuxime or ciprofloxacin in bacterial exacerbation of chronic bronchitis. *J Chemther* 1995;7:432-441.

54. Rebuck AS, Chapman KR, Abboud R, et al. Nebulized anticholinergic and sympathomimetic treatment of asthma and chronic obstructive airways disease in emergency room. *Am J Med* 1987;82:59-64.

# Chapter 9

# Secondary Prevention of CAD: An Integrative Medicine Approach

Martin J. Sullivan, MD, USA

Atherosclerosis leading to coronary artery disease (CAD) continues to be the most important single source of morbidity and mortality in North America. Significant advances have been made in the identification of risk factors, elucidation of pathophysiology, treatment of acute coronary syndromes, use of surgical and interventional techniques, and application of pharma-

cologic strategies for the reduction of recurrent events. Although these advances have made a major difference in short-term outcomes, it is likely that long-term outcomes are dependent on atherosclerosis regression. French et al (1), examine twenty-year outcomes in patients under the age of forty who underwent bypass grafting in New Zealand. As illustrated in Figure 9.1,

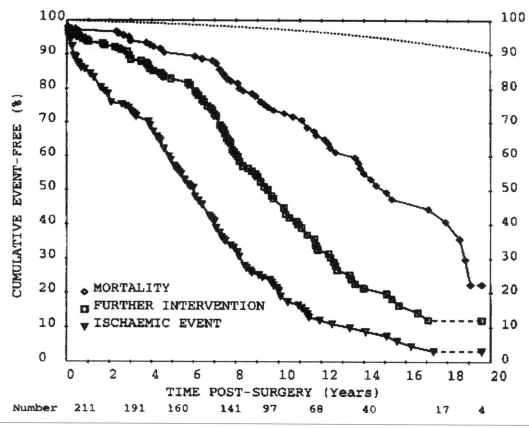

**Figure 9.1** Graph showing actuarial outcome after CABG in patients < 40 years old. The percentage of patients free of recurrent ischemia, reintervention, and death at yearly postoperative intervals is shown. The numbers of patients at each time are shown. Age-matched control subjects, dotted line.

Reprinted, by permission, from JK French et al., 1995, "Late outcome after coronary artery bypass graft surgery in patients," *Circulation* 92(9):II-14-II-19.

at twenty-year follow-up there was 20% survival and 0% event-free survival. The results clearly illustrate the limitations of acute interventions alone in the long-term management of CAD, especially in younger patients. It appears that, in addition to employing effective acute intervention, the best strategy for managing CAD is secondary prevention aimed at either delaying or reversing atherosclerosis progression.

Antihyperlipidemic agents, β-blockers, aspirin, and ACE inhibitors are effective in secondary prevention of CAD, and clearly play an important role in therapy. However, existing studies indicate that a more effective approach involves the addition of intensive lifestyle modification (diet, exercise, stress management) to a therapeutic regimen. Lifestyle interventions have been proven to significantly reduce future events and delay underlying disease progression (2-9). Although it seems clear from the outcomes that these interventions should be the cornerstone of therapy in this disorder, and evidence supporting this approach continues to accumulate, the vast majority of patients with coronary artery disease receive no lifestyle prevention or rehabilitation services (10,11). This phenomenon seems the result of a number of factors involving patient education, physician preferences, third-party reimbursement, and infrastructure.

It seems at this point that implementation of widespread secondary prevention in CAD is more of a cultural and educational issue than it is about scientific knowledge. This is an area where the emergence of the discipline of Integrative Medicine may offer new avenues to increase the use of lifestyle interventions in patients with CAD. Integrative Medicine is a rapidly emerging new field that seeks to combine conventional therapies with evidence-based complementary and alternative medicine techniques and a patient-centered mind-body-spirit approach (See Figure 9.2). This patient-centered Mind-Body-Spirit approach includes a focus on lifestyle (diet, exercise, stress management, self-care), and has very important implications for secondary prevention of CAD. The importance of Integrative Medicine in increasing use of lifestyle intervention in CAD lies in three factors: 1) its growing acceptance by the public, 2) generating interest in creating new systems of medical care, and 3) a growing physician educational component. There has been a huge upsurge in interest in complementary and alternative medicine (CAM) over the past five years by both the public and by health care providers. Eisenberg et al (12) examined patient use of CAM in 1992, and have demonstrated that 32% of the public used these services, with some 400 million patient vis-

its. A repeat survey in 1998 demonstrated a rise in use to 40%, with an estimated 600 million visits and expenditures of $34 billion (12). Why the recent dramatic increase in use? Astin (13) has explored the reasons for this interest in a recent healthcare survey in which 40% of respondents used CAM techniques. Patients reported that the primary reason for use was perceived efficacy – they felt that CAM was beneficial. Other reasons were cultural congruence with their CAM care provider (better understanding in the provider-patient interaction) and the use of a mind-body-spirit approach. Over 95% of patients used conventional medicine, and were generally satisfied with it, while at the same time they used CAM. They tended to have medical diagnoses that were chronic and not easily or totally alleviated by conventional therapy. Patients with more education and more symptoms were more likely to use CAM, as were those who reported a life-changing event. This growing interest by the public is embedded in a cultural shift that will increase use and acceptability of lifestyle changes by the public over the next decade. As this occurs in conjunction with better physician education and the growth of Integrative Medicine, it is likely that the use of lifestyle therapies in CAD will increase. In turn, this increased interest by patients and physicians will hopefully initiate new infrastructure and reimbursement models which will make widespread application of lifestyle interventions a reality.

## Lifestyle Factors in CAD

At least half of what influences the health status of the population is rooted in the lifestyle of individuals and in the environments in which they live (14). It is estimated that only 10% of the variability in health outcomes are linked to specific medical treatment interventions; the rest is linked to lifestyle, environment, and genetics. This concept is supported by the Cornell China Project (15). This study examined health records in 220 localities in China over a three-year period and found a very low incidence of coronary artery disease in Chinese men (risk ratio of 0.06 compared to contemporary norms for U.S. men) in their survey. They examined several geographic locations in which evidence of CAD could not be found in populations of several hundred thousand individuals. These results, when combined with those of the Honolulu Heart Study (16) and others (17-19), demonstrate the critical role of cultural factors in the genesis of CAD.

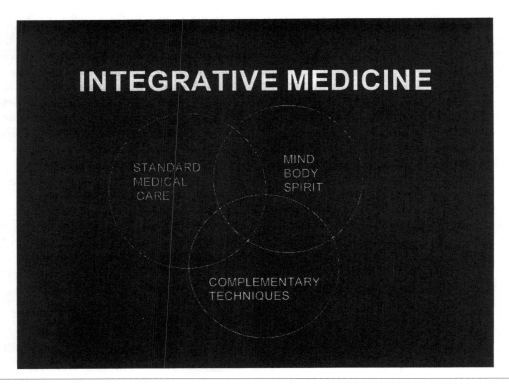

**Figure 9.2**   The three elements of integrative medicine

It has long been established that diet and smoking are related to CAD (20-28). More recent studies have refined the components of diet which are related to CAD incidence (25-26). While early studies focused on total fat and saturated fat, more recent studies have explored the protective roles of monounsaturated fatty acids, vegetable and cereal intake, and dietary vitamins (23,25,26). Over the past decade, more information linking sedentary lifestyle to CAD has accumulated (29,30). It now appears that even short intervals of regular exertion at low levels of aerobic activity confer significant health benefits when compared to a completely sedentary lifestyle.

It has only been recently that the weight of evidence clearly points to psychosocial factors as causative for CAD (31-37). Although early studies demonstrated a link between CAD and Type A behavior, more recent studies have not shown that all Type A's are at risk (33). It now appears that hostility is an important risk-conferring behavior in Type A individuals (33). There have been numerous articles demonstrating that social isolation is linked to CAD (32,33). Over the last five years, several well-done studies have shown a clear link between depression and CAD (33-37), often with risk ratios for CAD

of 3-4 for those who have major depression. This hazard ratio would be equal to or greater than that conferred by any other single risk factor.

Studies in high-risk westernized populations clearly demonstrate strong relationships between lifestyle and CAD. Diet, physical inactivity, and psychosocial factors, including social isolation, depression, and hostility are dependent on culture, and may possibly be changed significantly over time in a given population. The finding in cross-cultural studies that some populations have very low incidences of CAD supports the concept that atherosclerosis may be largely an unintended result of our current culture. Although public health initiatives have improved many of these factors (diet and toxic exposures), there have been significant limitations in advancing others (weight, exercise, stress, and smoking).

## Lifestyle Interventions in CAD

From the 1960's to the early 1980's, lifestyle changes in CAD focused primarily on exercise training of patients who were status post myocardial infarction.

This is supported by numerous studies demonstrating reduced mortality after exercise training in this population (37-39), Until the late 1980s, most investigators thought atherosclerosis was a relentlessly progressive process which could not be altered by modifying risk factors. As stated in the *British Medical Journal* in 1977, "Only the optimists among us believe that obstructive atheroma in the coronary arteries of our patients with angina might regress if we could persuade them to reduce the load of adverse factors in their lifestyle" (40). The first indication of coronary lesion regression came from case studies in the 1970's and the early 1980's. In these studies, patients who underwent serial angiography had less than 6% regression with standard medical therapy (41,42).

At present, numerous studies have examined the effect of lifestyle interventions in patients with CAD, demonstrating important reductions in symptoms and recurrent events (2-9). In addition, at least four dozen clinical trials (43-65), many using serial angiography, have demonstrated that pharmacologic lipid-lowering intervention programs can improve coronary luminal diameter, improve myocardial blood flow, reduce myocardial ischemia and infarction, and reduce coronary events in patients with coronary artery disease. Even though the changes in coronary lesions are small, they translate into significant improvement in outcome. This is likely due to prevention of plaque rupture, which is known to cause most acute cardiac events. Although pharmacologic management of lipids is an important therapeutic focus in managing patients with CAD, it should be viewed as part of a comprehensive risk reduction program. Pharmacotherapy can have major effects on LDL-cholesterol, and yet is not more effective (and in some comparisons is less effective) in reducing events or angiographic disease progression when compared to lifestyle interventions. In addition, pharmacologic therapy is often more costly than lifestyle management.

The **St. Thomas' Atherosclerosis Regression Study (STARS)** (6) examined the effects of dietary changes with or without cholestyramine versus usual care in men with angina or previous myocardial infarction. By decreasing total cholesterol and LDL more than control subjects, the progression of coronary atherosclerosis declined from almost half (46%) in those receiving usual care to only 12% in those receiving diet and cholestyramine and 15% of those receiving diet alone. Regression was seen in 4% of the usual care group and in 33% and 38% of the diet plus cholestyramine and diet alone groups, respectively. Although the addition of

Cholestyramine further reduced LDL-C when compared to diet alone, it did not improve angiographic or clinical outcomes. As in previous studies, lesions with greater than 50% stenosis demonstrated the most improvement. In addition to demonstrating anatomic effects of these diet-based therapies, the two treatment groups had fewer clinical cardiac events than the usual care group (p<0.05), and had less angina compared to baseline (p<0.05), while angina in controls did not change.

The blinded, randomized, controlled **Lifestyle Heart Trial** (2,3), is an example of an Integrative Medicine approach to CAD. It examined symptoms, risk factors, and coronary anatomy before and at one and five years after a comprehensive set of diet, exercise and behavioral interventions in the treatment group. All participants in this study had significant coronary atherosclerosis, a left ventricular ejection fraction greater than 25%, and were not taking lipid-lowering medications. The treatment group (N=22) was assigned to a low fat (10% of calories from fat) vegetarian diet, one hour a day of stress management, and three hours or more of aerobic exercise per week. Controls (N=19) were given usual care and were counseled to follow a 30% fat diet and exercise. At one and five years, compliance was quite good in treated patients for diet (~9% calories from fat), exercise (3-4 hrs/week), and stress management (5-8 hrs/week). By five years, nine of the control and no treatment patients were taking lipid-lowering medications. Of note, at 5 years controls also exercised (~3 hrs/week) and modified diet (~25% of calories from fat), while not participating in stress reduction to any significant degree. Although LDL was much lower in treated patients at one year (86 + 9 vs. 141 + 15 mg/dl p<0.05), there was no difference in LDL at year five.

At one year, the incidence of angina dropped 91% in the treatment group and increased 165% in controls (1). At five-year follow-up there were 25 events in 108 person years of observation in treated vs. 45 events in 78 person years in control patients (p<0.001); 10 of 28 treatment and 19 of 20 controls underwent PTCA or CABG procedures (p<0.01). The change in average stenosis severity in CAD lesions mirrored the clinical improvements, as illustrated in Figure 9.3. The average percent diameter stenosis decreased from 41% to 37% in treated patients while an increase was seen in the control group, from 41% to 52% (p=0.001). It is interesting to note that there was significant disease progression in controls despite their risk factor changes, which would be considered average for clinical populations with CAD. The Lifestyle Heart Trial

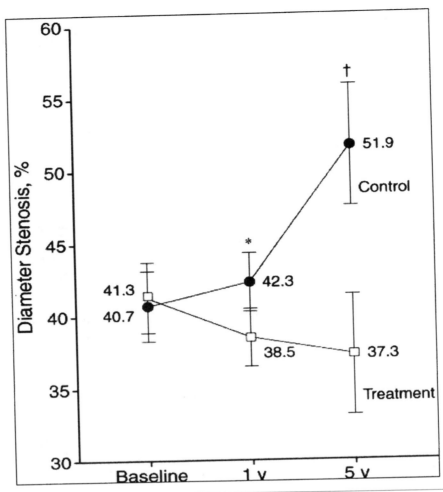

**Figure 9.3**    Average percent diameter stenoses for index lesions at baseline and one- and five-year follow-ups in control and treatment patients in the Lifestyle Heart Trial.
Reprinted, by permission, from D Ornish et al., 1998, "Intensive lifestyle changes for reversal of coronary artery disease," *JAMA* 280 (23):2001-2007.

was the first study to demonstrate that lesion progression could be slowed using lifestyle changes alone and, although small in size, has important ramifications for treatment in this disorder.

Compliance with the treatment program correlated with lesion changes in a dose-response fashion as illustrated in Figure 9.4, and yet changes in LDL-cholesterol or in trial LDL-cholesterol did not correlate with angiographic changes. This finding serves to emphasize the concept that factors other than serum lipids may have a major role in the atherosclerotic process. Also of note is the finding that although serum LDL and exercise levels were not different in the two groups at five years, treated patients had marked reductions in both events and atherosclerosis progression compared to controls. Although this is very likely due in part to lower LDL-C levels at

one year, it is interesting to consider the role of the psychosocial arm of the Lifestyle Heart Trial intervention. A recent study by Blumenthal et al (7) raises the possibility that stress reduction alone may have powerful effects on reducing morbidity. In this study, patients with CAD and angina were randomized to exercise or stress management interventions and compared with a matched control group which received usual care only. As illustrated in Figure 9.5, there was a 70% reduction in events in the stress management group as compared to controls. In the psychosocial intervention group this event reduction was accompanied by reductions in ischemia as measured by ambulatory Holter monitor and by radionuclide angiography during laboratory-induced mental stress. These results suggest that psychosocial interventions may play an important role in the

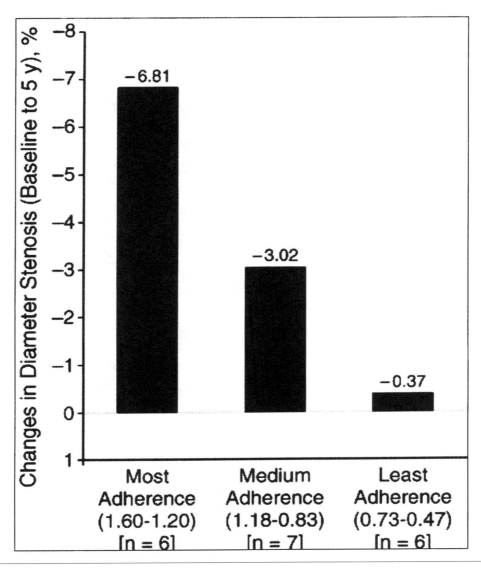

**Figure 9.4**   Relationship of change in diameter stenosis with program adherence in the treatment group at five year follow-up in the Lifestyle Heart Trial.
Reprinted, by permission, from D Ornish et al., 1998, "Intensive lifestyle changes for reversal of coronary artery disease," *JAMA* 280 (23):2001-2007.

management of CAD and certainly deserve careful study and consideration in the future.

The **Stanford Coronary Risk Intervention Project (SCRIP)** (8) also demonstrated the beneficial impact a multi-disciplinary approach could have on CAD. This study randomized 300 men and woman to usual care of their own physician or multifactor risk reduction that included diet education, exercise, weight loss, smoking cessation, and lipid lowering medical therapy. A significant increase in the use of lipid lowering therapy was seen in the treatment group when compared to controls. In the intervention group, significant changes versus the usual care patients occurred in LDL cholesterol and apolipoprotein B (-22%), HDL cholesterol (+12%), plasma triglycerides (-20%), body weight (-4%), and exercise capacity (+20%). The rate of coronary artery narrowing was 47% less than that for usual-care subjects (p<0.02). Further analysis of the coronary lesions found that new lesions tended to occur in the usual care patients rather than the risk reduction patients (new lesions/patient 0.47 vs. 0.30, p=0.06). Although there was no significant difference between groups in the overall mortality or cardiac death, there was a significant difference when comparing the combined end-point of cardiac deaths and hospitalizations for non fatal myocardial infarction, PTCA, and CABG (25 vs. 44, p=0.05).

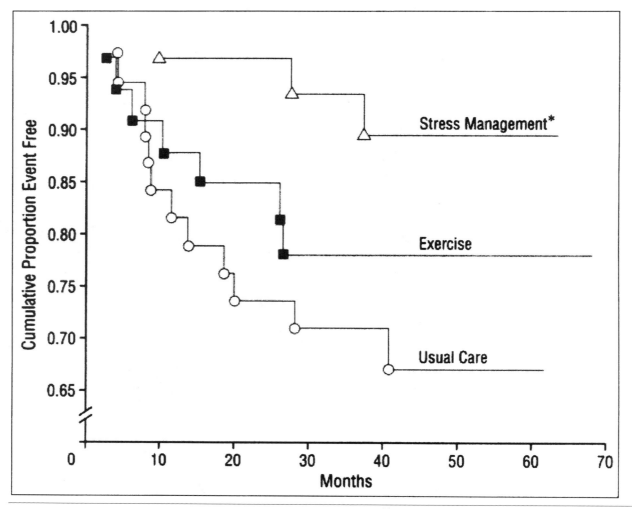

**Figure 9.5**   Five-year cumulative event-free survival in patients with CAD and angina randomized to stress management or exercise interventions compared with a usual care control group.
Reprinted, by permission, from JA Blumenthol et al., 1997, "Stress management and exercise training in cardiac patients with myocardial ischemia," *Archives of Inernal Medicine* 157(19):2213-2223.

Schuler et al (4) has examined the effects of intensive exercise and a 20% fat diet in patients with coronary artery disease. The study design gave controls a one-week hospitalization for instructions about the need for regular exercise and low fat diet (AHA phase 1 diet) and then discharged to the care of their private physician. The intervention group received three weeks of in-hospital instruction on a diet with less than 20% of calories from fat and less than 200mg cholesterol per day. In addition, they were asked to exercise at home on a bicycle ergometer for a minimum of 30 minutes a day with two 60-minute group exercise sessions per week. Patients were seen at the clinic at least four times a year. In

The **Heidelberg Study** (4), 111 male patients were randomized to these two arms. In the intervention arm there was delayed lesion progression by quantitative coronary angiography at one year. By decreasing total cholesterol by 11% and LDL by 9% with no change in HDL in treated patients, there was an increase in regression when compared to controls (32% vs 17%, p<0.05) and a decrease in progression (23% vs 48%, p<0.05) of coronary lesions. In addition, myocardial ischemia as measured by quantitative Thallium scanning after the intervention improved while there was no change in controls. These investigators also reported that exercise may have increased collateral formation in treated patients.

Another important dietary intervention was examined in the **Lyon Diet Trial**, (5,23) which randomized patients after myocardial infarction to a Step I AHA diet or a Mediterranean diet that emphasized use of monounsaturated fats and increases in fruits and vegetables. Both groups consumed 30% of calories from fat. There was no difference in serum LDL or HDL in the two groups at baseline or at one-year follow-up. Of note, serum Tocopherol levels were higher in the Mediterranean diet group during follow-up, suggesting higher dietary Vitamin E and therefore higher antioxidant intake. Despite no differences in blood cholesterol levels, there was a 70% reduction in events in patients in the treatment group when compared to controls during long-term follow-up. (Figure 6) This study clearly delineates the importance of diet in treating patients with CAD independent of changes in serum lipids. The magnitude of event reduction in this study exceeds that seen with lipid lowering pharmacotherapy (~30-40%), and highlights the concept that the goal in the treatment of CAD is not just manipulation of serum lipids but the reduction of events and delayed progression of disease. These results indicate that major event reduction can occur in CAD with diet alone without changes in LDL-C or HDL-C.

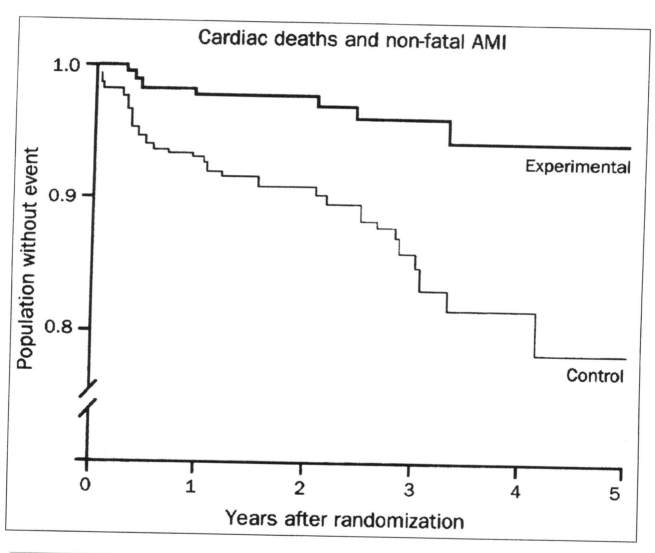

**Figure 9.6**   Event-free survival in patients randomized to Mediterranean diet versus usual care.
Reprinted with permission from Elsevier Science (The Lancet), 1997, 353:1454-1459.

## Implementing Secondary Prevention in CAD

The data at this point are clear and compelling: lifestyle interventions are effective therapies in patients with coronary artery disease. They increase quality of life, reduce symptoms and objective evidence of ischemia, reduce morbidity, and delay progression of atherosclerosis (2-9). Although meta-analysis in this area is subject to difficulties in interpretation, one such analysis found that treatment reduced the odds for coronary lesion progression by 49%, increased the odds for no change by 33%, and increased the odds for coronary artery regression by 219%. Cardiovascular events declined by 47% (66).

Whereas ten years ago the role of secondary prevention in CAD was unclear, intensive risk factor reduction has now emerged as important therapy in this disorder. The evidence for secondary prevention as a means of limiting coronary artery atherosclerosis, decreasing recurrent myocardial infarction, and improving survival has grown to the point that standard of care dictates cardiologists incorporate these interventions into their practice. In 1994, the AHA recommended patients with known coronary artery disease undergo a comprehensive risk factor reduction program centered on lipid lowering therapy, blood pressure control, smoking cessation, diet, exercise, weight reduction, and stress reduction (67). Although the guidelines here are clear, medicine has been slow to respond in implementing effective strategies to meet these goals.

Several studies have examined the current implementation rates of secondary prevention strategies in patients with CAD (10,11,68). Across geographic locations and practice types, the results are consistent in showing very low implementation rates. In 1991, Cohen et al (10) reported that only 25% of patients with CAD had either pharmacological or dietary therapy for hyperlipidemia one month after catheterization. Less than 20% of eligible patients participate in cardiac rehabilitation, largely due to low physician referral rates (10). A 1998 study of hospitalized patients with CAD showed that less than 15% of patients had received any formalized lifestyle intervention (stop smoking consult, cardiac rehabilitation, nutrition consult, or psychological referral) (11). There was a 1% rate of referral for exercise therapy with less than 50% of patients receiving appropriate lipid-lowering therapy.

## Integrative Approaches to Change

Why have lifestyle approaches to secondary prevention in CAD not become standard of care? Several issues seem to play a role in delaying implementation, including: 1) lack of reimbursement, 2) patient education and motivation (69), and 3) physician interest (10,11). In order for lifestyle interventions to be widely utilized, changes will need to be made in all three areas, and these areas are interdependent. It seems that patient interest in integrative approaches is clearly growing, and that this growth is related to a shift in cultural values (70). Strides in reimbursement are not apparent now, although several initiatives are promising reform in this arena. Physician interest seems higher now as a result of educational efforts and higher patient interest. The phenomenon of Integrative Medicine offers an additional impetus to change, which may improve all three of these areas in the next decade. Clearly, the best therapy for CAD is a combination of the best acute care, interventions, and pharmacotherapy combined with the effective use of diet, exercise, and psychosocial interventions (71). As the prevailing culture and the medical culture move toward more integrative approaches, it is likely that this combined approach will be adopted as standard of care for CAD.

## References

1. French JK, Scott DS, Whitlock RM, Nisbet HD, Vedder MK, Alan R, Smith WM. Late outcome after coronary artery bypass graft surgery in patients <40 years old. *Circulation* 1995; 92(9):II-14-II-1.
2. Ornish D, Scherwitz L, Billings J, Gould K, Merritt T, Sparler S, Armstrong W, Ports T, Kirkeeide R, Hogeboom C, Brand R. Intensive lifestyle changes for reversal of coronary artery disease. *JAMA* 1998;280(23):2001-2007.
3. Ornish D, Brown SE, Scherwitz LW. Can lifestyle changes reverse coronary heart disease? The Lifestyle Heart Trial. *Lancet* 1990;336:129-33.
4. Schuler G, Hambrecht R, Schlierf G. Myocardial perfusion and regression of coronary artery disease in patients on a regimen of intensive physical exercise and low fat diet. *J Am Coll Cardiol* 1992;19:34-42.

5. DeLorgeril M, Renaud S, Mamelle N, Salen P, Matin JL, Monjaud I, Guidollet J, Touboul P, Delaye J. Mediterranean alpha-linolenic acid-rich diet in secondary prevention of coronary heart disease. *Lancet* 1994;343(8911):1454-1459.

6. Watts GF, Lewis B, Brunt JNH. Effects on coronary artery disease of lipid-lowering diet, or diet plus cholestyramine, in the St. Thomas' Atherosclerosis Regression Study (STARS). *Lancet* 1992;339:563-69.

7. Blumenthal JA, Jiang W, Babyak MA, Krantz DS, Frid DJ, Coleman RE, Waugh R, Hanson M, Appelbaum M, O'Connor C, Morris JJ. Stress management and exercise training in cardiac patients with myocardial ischemia. Effects on prognosis and evaluation of mechanisms. *Arch In Med* 1997;157(19):2213-2223.

8. Haskell WL, Alderman EL, Fair JM, Maron DJ, Mackey SF, Superko HR, Williams PT, Johnstone IM, Champagne MA, Krauss RM, Farquhar JW. Effects of intensive multiple risk factor reduction on coronary atherosclerosis and clinical cardiac events in men and women with coronary artery disease: The Stanford Coronary Risk Intervention Project (SCRIP). *Circulation* 1994;89:975-990.

9. Connor WE; Connor SL; Katan MB; Grundy SM; Willett WC. Should a low-fat, high-carbohydrate diet be recommended for everyone? *NEJM* 1997;337(8):562-563.

10. Cohen MV, Byrne M, Levine B, Gutowski T, Adelson R. Low rate of treatment of hypercholesterolemia by cardiologists in patients with suspected and proven coronary artery disease. *Circulation* 1991;83:1294-1304.

11. Frolkis J, Zyzanski S, Schwartz J, Suhan P. Physician noncompliance with the 1993 national cholesterol education program (NCEP-ATPII) guidelines. *Circulation* 1998;98(9):851-855.

12. Eisenberg DM, Davis RB, Ettner SL, Appel S, Wilkey S, Van Rompay M, Kessler RC. Trends in alternative medicine use in the United States, 1990-1997: results of a follow-up national survey. *JAMA* 1998;280(18):1569-75

13. Astin JA. Why patients use alternative medicine: results of a national study. *JAMA* 1998;279(19):1548-1553.

14. McGinnis, M. and Foege. "Actual Causes of Death in the United States." Journal of the America Medical Association, November 10, 1993, Vol. 270, No. 18, pp. 2207-2212.

15. Campbell TC, Parpia B, Chen J. Diet, lifestyle, and the etiology of coronary artery disease: the China study. *Am J Cardiol* 1998;82(10B):18T-21T.

16. Reed D, Yano K. Predictors of arteriographically defined coronary stenosis in the Honolulu Heart Program. Comparisons of cohort and arteriography series analyses. *Am J Epidemiol* 1991;134(2):111-22.

17. Marmot MG, Syme SL, Kagan A et al. Epidemiologic studies of coronary heart disease and stroke in Japanese men living in Japan, Hawaii and California: prevalence of coronary and hypertensive heart disease and associated risk factors. *Am J Epidemiol* 1975;102:514-25.

18. Shaper AG. Communities without hypertension. In: Shaper AG, Hutt MSR, Fejfar Z. Cardiovascular disease in the tropics. London: British Medical Association, 1974;77-83.

19. Malmros H. The relation of nutrition to health. A statistical study of the effect of wartime on arteriosclerosis, cardiosclerosis, tuberculosis and diabetes. *Acta Med. Scand* 1950;Suppl: 246:137-50.

20. Neaton JD, Kuller LH, Wentworth D, Borhani NO. Total and cardiovascular mortality in relation to cigarette smoking, serum cholesterol concentration, and diastolic blood pressure among black and white males followed up for five years. *Am Heart J* 1984;108(3,pt.2):759-769.

21. Keys A, ed. Coronary heart disease in seven countries. *Circulation* 1970;41(Suppl 1):I-1-I-198.

22. Keys A, Aravanis C, Van Buchem FSP et al. The diet and all-causes death rate in the Seven Countries Study. *Lancet* 1981;2:58-61.

23. de Lorgeril M, Salen P, Caillat-Vallet E, Hanauer MT, Barthelemy JC, Mamelle N. Control of bias in dietary trial to prevent coronary recurrences: The Lyon Diet Heart Study. *Eur J Clinl Nutr* 1997;51(2):116-122.

24. Carlson LA, Bottiger LE. Ischaemic heart-disease in relation to fasting values of plasma triglycerides and cholesterol: Stockholm Prospective Study. *Lancet* 1972;1:865-868.

25. Rimm E, Ascherio A, Giovannucci E, Spiegelman D, Stampfer M, Willett W. Vegetable, fruit, and cereal fiber intake and risk of coronary heart disease among men. *JAMA* 1996;275(6):447-451.

26. Hu FB, Stampfer MJ, Manson JE, et al. Dietary fat intake and the risk of coronary artery disease in women. *N Engl J Med* 1997;337:1491-1499.

27. Rosenman RH, Brand RJ, Jenkins D et al. Coronary heart disease in the Western Collaborative Group Study. *JAMA* 1975;233(8):872-877.

28. Hubert HB, Feinleib M, McNamara PM, Castelli WP. Obesity as an independent risk factor for cardiovascular disease: a 26-year follow-up of participants in the Framingham Heart Study. *Circulation* 1983;67:968-77.

29. Ekelund L-G, Haskell WL, Johnson SL, Whaley FS, Criqul MH, Sheps DS. Physical fitness as a predictor of cardiovascular mortality in asymptomatic North American men. *N Engl J Med* 1988;319:1379-1384.

30. Haskell WL. Health consequences of physical activity: understanding and challenges regarding dose response. *Med Sci Sports Exerc* 1994;26:649-60.

31. Reed D, McGee D, Yano K, Feinleib M. Social networks and coronary heart disease among Japanese men in Hawaii. *Am J Epidemiology* 1983;117(4):384-396.

32. Williams RB, Barefoot JC, Califf RM et al. Prognostic importance of social and economic resources among medically treated patients with angiography documented coronary artery disease. *JAMA* 1992;267(4):520-524.

33. Pandya D. Psychological stress, emotional behaviour and coronary artery disease. (Review) *Comprehensive Therapy* 1998;24(5):265-271.

34. Brezinska V, Kittel F. Psycosocial factors of coronary heart disease in women: a review. (Review) *Social Science and Medicine* 1996;42(10): 1351-1365.

35. Barefoot, JC, Schroll, M. Symptoms of depression, acute myocardial infarction, and total mortality in a community sample. *Circulation* 1996; 93: 1976-1980.

36. Ford DE, Mead LA, Chang PP, Cooper-Patrick L, Wang NY, Klag J. Depression is a risk factor for coronary artery disease in men: the precursors study. *Arch Int Med* 1998;158(13):1422-1426.

37. Carney, Freedland, Rich et al. Depression as a risk factor for cardiac events in established coronary heart disease: A review of possible mechanisms. *Annals of Behavioral Medicine* 1995; 17: 142-129.

38. O'Connor GT. An overview of randomized trails of rehabilitation with exercise after myocardial infarction. *Circulation* 1989;80:235-244.

39. Miller TD, Balady GJ, Fletcher GF. Exercise and its role in the prevention and rehabilitation of cardiovascular disease. *Ann Behav Med* 1997;19(3):220-229.

40. Anonymous. Regression of atheroma. *Br Med J* 1977;2:1-2.

41. Gensini GG, Esente P, Kelly A. Natural history of coronary disease in patients with and without bypass graft surgery. *Circulation* 1974; 49(Suppl.2):II-98 - II-102.

42. Landmann J, Kolsters W, Bruschke AVG. Regression of coronary artery obstructions demonstrated by coronary arteriography. *Euro J Cardiol* 1976;4:475-79.

43. Sacks FM, Pfeffer MA, Moyé LA, Rouleau JL, Rutherford JD, Cole TG, Brown L, Warnica 44. J, Arnold JMO, Wun C-C, Davis BR, Braunwald E., for the Cholesterol and Recurrent Events Trial Investigators. The effect of pravastatin on coronary events after myocardial infarction in patients with average cholesterol levels. *N Engl J Med* 1996;335:1001-1009.

45. Cashin-Hemphill L, Mack WJ, Pogoda JM. Beneficial effects of colestipol-niacin on coronary atherosclerosis: a 4-year follow-up. *JAMA* 1990;264:3013-17.

46. Brown G, Albers JJ, Fisher LD. Regression of coronary artery disease as a result of intensive lipid-lowering therapy in men with high levels of apolipoprotein B. *N Engl J Med* 1990;323:1289-98.

47. Kane JP, Malloy MJ, Ports TA. Regression of coronary atherosclerosis during treatment of familial hypercholesterolemia with combined drug regimens. *JAMA* 1990;264:3007-12.

48. Buchwald H, Varco RL, Matts JP. Effect of partial ileal bypass surgery on mortality and morbidity from coronary heart disease in patients with hypercholesterolemia: report of the Program on the Surgical Control of the Hyperlipidemias (POSCH). *N Engl J Med* 1990;323:946-55.

49. Waters D, Higginson L, Gladstone P, Kimball B, Le May M, Boccuzzi SJ, Lesperance J, the CCAIT Study Group. Effects of monotherapy with an HMG-CoA reductase inhibitor on the progression of coronary atherosclerosis as assessed by serial quantitative arteriography: The Canadian Coronary Atherosclerosis Intervention Trial. *Circulation* 1994;89:959-968.

50. Waters D, Higginson L, Gladstone P, Kimball B, LeMay M, Lesperance J. Design features of a controlled clinical trial to assess the effect of an HMG CoA reductase inhibitor on the progression of coronary artery disease. *Controlled Clinical Trials* 1993;14:45-74.

51. Pitt B, Mancini GBJ, Ellis SG, et al., for the PLAC-I Investigators. Pravastatin limitation of

atherosclerosis in the coronary arteries (PLAC-I): reduction in atherosclerosis progression and clinical events. *J Am Coll Cardiol* 1995;26:1133-1139.

52. Jukema JW, Bruschke AVG, van Boven AJ, Reiber JHC et al. Coronary artery disease/myocardial infarction: effects of lipid lowering by pravastatin on progression and regression of coronary artery disease in symptomatic men with normal to moderately elevated serum cholesterol levels: the regression growth evaluation statin study (REGRESS). *Circulation* 1995;91:2528-2540.

53. Rossouw JE. Lipid-lowering interventions in angiographic trials. *Am J Cardiol* 1995;76:86C-92C.

54. Scandinavian Simvastatin Survival Study Group. Randomised trial of cholesterol lowering in 4444 patients with coronary heart disease: the Scandinavian Simvastatin Survival Study (4S). *Lancet* 1994;344:1383-1389.

55. The Scandinavian Simvastatin Survival Study Group. Design and baseline results of the Scandinavian Simvastatin Survival Study of patients with stable angina and/or previous myocardial infarction. *Am J Cardiol* 1993;71:393-400.

56. Kjekshus J, Pedersen TR, for the Scandinavian Simvastatin Survival Study Group. Reducing the risk of coronary events: evidence from the Scandinavian Simvastatin Survival Study (4S). *Am J Cardiol* 1995;76:64C-68C.

57. Pearson TA, and Swan HJC. Lipid lowering: the case for identifying and treating the high-risk patients. *Cardiology Clinics* 1996;14:117-130.

58. Scandinavian Simvastatin Survival Study Group. Baseline serum cholesterol and treatment effect in the Scandinavian Simvastatin Survival Study (4S). *Lancet* 1995;345:1274-1275.

59. Sacks FM, Pfeffer MA, Moye LA, Rouleau JL, et al, for the Cholesterol and Recurrent Events Trial Investigators. The effect of pravastatin on coronary events after myocardial infarction in patients with average cholesterol levels. *N Engl J Med* 1996; 335:1001-1009.

60. Sacks FM, Pfeffer MA, Moye L, et al. Rationale and design of a secondary prevention trial of lowering normal plasma cholesterol levels after acute myocardial infarction: the Cholesterol and Recurrent Events trial (CARE). *Am J Cardiol* 1991;68:1436-1446.

61. Tonkin AM, for the LIPID Study Group. Management of the Long-term Intervention with Pravastatin in Ischaemic Disease (LIPID) study after the Scandinavian Simvastatin Survival Study (4S). *Am J Cardiol* 1995;76:107C-112C.

62. Treasure CB, Klein JL, Wientraub WS, Talley DJ, et al. Beneficial effects of cholesterol-lowering therapy on the coronary endothelium in patients with coronary artery disease. *N Engl J Med* 1995;332:481-487.

63. Anderson, TJ, Meredith IT, Yeung AC, Frei B, Selwyn AP, Ganz P. The effect of cholesterol-lowering and antioxidant therapy on endothelium-dependent coronary vasomotion. *N Engl J Med* 1995;332:488-493.

64. Leung WH, Lau CP, Wong CK. Beneficial effect of cholesterol-lowering therapy on coronary endothelium-dependent relaxation in hypercholesterlaemic patients. *Lancet* 1993;341:1496-1500.

65. Pearson TA. Primary and secondary prevention of coronary artery disease: trials of lipid lowering with statins. *Am J Cardiol* 1998;82(10A):28S-30S.

66. Gould AL, Rossouw JE, Santanello NC, Heyse JF, Furberg CD. Cholesterol reduction yields clinical benefit: impact of statin trials. *Circulation* 1998;97:946-952.

67. Whellan DJ, Molloy M, Quillian R, Norris J, Sullivan MJ. Coronary Artery Disease: The Basis for Secondary Prevention. In: Interventional Cardiovascular Medicine: Principles and Practices, 2nd Edition, Stack R, Oneill W, and Roubin G (Eds). Churchill-Livingstone; New York, New York. In press.

68. Pearson T, Rapaport E, Criqui M, Furberg C, et al. Optimal risk factor management in the patients after coronary revascularization: a statement for healthcare professionals from an American Heart Association writing group. *Circulation* 1994;90:3125-3133.

69. Marcelino JJ, Feingold KR. Inadequate treatment with HMG-CoA reductase inhibitors by health care providers. *Am J Med* 1996;100(6):605-610.

70. Illich, Ivan. Limits to medicine: Medical Nemesis: The Expropriation of Health. Harmondsworth; New York: Penguin Books, 1977, c1976.

71. Ray PH. The rise of integral culture. *Noetic Sci Rev* 1996;Spring:4-15.

72. Merz C N B, Rozanski A. Remodeling cardiac rehabilitation into secondary prevention programs. *Am Heart J* 1996;132(2):418-427.

PART IV

# Integrating New Technologies In Cardiopulmonary Rehabilitation

# Chapter 10

# Cardiac Pacemakers
# and Exercise Rehabilitation

Dawn M. Hamilton, MSc, Mike King, MA, Catherine T. Sharp, MPAS, Robert G. Haennel, PhD, Canada

## Introduction

Cardiac pacing is a rapidly growing and ever changing field. Recent advances in the field have resulted in wider use of permanent pacemakers capable of a pacing rate that responds to various metabolic and physical stimuli (1). While rate-responsive pacemakers approximate the heart's normal response to exercise, no pacemaker has yet been able to perfectly mimic normal heart function. The many different types of pacemakers currently in use and the rising rate of pacemaker implantation (2) underscores the need for the health professional to understand pacing technology and the impact it has on the principles of exercise testing and prescription. Therefore, this paper provides an overview of the various types of pacemakers and examines their influence on the patients' exercise responses in an effort to provide practitioners with guidelines for exercise testing and prescription for pacemaker dependent patients.

## Basic Science

### Pacemaker Design

A pacemaker consists of a pulse generator, a long life battery (typically lithium iodide) and electrical microcircuitry for timing, sensing, and pacing functions. These components are encased in a titanium or stainless steel "can" which is implanted in a subcutaneous pocket in the chest or abdominal wall. A coated lead wire connected to the can is threaded through a vein (typically the subclavian vein) and into the right atrium via the superior vena cava. The

tip of the lead may be implanted in the atrium, it may pass through the tricuspid valve to be implanted in the right ventricle, or leads may be implanted in both right atrium and right ventricle. Some newer pacemakers have a single lead that is implanted in the ventricle with an extra electrode on the portion of the lead that passes through the atrium (known as a single-pass or floating lead). (figure 10.1) The lead wire acts as an interface between the heart and the pacemaker, with one or two electrodes at the tip that deliver the electrical impulse and sense intrinsic myocardial electrical activity. Typically, a pacemaker is indicated for patients with sinoatrial disease and/or complete heart block, but pacemakers have also been successful in treating second-degree (Mobitz Type II) heart block and congestive heart failure (1,3). As indicated by the pacemaker code (table 10.1), pacemakers may have several functions, and may be single or dual chamber devices.

### Single Chamber Pacemakers

A VVI (see pacemaker codes in table 10.1) pacemaker paces and senses in the ventricle, and inhibits pacing when intrinsic cardiac activity is sensed. An AAI pacemaker paces and senses the atrium, and inhibits pacing when intrinsic activity is sensed. Both systems pace at a fixed rate, firing if the patient's intrinsic rate falls below the lower rate limit and inhibiting pacing if the patient's intrinsic rate is faster than the set rate. Since VVI pacemakers do not sense activity in the atrium, atrial contraction can occur anywhere in the cardiac cycle with no relation to ventricular pacing. This is a major limitation of VVI pacing, with ensuing loss of AV (atrioventricular) synchrony, absence of atrial

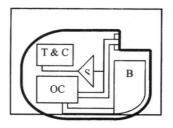

Pacemaker body:

T&C = timing and control; B = battery; S = sensor function which alters timing of stimulation depending on feedback from lead wires; OC = output circuit controlling amplitude and duration of electrical stimulation.

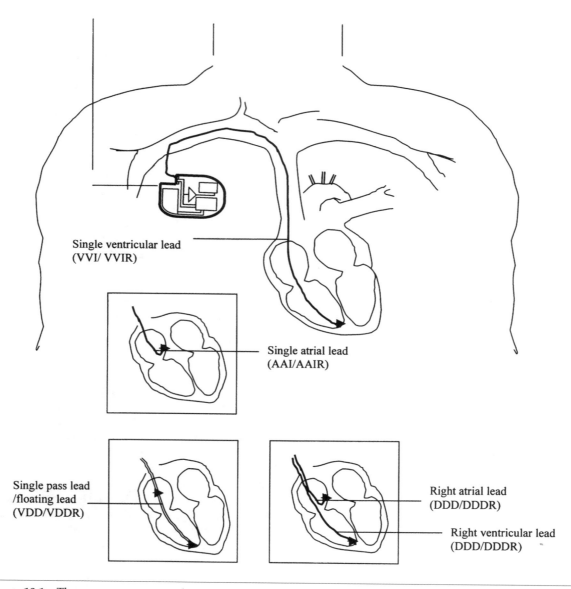

Single ventricular lead (VVI/ VVIR)

Single atrial lead (AAI/AAIR)

Single pass lead /floating lead (VDD/VDDR)

Right atrial lead (DDD/DDDR)

Right ventricular lead (DDD/DDDR)

**Figure 10.1**  The permanent pacemaker. A permanent pacemaker consists of a pacemaker body or can, connected to the myocardium by one or more leads.

**Table 10.1 NASPE/BPEG Pacemaker Code\***

| First letter | Second letter | Third letter | Fourth letter | Fifth letter |
|---|---|---|---|---|
| Chamber(s) paced | Chamber(s) sensed | Response to sensing | Programmability/ rate modulation | Antitachycardia features |
| A = Atrium | A = Atrium | I = Inhibited | P = Programmable | P = Pacing |
| V = Ventricle | V = Ventricle | T = Triggered | M = Multi-programmable | S = Shock |
| D = Dual (A & V) | D = Dual (A & V) | D = Dual (I & T) | C = Communicating | D = Dual (P & S) |
| 0 = none | 0 = none | 0 = none | R = Rate responsive | 0 = none |
|  |  |  | 0 = none |  |

\* This five-letter code to describe pacemaker function was developed in 1987 by the North American Society for Pacing and Electrophysiology and the British Pacing and Electrophysiology Group.

contribution to end-diastolic volume, and intermittent valvular regurgitation (3). The resultant decrease in stroke volume, cardiac output ($Q_c$), and blood pressure may cause the patient to experience some of the clinical signs of pacemaker syndrome: fatigue, dyspnea, lightheadedness, syncope, and impaired exercise capacity (4,5). Because of this, VVI pacemakers are rarely used for patients who have a properly functioning sinus node. However, the VVI mode is useful for patients with intermittent conduction blocks, and for those with chronic atrial fibrillation(6), with or without AV node ablation. The AAI pacemakers have been found to result in a better quality of life when compared to VVI in patients who have sinus node dysfunction (i.e., sick sinus syndrome) but intact AV conduction. This is because the AAI mode preserves both AV synchrony and an intrinsic rate response to exercise (7).

## Rate Responsiveness

If the pacemaker is equipped with a rate-adaptive feature, the pacemaker code will have an R in the fourth position. Although rate-responsive pacemakers are normally also programmable, the letter R takes precedence over the hierarchy of programmability indicators (1). The rate responsive feature was designed to help patients with chronotropic incompetence (the inability of the HR [heart rate] to keep pace with increasing metabolic demands during activity). Although there is no universally established definition of chronotropic incompetence, most investigators use the definition traditionally applied to patients with ischemic heart disease (i.e.,

HRmax < 2 standard deviations of age-predicted maximum), with a HRmax < 100 beats/min representing "severe" chronotropic incompetence (8). Rate modulated pacing has been shown to produce greater $Q_c$ (approx. 20%) than VVI pacing in patients with complete AV block (9). Rate adaptive sensors have also been reported to improve exercise duration,10 $\dot{V}O_2$max (10-12), anaerobic threshold (10-12) peak heart rate (HR) (10,11,13) and quality of life (14). The rate responsive feature may be used in both single and dual chamber pacemakers, controlled by various types of sensors that respond to physiological, mechanical, or electrical signals so that the pacing rate is adjusted in a "physiologic" manner (5). For safety, these pacemakers have a programmed maximum sensor rate to prevent inappropriately fast pacing rates. While rate responsiveness is an improvement over fixed-rate pacemakers, VVIR pacemakers still have the drawback of not maintaining AV synchrony.

## Dual Chamber Pacemakers

Dual chamber pacemakers (DDD and DDDR) have lead wires in both the atrium and ventricle, giving them the capacity to sense and pace both chambers (15). The response to sensing is dual, in that they can inhibit pacing when intrinsic activity is sensed, or trigger when either the atria or the ventricles do not respond on their own. These devices are also multi-programmable in that they can be used in atrial only, ventricular only, or dual chamber modes. The DDD pacemaker has a programmed low rate, high rate, and AV interval. If the intrinsic atrial rate falls below the lower threshold, the atrial pacemaker takes over. If the intrinsic atrial rate is above the lower threshold, the atrial pacemaker is inhibited and the pacemaker starts a countdown of the programmed AV interval. If the ventricle responds before the AV interval expires, the ventricular pacemaker is inhibited. However, if the AV interval expires without an intrinsic ventricular response, the pacemaker triggers an impulse in the ventricle (6). The main advantages of dual chamber pacemakers are that they maintain AV synchrony and more closely mimic the normal cardiac cycle. The addition of a rate-responsive feature (DDDR) overcomes chronotropic incompetence, and produces a significantly greater exercise duration (16-18), $Q_c$ at rest (16) and during exercise (17), as well as a decreased severity of tricuspid and mitral regurgitation versus VVIR pacing (4).

Dual chamber pacing is not indicated for all patients. Patients with a history of chronic atrial fibrillation do not require a lead to be placed in the atrium. For these patients, a single lead in the ventricle that provides a regular ventricular rate and does not respond to the chaotic electrical events of the atria is preferred. However, patients with paroxysmal atrial tachyarrhythmias can benefit from DDD pacing. These patients should be implanted with a pacemaker that has a mode switching feature to prevent occasional tracking of rapid atrial rates to the ventricle. Automatic mode switching is a feature that allows the pacemaker to shift from DDD to a non-atrial tracking mode (VVI) whenever the patient's atrial rate exceeds a pre-programmed level. Patients with existing sinoatrial disease are more susceptible to the development of atrial flutter and/or fibrillation. While deterioration of sinoatrial function associated with age is slow, the use of beta blockers and some antiarrythmic medications may further depress sinoatrial function and increase the chance of developing atrial tachyarrhythmias (19). For these patients, VVI or VVIR pacing is preferable. Other patients with sinus node brady-dysrhythmias and normal intrinsic conduction have been found to have better cardiac hemodynamics with AAIR pacing as compared to DDDR pacing (20). However, because of the concern that patients may subsequently develop AV block, these pacemakers are under utilized. In addition, if the patient has a dual chamber pacemaker, a simple programming change is all that is required for the pacemaker to pace in the DDDR mode instead of the AAIR mode if a patient's intrinsic conduction deteriorates.

## Sensors Used for Rate Modulation

Rickards and Donaldson (22) suggested that sensors used for rate adaptive pacing could be classified according to their ability to mimic the normal sinus node (i.e., physiologic) verses those sensors which are simply a surrogate for metabolic demand (i.e., non-physiologic).

## Physiologic Sensors

These sensors detect internal changes that occur as a consequence of exercise. These types of sensors include pH, $O_2$ saturation, ventricular volume changes, myocardial contractility, endocardial acceleration, minute ventilation and QT. Many of these sensors failed in mass production because of the need for a specialized lead interface. Others such as the myocardial contractility sensor (Biotronik) and the endocardial acceleration sensor (SORIN) are still being tested. Presently, the QT and minute ventilation sensors are those most commonly in use.

### The QT Sensor

It has long been known that the QT interval varies as a function of HR. Early investigators (23,24) reported that increases in HR contributed up to 75% of the QT shortening during exercise, while sympathetic activity (in particular circulating catecholamines) was responsible for the remainder of the shortening. Thus, the QT sensor detects QT shortening, corrects for the effect of rate, and adjusts the pacing rate according to sympathetic stimulation (23,25). The QT sensor produces a workload-appropriate rate response (26), but the response time is slower than that of other types of sensors. However, this gradual increase in rate allows for longer diastolic filling times. Thus, the relative contributions of stroke volume and HR to increased $Q_c$ with exercise are more similar to the healthy heart than with other sensors (27). The QT sensor also has a more physiologic response to stress and other emotional changes, sensing the QT changes caused by the increase in circulating catecholamine during stress (25).

Inappropriate rate changes that plague the QT sensor can be the result of plasma levels of electrolytes, minerals and drugs that alter the QT length. Hypercalcemia shortens the QT length and hypocalcemia prolongs the QT, which may cause inappropriately fast or slow heart rate responses (28). The use of diuretics may prolong the QT interval, thus blunting the heart rate responses (29). Beta blockers may decrease QT interval (30), thus any dose changes may effect the heart rate response. Procainamide, Quinidine and other antiarrhythmic agents may also lengthen the QT interval and blunt heart rate responses (30).

It is also important to note that most QT sensors employ a unipolar pacing spike in the right ventricle to initiate the QT measurement. Therefore, clinicians must be aware of the hazards of myopotential oversensing in pacemaker dependent patients who begin to use large muscles in the upper torso. Myopotential oversensing of electrical activity that is non-heart related can lead to failure to deliver an impulse, and possible ventricular standstill during vigorous exercise.

To address the problem of the slow rate response, newer QT sensors utilize algorithms with curvilinear rate response curves to decrease the lag time in rate response at the onset of exercise. Although significantly improved, the speed of rate response is still comparatively slow and remains one of the main limitations of the QT sensor (25).

### The Minute Ventilation Sensor

The minute ventilation sensor is based on the normal linear relationship between workload, HR, ventilation, and $\dot{V}O_2$ below the anaerobic threshold (31). Minute ventilation is estimated continuously through measurements of the frequency and amplitude of transthoracic impedance. Transthoracic impedance is measured by passing a low level current between the pacing lead and the pulse generator, where inflation and deflation of the lungs produces a change in bioelectrical resistance. Minute ventilation appears to provide a reasonable rate response over the entire range from rest to peak exercise (31-33), and correlates well with $\dot{V}O_2$, respiratory quotient, tidal volume and respiratory rate (32,34,36).

While the demonstrated HR–respiratory rate correlation is significant (33), respiratory rate is not ideal in predicting HR. Indeed, the respiratory rate dependent pacemakers have a maximum sensitivity in the medium to high workload range and do not appear to respond appropriately to non-exercise related stresses (37,38). Minute ventilation has a medium speed of rate response. Although neural activity results in an almost instantaneous change in respiration at the onset of exercise, the average algorithm used by the pacemaker to calculate minute ventilation changes has led to a delay of approximately 30 - 45 seconds before a rate response can be observed (34,38,39). Further, respiratory rate tends to remain high during the recovery from exercise, resulting in an inappropriately high pacing rate for 1–2 minutes after exercise is stopped (40). Minute ventilation sensing can be affected by such disorders as heart failure, pulmonary disease (28,41), pleural or pericardial effusions, and cardiomyopathy (42). Also, shallow breathing patterns often seen in elderly individuals, coughing, continuous talking during exercise (28), and obesity (41) may effect ventilation and thus the HR responses.

### Non-Physiologic Sensors

These sensors detect changes in body movement. While body motion is a crude surrogate of metabolic demand, the rapid onset of the rate response and the relative simplicity of implementation (no need for a special lead interface), have resulted in motion sensors being widely used. Two common motion sensors are the activity sensor and the accelerometer.

### The Activity Sensor

The activity sensor has a piezoelectric crystal attached to the inside of the pacemaker casing facing the pectoral muscle. Body movement causes pressure or vibrations on the casing and subsequent deformation of the crystal. This deformation of the crystal is then translated into an electrical signal that is processed by the rate response algorithm, which in turn, produces the appropriate rate response (43). A drawback of the activity sensor is its susceptibility to extraneous vibrations, such as those produced by riding in a car (43-45). In addition, activity sensors often result in an excessive HR response to tempo changes, staircase decent, and upper arm activity (45-47). The rapid and large initial HR response to exercise has been found to minimize diastolic filling time at a given workload, thus compromising the expected increase in stroke volume during submaximal exercise (27). Further, the activity sensor may under-respond to activities in which there is minimal thoracic movement such as smooth calisthenics movements, treadmill gradient change, and cycle ergometer exercise (39,48,49). The piezoelectric crystal may also lack specificity because it only detects vibrations greater than 10 Hz when in fact most body movements associated with activities of daily living occur in the frequency of 1 to 4 Hz (17). Despite these drawbacks, the activity sensor offers the best approximation to sinus rhythm in the speed of onset of rate response (44), and is preferred for exercise that is light and/or of short duration because of its rapid rate acceleration (45).

### The Accelerometer

This sensor differs from the activity sensor in that the crystal is attached to a circuit board suspended inside the pacemaker, and movement is sensed in the anterior-posterior plane (50). Horizontal acceleration due to rhythmic movement (i.e., walking) is averaged over time, and the pacing rate is set using various algorithms to produce a pacing rate proportional to the activity (51). The design of the accelerometer is presumed to yield better proportionality in rate response as it detects movement in the low frequency range more common to activities of daily living (43). Other advantages of accelerometers are their ability to differentiate workload levels produced by variations in slope, thus providing a rate response to exercise closer to the sinus rate (52-56) and more proportional to increases in metabolic demand than activity sensors (52,55,57). The HR responses to stair climbing and descent are also more appropriate with an accelerometer, producing a greater HR increase during ascent than descent (53,54,58). Lau (43) suggests, however, that both activity sensors and accelerometers underestimate the normal sinus response during stair climbing and cycle ergometry.

### Dual Sensors

The idea of combining sensors to optimize the rate response over the entire physiological range was first introduced by Stangl et al. (59) who suggested that no single parameter could be used to produce an appropriate rate response at both low and high exercise intensities. Typically these dual sensor devices combine the rapid response of an activity sensor with a slower, more physiologic sensor, such as QT or minute ventilation (28). Input from each sensor is cross-checked with the other to confirm the need for a rate response, thus avoiding inappropriate rate increases that plague individual sensors (e.g., environmental vibrations or drug-induced QT shortening) (60). The contribution of each sensor to the overall rate response can also be programmed. For example, the Topaz™ (Vitatron Medical B.V., Netherlands), a dual sensor pacemaker that combines the QT and activity sensors, may be programmed to respond to input from either of the two individual sensors or a blended input. The resulting signal is a proportion of the activity sensor signal (0, 25%, 50%, 75%, 100%), and an inverse proportion of the QT sensor signal (100%, 75%, 50%, 25%, 0), thus allowing for five different sensor combinations (45).

The multiple programming options of dual sensor devices were designed to enhance the overall rate response from rest though to peak exertion. Dual sensor pacemakers have been found to improve the speed and proportionality of the rate response compared to single sensor devices (44,61), deliver more appropriate pacing rates for ascending and descending stairs (46), and simulate the physiologic increase in stroke volume and $Q_c$ in response to the onset of exercise (27,61).

## Clinical Applications

### Exercise Testing

Prior to a pacemaker-dependent patient starting a cardiac rehabilitation program or being given a recommendation for home exercise, an exercise test should be performed to evaluate pacemaker function, establish the patient's physiological response to exercise, and to monitor for signs and symptoms of exertional intolerance. Before selecting the test protocol and modality it is important to know the type of pacemaker, mode, type of sensor(s), and programmable features of the device. For example, individuals with VVI pacemakers may have little or no chronotropic reserve. Relative to healthy individuals, these patients also have altered cardiac hemodynamics. VVI pacing results in a higher heart rate (HR) and lower stroke volume at rest, and lower peak oxygen uptake ($\dot{V}O_2$max) and Qc during exercise (62). These patients should have an extended warm-up to avoid dyspnea and premature fatigue, and may have a markedly reduced functional capacity compared to those with rate responsiveness and AV synchrony (3). With rate adaptive devices, the type of sensor(s) should be considered. For example, activity sensors often respond sluggishly to kinesiologically smooth activities such as changes in workloads during cycle ergometry work (63), or grade changes in treadmill protocols (39,64). The patient may be carrying the manufacturer's information card indicating the type and mode of their pacemaker. If not, this information should be obtained from the pacemaker clinic prior to the test.

Most pacemaker recipients exercise in the 3 to 5 METs range, which is missed by most traditional exercise testing protocols (8). Because of this, several researchers have suggested the use of a low level exercise protocol with very small metabolic increases to evaluate pacemaker patients (65,66). This is especially important if the implanted device does not have rate modulation, or if AV synchrony is compromised (i.e., with VVI/VVIR pacing modes). Treadmill protocols such as the modified Bruce or Balke type protocols have been recommended in the past (3), but there are disadvantages to each. The initial stages of the modified Bruce and the entire Balke-Ware protocol depend on grade changes only, so these protocols are not appropriate for patients with activity sensors. The chronotropic assessment exercise protocol (CAEP) (66), which is employed by many pacemaker clinics, utilizes both grade and speed in small load increments to assess performance and the patient's overall chronotropic response. These features have made the CAEP the most appropriate and widely accepted testing protocol for pacemaker recipients (table 10.2).

The CAEP protocol, similar to the Bruce, results in a significant linear relationship between HR reserve (HRR) and metabolic reserve ($\dot{V}O_2R$) throughout the exercise, with a slope close to 1 and a y-intercept close to zero. Despite differences in functional ability and age, the percent HRR and percent $\dot{V}O_2R$ should be almost identical at each stage of the exercise (8). A diagnosis of chronotropic incompetence is made when the %HRR is significantly less than % $\dot{V}O_2R$ during exercise.

$$\%HR \text{ Reserve} = [(HR_{stage} - HR_{rest}) / (HR_{max} - HR_{rest})] \times 100$$

$$\%\dot{V}O_2 \text{ Reserve} = [(METS_{stage} - METS_{rest}) / (METS_{max} - METS_{rest})] \times 100$$

Prior to the graded exercise test, baseline measures should include HR, blood pressure, and if available, $\dot{V}O_2$. Continuous ECG monitoring is recommended, with HR, blood pressure (BP), $\dot{V}O_2$, and rating of perceived exertion (RPE) recorded at the end of every stage. For paced patients with coronary artery disease, the pacemaker should be programmed so that the upper rate limit is at least 10 bpm below the patient's ischemic threshold (3). For patients with concurrent significant left ventricular dysfunction, careful assessment of the physiological responses at the upper rate limit is needed to ensure that systolic blood pressure is maintained at a safe level. During the exercise test the normal indications for terminating exercise

**Table 10.2  The Chronotropic Assessment Exercise Protocol (CAEP)**

| Stage | Speed (MPH) | Grade (%) | Time (min) | Cumulative time | METs |
|---|---|---|---|---|---|
| Warm-up (0) | 1.0 | 0 | — | — | 1.5 |
| 1 | 1.0 | 2 | 2 | 2 | 2.0 |
| 2 | 1.5 | 3 | 2 | 4 | 2.8 |
| 3 | 2.0 | 4 | 2 | 6 | 3.6 |
| 4 | 2.5 | 5 | 2 | 8 | 4.6 |
| 5 | 3 | 6 | 2 | 10 | 5.8 |
| 6 | 3.5 | 8 | 2 | 12 | 7.5 |
| 7 | 4 | 10 | 2 | 14 | 9.6 |
| 8 | 5.0 | 10 | 2 | 16 | 12.1 |
| 9 | 6.0 | 10 | 2 | 18 | 14.3 |
| 10 | 7.0 | 10 | 2 | 20 | 16.5 |
| 11 | 7.0 | 15 | 2 | 22 | 19.0 |

testing apply (3), with some additional considerations.

In the pacemaker dependent patient, the left bundle branch block pacing artifact often obscures ECG evidence of ischemia. If the patient has symptoms of angina, a diagnosis of ischemia is best determined by stress echocardiography or myocardial perfusion imaging techniques, such as sestamibi or thallium scanning (3). Often, even though patients may be paced at rest, the myocardium may respond to exercise producing an intrinsic rhythm which overrides the pacemaker. If a series of intrinsic beats are seen, normal ECG interpretations apply.

At the upper rate limit, patients with dual chamber pacemakers tracking intrinsic atrial rhythms may show 2:1 block or pacemaker psuedo-Wenckebach patterns (22). This is caused by atrial sinus beats falling in the total atrial refractory period set by the pacemaker. The total atrial refractory period is a programmed feature of the dual chamber pacemaker, which prevents ventricular tracking of rapid atrial rates which can occur in atrial fibrillation or atrial tachycardia (22). This response is a complex program feature; however, it is critical to understand when this feature is functioning correctly. For example, if a patient's exercising HR exceeds the upper rate limit, the pacemaker should demonstrate a psuedo-Wenckebach pattern (i.e., 5 out 6 beats conducted), complete with a prolonged atrioventricular delay when the atrial rates are at or near the upper rate limit. This pattern maintains a higher HR without risking rapid ventricular responses. If the patient shows a 2:1 block at or near the upper rate limit, the pacemaker may not be programmed optimally for a patient who participates in an exercise program. The 2:1 response pattern of pacemaker blocking can lead to rapid rate drop and may cause dizziness, fainting and marked feelings of distress especially when the rise in HR has occurred as an appropriate response to exercise (22), Patients demonstrating either a 2:1 block pattern, or a pseudo-Wenckebach pattern at low levels of exertion, in the absence of atrial fibrillation and atrial tachycardias, should be referred to their pacemaker clinic to determine if a higher upper rate limit should be programmed.

Two simple field tests, the six-minute walk test and the shuttle walk, have been recommended for pacemaker dependant patients as simple tests of functional ability (67,68). Although these authors claim that these walking tests give enough information to program pacemakers, others have said that the six-minute walk is inadequate for pacemaker patients (69). We recommend a graded exercise test such as the CAEP treadmill protocol for

evaluating pacemaker function and exercise prescription. The walking tests may however, be useful as pre-post measures to document functional improvements for those exercise centers that do not have access to conventional graded exercise testing.

## Exercise Prescription

The health benefits of regular physical activity are numerous, and may have an even greater effect on those who are sedentary or have a chronic disease than on the healthy population. Therefore, it is essential that the health professional encourage pacemaker patients to engage in regular, moderate physical activity (3). Even chronotropically incompetent patients (i.e., with a VVI pacemaker) can increase cardiovascular function and $\dot{V}O_2max$ (70) through peripheral adaptations such as increased capillary and mitochondria density in skeletal muscle (3). However, these functional increases tend to be smaller than those seen in patients with rate responsive devices (71). In addition, exercise training can help reduce coronary artery risk factors (e.g., cholesterol modification and hypertension reduction). Other significant benefits of exercise are: decreased anxiety and depression, enhanced feelings of well-being and improved performance of work and other daily activities (3).

For pacemaker dependent patients, the principles of exercise prescription are identical to those used for post myocardial infarction patients, with some extra considerations. The data from the graded exercise test should be reviewed first, with the maximum workload achieved (METs), ECG responses, and symptoms taken into consideration when developing the prescription. As always, a warm-up and cool-down period of 5 to 15 minutes of aerobic activity at a low intensity level is recommended. In general, activities should be selected so that the intensity can be closely monitored during exercise (5). Initial ECG telemetry monitoring may be useful to ensure proper functioning of the pacemaker and to evaluate and make adjustments if necessary to the exercise prescription. Full knowledge of the pacemaker's function and programming is essential. Because there is some danger of dislodging newly implanted leads, upper body exercises should be avoided for the initial 4 to 6 weeks following implantation. After that, routine activities involving the upper extremities are permitted. Muscular strength and endurance exercises involving the upper extremities should be performed with slow and controlled movements, at a low to moderate intensity, 2 to 3 days per week. Vigorous upper body activities or contact sports are not advised (3).

The intensity of aerobic exercise is typically prescribed at 65 to 90% of $HR_{max}$, or 50 to 85% of $\dot{V}O_2$reserve or HR reserve (where training HR = $(HR_{max} - HR_{rest}) (50-85\%) + HR_{rest}$). For individuals with very low levels of fitness the exercise intensity may be set lower, between 40-50% $\dot{V}O_2$reserve or HR reserve (3). The %HRmax and %HR reserve methods are commonly used to identify a training intensity for cardiac patients. Both HR methods assume chronotropic competence, where the percent HR and metabolic reserves are numerically similar at each stage in an exercise test (66). When prescribing an exercise intensity for paced patients however, one cannot assume that they are chronotropically competent. Therefore, it is recommended that the prescribed exercise intensity be based on the %$\dot{V}O_2$ reserve, with the assigned training HR range reflecting the desired metabolic load (as measured at each stage during the exercise test). The RPE is a useful adjunct to the exercise prescription, and should generally be kept between 11 (fairly light) and 15 (hard) on the original Borg scale (3). Alternately, if the graded exercise test incorporated indirect calorimetry, setting the maximum exercise intensity at a HR 10 beats/minute below the anaerobic threshold has also been shown to yield improvements in functional ability in patients with rate responsive devices (72). Given that the majority of pacemaker recipients are elderly and perhaps unaccustomed to exercise, it may be appropriate to keep the initial exercise sessions short (i.e., 15 minutes or less). Where necessary, interval activity may be used, but the duration of the intervals must be long enough to allow for the delayed response of some sensor-driven pacemakers (i.e., QT sensor or minute ventilation sensor). A target of 20 to 40 minutes per aerobic training session, 3 to 5 times per week may be used as training objective.

For the patient with a non rate-responsive device (i.e., VVI pacemakers) there may be little or no rise in HR with exercise. For these patients, it has been suggested that the blood pressure response to exercise can be used to prescribe intensity by modifying the standard HR reserve equation to systolic blood pressure (SBP), where the training SBP = $(SBP_{max}-SBP_{rest}) \times (50–80\%) + SBP_{rest}$ (70). The resting blood pressure should be the lower of either the readings noted in a recent physical examination or the readings taken just before the exercise test. Typically, both HR and blood pressure are higher prior to an exercise test because of the stress associated with anticipation of the test (8). Excessively high

values will not provide an ample range for exercise training. If the CAEP protocol is used, MET levels achieved at the prescribed blood pressure range are easily determined, and appropriate activities can then be identified from MET tables. Chronotropically incompetent patients need to have systolic pressure monitored throughout exercise to ensure a safe intensity level is maintained. Such patients also require a longer warm-up period, and should work at half the prescribed intensity for the first 5 to 10 minutes to avoid dyspnea or premature fatigue (3,70). The patient's perceived exertion may also be considered as a subjective measure of intensity with a target range that reflects the desired metabolic load. If an initial exercise test has not been performed, an RPE of 11-15 on the original Borg scale may be used (3). A gradual cool-down involving repetitive action of large muscle groups is recommended to prevent post-exercise syncope. Finally, it should be remembered that VVI paced patients may have greatly reduced exercise capacity when compared to those with rate modulation and AV synchrony.

It is prudent to be reminded of the characteristic responses of each different type of sensors when designing an exercise program for patients with rate adaptive pacemakers. Motion sensors, especially the activity sensors, do not respond well to cycling or to grade changes on a treadmill. For patients with activity sensors, exercise on the treadmill should use speed changes more than gradient changes, and if cycling is desired, a combined arm - leg ergometer may yield a more appropriate HR response (73). Accelerometers respond better to treadmill slope changes, cycle ergometry, and staircase climbing than do activity sensors, however it would still be wise to follow the above recommendations for all motion-type sensors.

The QT sensors have a slow initial rate response to activity, so a long, low-intensity warm-up is even more important than usual. Activities such as stair climbing, weight lifting, or any activity that involves rapid changes in acceleration may be inappropriate because of the paradoxical increase in HR that may occur after the completion of exercise (47,74). Vigorous muscle activity of the upper torso should be avoided by those with QT sensors because of the possibility of myopotential oversensing, which could, in extreme instances, lead to ventricular standstill.

For the patient with a minute ventilation sensor, a prolonged warm-up remains important due to the delayed response often associated with this sensor (35,75). It is also important to remind the patient to avoid shallow breathing and continuous talking during exercise so that the pacemaker can respond appropriately (28).

## Monitoring Exercise

Although monitoring of pacemaker function is the role of pacemaker clinics, the ability to regularly monitor paced patients during exercise sessions may assist in identifying problems not seen in periodic clinic visits. For the pacemaker patient, participation in a cardiac rehabilitation program is ideal because of the individual supervision and monitoring available in such a program.

When monitoring these patients, one should be aware that a patient's ECG will vary depending on the pacing system. Atrial pacing will produce a pacemaker spike before the P wave and should be followed by a normal QRS complex. The P waves may appear inverted or irregular and the PR interval may vary, depending on the location of the atrial lead placement. When atrial pacing is used, periodic ECG strips or telemetry recordings should be used to ensure that the patient continues to have normal AV conduction.

In single-chamber ventricular pacing systems, AV conduction is not maintained; therefore, there is no relationship between atrial and ventricular depolarization. Traditional ventricular pacing artifact produces a wide left bundle branch pattern as the impulse originates in the right ventricular apex and does not depolarize the ventricles along the normal electrical pathways. Chronic atrial fibrillation is a common reason for implantation of a ventricular device; however, development of atrial fibrillation post implantation is also common. In the absence of AV synchrony, the atrium may become irritated and enlarged by coincidental atrial and ventricular contractions. The loss of the atrial contribution to ventricular filling and the reduced $Q_c$ may produce the symptoms of pacemaker syndrome in some patients (5). These symptoms can be subtle and often quite nonspecific, and may include lethargy, fatigue, hypotension, dyspnea, syncope, depression, and impaired functional capacity. These signs and symptoms may also signal sub optimal pacemaker function. Patients exhibiting these symptoms should be referred to their pacemaker clinic for evaluation.

Periodic ECG or telemetry readings should also be performed on ventricularly paced patients to ensure that retrograde ventriculo-atrial conduction does not occur. Retrograde conduction could result in overdrive suppression of the sinus node and force the heart to pace at the lower rate setting of the device. This may lead to symptomatic bradycardia, as the sinus node is continually bombarded by a retrograde depolarization wave front, and is not able to spontaneously depolarize and coordinate the heart rhythm. Although it is the place of the pacemaker clinic or cardiologist to resolve this type of problem, the exercise professional should be aware of this possibility when the patient is constantly paced at the lower rate limit. A quick check of the ECG can reveal retrograde conduction, and the patient should then be referred back to the pacemaker clinic.

In monitoring patients with dual chamber pacing systems, the ECG will differ depending on the pacing need. If both the atrium and the ventricle are electrically silent, a pacemaker spike will appear before both complexes. If the atrium is viable, dual chamber sensing and pacing can be differentiated from ventricular pacing because a uniform relationship between the P wave and QRS complex will be maintained. Complications specific to dual chamber pacing are tracking of supraventricular tachycardias and re-entry phenomenon. Periodic or "paroxysmal" atrial fibrillation or chronic atrial fibrillation that may develop post-implantation will be sensed in the atrium and may produce an inappropriately fast ventricular rhythm. Fortunately, new mode switching devices prevent this response. The conversion to sinus rhythm and restoration of dual chamber pacing is beneficial to the patient's exercise tolerance and general well being. Retrograde ventriculo-atrial conduction in dual chamber pacing can produce pacemaker mediated tachycardia, an endless loop arrhythmia (76), whereby a slow retrograde conduction falls outside the post ventricular atrial refractory period, thus stimulating the atrium. This produces an inverted P wave on a standard strip (76), which is sensed, and conducted to the ventricle, causing a rapid ventricular rate. If pacemaker mediated tachycardia is suspected, the episode should be documented with an ECG strip, and the pacemaker clinic notified immediately.

Patients with QT sensors need to be monitored very closely because of the many things that can affect this sensor. Patients should be cautioned to report any changes in medication or missed medications due to the effect that some medications have on the QT length, which may result in inappropriately high or low responses during exercise (30). It is also prudent to remember that the QT sensor is affected by emotional factors. If the patient experiences angina and becomes frightened or anxious, the increased catecholamine levels could, in turn, trigger an increased heart rate and ultimately exacerbate the angina. The potential complications from such a positive feedback loop underscores the need for those involved in exercise prescription and monitoring to be aware of the nature of the sensor(s) used in rate modulated pacing (73).

## Summary

A basic understanding of the functioning of the various types of pacemakers is essential in order to safely prescribe activity for the pacemaker-dependent patient. Atrial, ventricular and dual chamber devices can produce varying exercise responses that must be considered when formulating the exercise prescription. The type of rate adaptive sensor(s) used also affects the nature of the heart rate response, and therefore, must also be considered. Although the value of exercise testing for ECG evidence of ischemia may be limited in paced patients, it is useful in determining exercise capacity and pacemaker function, and essential in formulating an exercise prescription. All pacemaker patients, even those who are chronotropically incompetent, will benefit from regular exercise and should be encouraged to be active within prescribed limits. Regular monitoring by knowledgeable professionals can help identify problems in pacemaker function and insure a safe exercise experience. Participation in a supervised exercise training program can greatly enhance the follow-up and management of paced patients as well as to afford them the opportunity to experience the physical and psychological benefits typically associated with exercise rehabilitation.

## References

1. Lau CP: Context of rate of adaptive pacing in the history of cardiac pacing. In: Lau CP ed. Rate Adaptive Cardiac Pacing: Single and Dual Chamber. New York: Futura Publishing Co. Inc, 1993:1-5.
2. Goldman BS, Nishimura S, Lau C: Survey of cardiac pacing in Canada (1993). *Can J Cardiol* 1996; 6:573-578.
3. American College of Sports Medicine: ACSM's Guidelines for Exercise Testing and Prescription, 6th ed. Philadelphia: Lipppincott Williams & Wilkins, 2000.
4. Lau CP: Hemodynamic basis of rate adaptive pacing: Rate modulation versus AV synchrony. In: Lau CP, ed. Rate Adaptive Cardiac Pacing: Single and Dual Chamber. New York: Futura, 1993:31-46.
5. West M, Johnson T, Roberts SO: Pacemakers and implantable cardioverter defibrillators. In: Durnstine JL, ed. ACSM's Exercise Management for Persons with Chronic Diseases and Disabilities. Champaign, IL: Human Kinetics, 1997:37-41.
6. Shaffer RB: Keeping pace with permanent pacemakers. *Dimensions of Critical Care Nursing* 1999; 18:2-8.
7. Lau CP, Tai YT, Leung WH, Wong CK, Lee P, Chung FL: Rate adaptive pacing in sick sinus syndrome: effects of pacing modes and intrinsic conduction on physiological responses, arrhythmias, symptomatology and quality of life. *European Heart Journal* 1994; 15:1445-55.
8. Lau CP: Normal exercise cardiopulmonary physiology and chronotropic incompetence. In: Lau CP, ed. Rate Adaptive Cardiac Pacing: Single and Dual Chamber. New York: Futura, 1993:7-23.
9. Lau CP, Wong CK, Leung WH, Liu WX: Superior cardiac hemodynamics of atrioventricular synchrony over rate responsive pacing at submaximal exercise: Observations in activity sensing DDDR pacemakers. *PACE* 1990; 13:1832-1837.
10. Benditt DG, Mianulli M, Fetter J, et al: Single-chamber cardiac pacing with activity-initiated chronotropic response: Evaluation by cardiopulmonary exercise testing. Circulation 1987; 75:184-191.
11. Humen DP, Kostuk WJ, Klein GJ: Activity-sensing, rate-responsive pacing: Improvement in myocardial performance with exercise. *PACE* 1985; 8:52-59.
12. Nishino M, Ito T, Miyawaki M, et al: Benefits of rate responsive pacing in patients with sick sinus syndrome. *Angiology* 1994; 45:353-360.
13. Hedman A, Hjemdahl P, Nordlander R, Astrom H: Effects of mental and physical stress on central haemodynamics and cardiac sympathetic nerve activity during QT interval-sensing rate responsive and fixed rate ventricular inhibited pacing. *European Heart Journal* 1990; 11:903-915.
14. Staniforth AD, Andrews R, Harrison M, Perry A, Cowley AJ: "Value" of improved treadmill

exercise capacity: lessons from a study of rate responsive pacing. *Heart* 1998;80:383-386.

15. Furman S, Gross J: Dual-chamber pacing and pacemakers. *Current Problems in Cardiology* 1990;121-179.

16. Sulke N, Chambers J, Dritsas A, Sowton E: A randomized double-blind crossover comparison of four rate responsive pacing modes. *JACC* 1991;17:696-706.

17. Jutzy RV, Florio J, Isaeff DM et al: Comparative evaluation of rate modulated dual chamber and VVIR pacing. *PACE* 1990;13:1838-1846.

18. Lemke B, Dryander SV, Jager D, Machraoui A, MacCarter D, Barmeyer J: Aerobic capacity in rate modulated pacing. *PACE* 1992;15:1914-1918.

19. Lau CP: Limitations of DDD pacing. In: Lau CP, ed. Rate Adaptive Cardiac Pacing: Single and Dual Chamber. New York: Futura, 1993:25-29.

20. Vardas PE, Simantirakis EN, Parthenakis FI, Chrysostomakis SI, Skalidis EI, Zuridakis EG: AAIR verses DDDR pacing in patients with impaired sinus node chronotropy: An echocardiographic and cardiopulmonary study. *PACE* 1997; 20: 1762-1768.

21. Lau CP: Atrial rate adaptive pacing for sinoatrial disease. In: Lau CP, ed. Rate Adaptive Cardiac Pacing: Single and Dual Chamber. New York: Futura, 1993:233-248.

22. Rickards AF, Donaldson RM: Rate-responsive pacing. *Clin Prog Pacing and Electrophysiol* 1983;1:12-19

23. Hedman A, Nordlander R, Pehrsson SK: Changes in QT and QaT intervals at rest and during exercise with different modes of cardiac pacing. *PACE* 1985; 8:825-831.

24. Fananapazir L, Bennett DH, Faragher EB: Contribution of heart rate to QT interval shortening during exercise. *Eur Heart J* 1983; 4:265-271.

25. Lau CP: Ventricular paced QT interval. In: Lau CP, ed. Rate Adaptive Cardiac Pacing: Single and Dual Chamber. New York: Futura, 1993:123-136.

26. Provenier F, Van Acker R, Backers J, Van WassenHove E, De Meyer V, Jordaens L: Clinical observations with a dual sensor rate adaptive single chamber pacemaker. *PACE* 1992; 15:1821-1825.

27. Haennel RG, Logan T, Dunne C, Burgess JJ, Busse EFG: Effects of sensor selection on exercise stroke volume in pacemaker dependent patients. *PACE* 1998; 21:1700-1708.

28. Katritsis D, Camm AJ: Adaptive rate pacemakers: Comparison of sensors and clinical experience. *Cardiology Clinics* 1992; 10:671-687.

29. Moses HW et al: A Practical Guide to Cardiac Pacing 4th ed. Boston: Little, Brown and Company, 1995:91.

30. Muus KP: AANA journal course: Update for nurse anesthetists - cardiac pacemakers. *AANA* 1993; 61:503-508.

31. Alt E, Heinz M, Hirgstetter C, Emslander HP, Daum S, Blomer H: Control of pacemaker rate by impedance-based respiratory minute ventilation. *Chest* 1987; 92:247-252.

32. Nappholtz T, Valenta H, Maloney J, et al: Electrode configurations for respiratory impedance measurement suitable for rate responsive pacing. *PACE* 1986; 9:960-964.

33. Rossi P, Plicchi G, Canducci G, et al: Respiratory rate as a determinant of optimal pacing rate. *PACE* 1983; 6:502-507.

34. Lau CP, Antoniou A, Ward DE, et al: Initial clinical experience with a minute ventilation sensing rate modulated pacemaker: Improvements in exercise capacity and symptomatology. *PACE* 1988; 11:1815-1822.

35. Kay GN, Bubien RS, Epstein AE, et al: Rate-modulated cardiac pacing based on transthoracic measurements of minute ventilation correlation with exercise gas exchange. *J Am Coll Cardiol* 1989; 14:1283-1289.

36. Lau CP, Ward DE, Camm AJ: Rate responsive pacing with a pacemaker that detects the respiratory rate: Clinical advantages and complications. *Clin Cardiol* 1988; 11:318-324.

37. Santomauro M, Fazio S, Ferraro S et al: Follow-up of a respiratory rate modulated pacemaker. *PACE* 1992; 5:17-21.

38. Mond H, Strathmore N, Kertes P et al: Rate responsive pacing using a minute ventilation sensor. *PACE* 1989; 12:3321-330.

39. Lau CP, Butrous GS, Ward DE, Camm AJ: Comparison of exercise performance of six rate-adaptive right ventricular cardiac pacemakers. *Am J Cardiol* 1989; 63:833-838.

40. Lau CP: Respiration. In: Lau CP, ed. Rate Adaptive Cardiac Pacing: Single and Dual Chamber. New York: Futura, 1993:101-121.

41. Rossi P: Rate-responsive pacing: Biosensor reliability and physiological sensitivity. *PACE* 1987; 10:454-466.

42. Camm AJ, Garratt C, Paul V: Single-chamber rate adaptive pacing. *J Electrophysiol* 1989; 3:181-189.

43. Lau CP: The sensing of body movement and acceleration forces. In: Lau CP, ed. Rate Adaptive Cardiac Pacing: Single and Dual Chamber. New York: Futura, 1993:73-97.

44. Leung SK, Lau CP, Tang MO, Leung Z: New integrated sensor pacemaker: Comparison of rate responses between an integrated minute ventilation and activity sensor and single sensor modes during exercise and daily activities and nonphysiological interference. *PACE* 1996; 19(pt II):1664-1671.

45. Clementy J, Barold SS, Garrigue S et al: Clinical significance of multiple sensor options: rate response optimization, sensor blending, and trending. *Am J Cardiol* 1999; 83:166D-171D.

46. Alt E, Combs W, Willhaus R, et al: A comparative study of activity and dual sensors: Activity and minute ventilation pacing responses to ascending and descending stairs. *PACE* 1998; 21:1862-1868.

47. Sulke AN, Pipilis A, Henderson RA, Bucknall CA, Sowton E: Comparison of the normal sinus node with seven types of rate responsive pacemaker during everyday activity. *Br Heart J* 1990; 64:25-31.

48. Lau CP, Mehta D, Toff WD et al: Limitations of rate response of an activity-sensing rate response pacemaker to different forms of activity. *PACE* 1988; 11:141-150.

49. McAlister HF, Sobermann J, Klementowicz P, et al: Treadmill assessment of an activity-modulated pacemaker: The importance of an individual programming. PACE 1989; 12:486-501.

50. Lau CP, Tai YT, Fong PC, et al: Clinical experience with an activity sensing DDDR pacemaker using an accelerometer sensor. *PACE* 1992; 15:334-342.

51. Alt E, Millerhagen JO, Heemels J: (1995). Accelerometers. In Ellenborgen KA, Kay GN, Wilkoff BL eds. Clinical Cardiac Pacing. Toronto, Ontario: W.B. Saunders Co, 1995:267-276.

52. Alt E, Matula M, Holzer K: Behavior of different activity-based pacemakers during treadmill exercise testing with variable slopes: A comparison of three activity-based pacing systems. *PACE* 1994; 17:1761-1770.

53. Bacharach DW, Hilden RS, Millerhagen JO, et al: Activity-based pacing: Comparison of a device using an accelerometer versus a piezoelectic crystal. *PACE* 1992; 15:188-196.

54. Millerhagen J, Bacharch D, Street G, et al: A comparison study of two activity pacemakers: An accelerometer versus piezoelectric crystal device. *PACE* 1991; 14:665.

55. Candinas RA, Gloor HO, Amann FW, Schoenbeck M, Turina M: Activity-sensing rate responsive verses conventional fixed-rate pacing: a comparison of rate behavior and patient well-being during routine daily exercise. *PACE* 1991; 14:204-213.

56. Garrigue S, Chaix C, Gencel L, et al: Scoring method for assessing rate adaptive pacemakers: Application to two different activity sensors. *PACE* 1998; 21:509-519.

57. Charles RG, Heemels JP, Westrum BL: Accelerometer-based adaptive-rate pacing: a multicenter study. *PACE* 1993; 16:418-425.

58. Candinas R, Jakob M, Buckingham TA, Mattmann H, Amann FW: Vibration, acceleration, gravitation, and movement: Activity controlled rate adaptive pacing during treadmill exercise testing and daily life activities. *PACE* 1997; 20:1777-1786.

59. Stangl K, Wirtzfeld A, Heinze R, Laule M, Seitz K, Gobl G: A new multisensor pacing system using stroke volume, respiratory rate, mixed venous oxygen saturation, and temperature, right atrial pressure and right ventricular pressure and dP/dt. *PACE* 1988; 11:712-724.

60. Lau CP: The combination of sensors and algorithms. In: Lau CP, ed. Rate Adaptive Cardiac Pacing: Single and Dual Chamber. New York: Futura, 1993:213-227.

61. Leung SK, Lau CP, Tang MO: Cardiac output is a sensitive indicator of difference in exercise performance between single and dual sensor pacemakers. *PACE* 1998; 21(Pt.I):35-41.

62. Miyazawa K, Yamaguchi J, Komatsu E, Kagaya S, Oda J: Cardiovascular response to exercise in pacemaker implanted patients with fixed heart rate. *Jpn Heart J*. 1989; 30:809-816.

63. Pashkow FJ: Patients with implanted pacemakers or implanted cardioverter defibrillators. In Wenger NK and Hellerstein HK eds. Rehabilitation of the Coronary Patient 3rd Edition. Churchill Livingstone New York 1992; 431-438.

64. Mehta D, Lau CP, Ward DE, et al: Comparative evaluation of chronotropic responses of QT sensing and activity sensing rate responsive pacemakers. *PACE* 1988; 11:1405-1412.

65. Alt E: A protocol for treadmill and bicycle stress testing designed for pacemaker patients. *Stimucoeur* 1987; 15:33-35.

66. Wilkoff BL, Corey J, Blackburn G: A mathematical model of the cardiac chronotropic response to exercise. *J Electrophysiol* 1989; 3:176-180.

67. Provenier F, Jordaens L: Evaluation of six minute walking test in patients with single chamber rate responsive pacemakers. *Br Heart J* 1994; 72:192-196.

68. Payne GE, Skehan JD: Shuttle walking test: a new approach for evaluating patients with pacemakers. *Heart* 1996; 75:414-418.

69. Lagenfeld H, Schneider B, Grimm W, et al: The six-minute walk – An adequate test for pacemaker patients? *PACE* 1990; 13(pt II):1761-1765.

70. Superko HR: Effects of cardiac rehabilitation in permanently paced patients with third-degree heart block. *J Cardiac Rehab* 1983; 3:561-568.

71. Lau CP: Comparative hemodynamic studies between different rate adaptive modes. In: Lau CP, ed. Rate Adaptive Cardiac Pacing: Single and Dual Chamber. New York: Futura, 1993:51-61.

72. Greco EM, Guardini S, Citelli L: Cardiac rehabilitation in patients with rate responsive pacemakers. *PACE* 1998; 21:568-575.

73. Sharp CT, Busse EF, Burgess JJ, Haennel RG: Exercise prescription for patients with pacemakers. *J. Cardiopulm Rehabil* 1998; 18:421-431.

74. Connelly DT, Rickards AF: Rate responsive pacing using electrographic parameters as sensors. *Cardiology Clinics* 1992; 10:659-667.

75. Lau CP, Wong CK, Leung WH, et al: A comparative evaluation of minute ventilation sensing and activity sensing adaptive-rate pacemakers during daily activities. *PACE* 1989; 12:1514-1521.

76. Corbelli R, Masterson M, Wilkoff BL: Chronotropic response to exercise in patients with atrial fibrillation. *PACE* 1990; 13:179-187.

Chapter 11

# Mechanical Ventilation During Exercise in COPD

Denis E. O'Donnell, MD, Katherine A. Webb, MSc, Susan M. Revill, PhD, Canada

Chronic obstructive pulmonary disease (COPD) is a heterogeneous disorder characterized by dysfunction of the small and large airways, as well as destruction of the lung parenchyma and vasculature, in highly variable combinations. Breathlessness and exercise intolerance are the most common symptoms of COPD and progress relentlessly as the disease advances. Exercise intolerance is multifactorial, but in more severe disease, ventilatory limitation is often the proximate exercising limiting event. Multiple factors determine ventilatory limitation and include integrated abnormalities of ventilatory mechanics and ventilatory muscle function as well as increased ventilatory demand and alterations in the neuroregulatory control of breathing. Theoretically, interventions that delay ventilatory limitation or that unload overburdened ventilatory muscles, should improve exercise performance. In this respect, several recent studies have shown that non-invasive ventilatory assistance (VA) effectively relieved dyspnea and improved exercise endurance in patients with severe COPD. In this review, we will describe the abnormalities of dynamic ventilatory mechanics and muscle function in COPD during exercise and how these collectively contribute to exercise intolerance. We will then describe how these mechanical derangements can be manipulated for the patients' benefit using optimized VA. Finally, we will outline how recent studies on the effects of acute VA during exercise have provided valuable insights into mechanisms of dyspnea and disability in patients with advanced disease.

## Exercise Limitation in COPD

Exercise limitation is multifactorial in COPD. Recognized contributory factors include (1) ventilatory limitation due to impaired respiratory system mechanics and ventilatory muscle dysfunction, (2) metabolic and gas exchange abnormalities, (3) peripheral muscle dysfunction, (4) cardiac impairment, (5) exertional symptoms, and (6) any combination of these interdependent factors(1-6). The predominant contributory factors to exercise limitation vary among patients with COPD, or indeed, in a given patient over time. The more advanced the disease, the more of these factors that come into play in a complex integrative manner. However, in such patients, the inability to further increase ventilation in the face of increasing ventilatory demands is often a primary contributing factor to exercise intolerance.

## Ventilatory Mechanics in COPD

Although the most obvious physiological defect in COPD is expiratory flow limitation due to combined reduced lung recoil and airway tethering as well as intrinsic airway narrowing, the most important mechanical consequence of this is a "restrictive" ventilatory deficit due to lung hyperinflation (7,8) (Figure 11.1). When expiratory flow limitation reaches a critical level, lung emptying becomes incomplete during resting tidal breathing, and lung volume fails to decline to its natural equilibrium point (i.e., passive functional residual capacity [FRC]). End-expiratory lung volume (EELV), therefore, becomes dynamically and not statically, determined and represents a higher resting lung volume than in health. In COPD, EELV is a continuous variable that fluctuates widely with rest and activity. When ventilation ($V_E$) increases in flowlimited patients during exercise, dynamic EELV increases even further above resting values: this is termed dynamic lung hyperinflation (DH) (figure 11.1). By contrast, in healthy, non-flow limited subjects, EELV may actually decline during the increased $V_E$ of exercise, particularly in younger individuals (9) (figure 11.1). This allows tidal volume ($V_T$) expansion within the linear portion of the respiratory system's pressure-volume relationship where "high-end" elastic loading is avoided. Expiratory muscle recruitment and reduced EELV also favourably affect diaphragmatic function in health (9). Many of these important advantages are lost in COPD patients because of DH. The pattern and extent of DH development

in COPD patients is highly variable: the average range of increase in EELV in published series is 0.3 to 0.6 L (10-13). However, some patients do not increase EELV during exercise whereas others show dramatic increases (i.e., >I L) (10-13). Patients with a more emphysematous clinical profile show rapid rates of dynamic hyperinflation early in exercise, with earlier attainment of critical ventilatory constraints, greater dyspnea levels, and reduced symptom-limited $\dot{V}O_2$max. Patients with a predominant "chronic bronchitis" clinical profile show comparable levels of DH from rest to peak exercise in absolute terms; but in these patients, the rate of DH accelerates later in exercise than in the emphysematous patients. Important determinants of DH include: (1) the level of baseline lung hyperinflation, (2) the extent of expiratory flow limitation, (3) ventilatory demand, and (4) breathing pattern for a given ventilation. While DH serves to maximize tidal expiratory flow rates during exercise, it has serious consequences with respect to dynamic ventilatory mechanics, inspira-

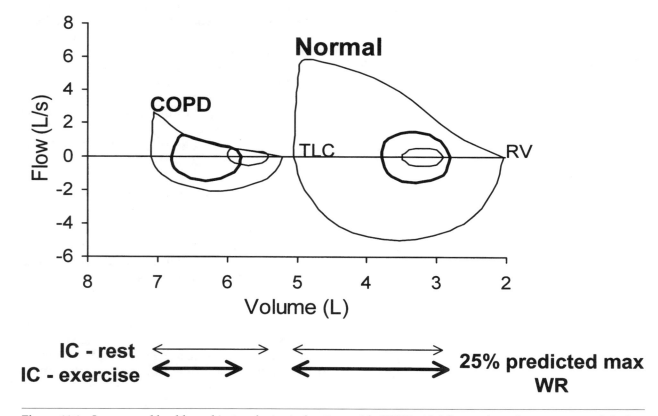

**Figure 11.1**   In a normal healthy subject and a typical patient with COPD, tidal flow-volume loops at rest and during exercise (peak exercise in COPD compared with exercise at a comparable metabolic load in the age-matched healthy person) are shown in relation to their respective maximal flow-volume loops.

tory muscle function, respiratory sensation and, probably, cardiac function (14).

## Dynamic Lung Hyperinflation and Restrictive Mechanics During Exercise in COPD

An important mechanical consequence of DH is the occurrence of severe mechanical constraints on tidal volume ($V_T$) expansion during exercise: $V_T$ is truncated from below by the increasing EELV and constrained from above by the relatively reduced inspiratory reserve volume (IRV) and the total lung capacity (TLC) enveloppe (14) (figures 11.1 and 11.2). Thus, at comparable low work rates in COPD patients, dynamic end-inspiratory lung volume (EILV) and $V_T$/inspiratory capacity ratios ($V_T$/IC) are greatly increased, and the IRV is diminished compared with healthy subjects (figures 11.1 and 11.2). To increase $V_E$ during exercise, such patients must rely on increasing breathing frequency; but this tachypnea, in turn, causes further DH in a vicious cycle (figure 11.2).

## Ventilatory Muscle Dysfunction in COPD

The behaviour of EELV during exercise is usually tracked by serial IC maneuvres (10-14). The smaller the IC becomes during exercise, the closer $V_T$ is positioned to TLC and the upper alinear extreme of the respiratory system's (combined chest wall and lung) pressure-volume relationships, where there is increased elastic loading of muscles already burdened by increased resistive work. The combined elastic and resistive loads on the ventilatory muscles substantially increase the mechanical work and the oxygen cost of breathing at a given ventilation in COPD compared with health. At a peak exercise $V_E$ of approximately 20 L/min, ventilatory work may approach over 200 joules/min and respiratory muscle $\dot{V}O_2$ exceeds 300 ml/min in COPD (15). The net effect of DH in COPD is, therefore, that the $V_T$ response to increasing exercise is progressively constrained despite inspiratory efforts that approach the maximum: the ratio of effort (i.e., tidal esophageal pressures relative to maximum [$Pes/PI_{max}$]) to tidal volume response ($V_T$/VC) are thus, significantly higher at any given work rate or ventilation in COPD compared with health (14) (figure 11.2).

Another more recently recognized mechanical consequence of DH is inspiratory threshold loading (ITL). Since in flow-limited patients, inspiration begins before tidal lung emptying is complete, the inspiratory muscles must first counterbalance the combined inward (expiratory) recoil of the lung and chest wall before inspiratory flow is initiated. This phenomenon (i.e., reduced lung emptying) is associated with air trapping and positive intrapulmonary pressures at the end of quiet expiration (autoPEEP or intrinsic PEEP). The ITL, which may be present at rest in some flow-limited patients with COPD, further increases with exercise and can be substantial (e.g., -6 to −14 cm $H_2O$) and may have important implications for dyspnea causation (14).

Lung hyperinflation during exercise is accommodated primarily by the expansion of the rib cage compartment which, in turn, shortens the accessory muscles of inspiration causing functional muscle weakness (11). DH also alters the length-tension relationship of the diaphragm, and compromises its ability to generate pressure (7). Attendant tachypnea and increased velocity of muscle shortening during exercise results in further functional inspiratory muscle weakness as well as contributes to reduced dynamic lung compliance (7). Because of weakened inspiratory muscles and the intrinsic mechanical loads already described, tidal inspiratory pressures represent a much higher fraction of their maximal force generating capacity than in health at a similar work rate or ventilation (14) (figure 11.2). DH may alter the pattern of ventilatory muscle recruitment to a more inefficient pattern with negative implications for muscle energetics (11).

The degree to which ventilatory pump failure contributes to ventilatory limitation in COPD is uncertain and has been the subject of extensive study (16-20). Theoretically, reduced ventilatory capacity due to reduced ventilatory muscle strength or fatigue in the setting of increased ventilatory muscle loading, should contribute to ventilatory limitation in many patients with advanced COPD (16-20). In addition to mechanical factors, respiratory muscles can become weakened in COPD because of the effects of malnutrition, excessive steroid usage, electrolytic disturbances, hypoxemia, hypercapnia, and acidosis. However, the evidence that a weakened ventilatory pump contributes to exercise intolerance is not conclusive (16-20). The prevalence of inspiratory muscle weakness in the COPD population has not been established and may not be as pervasive as previously thought. In fact, there is evidence that

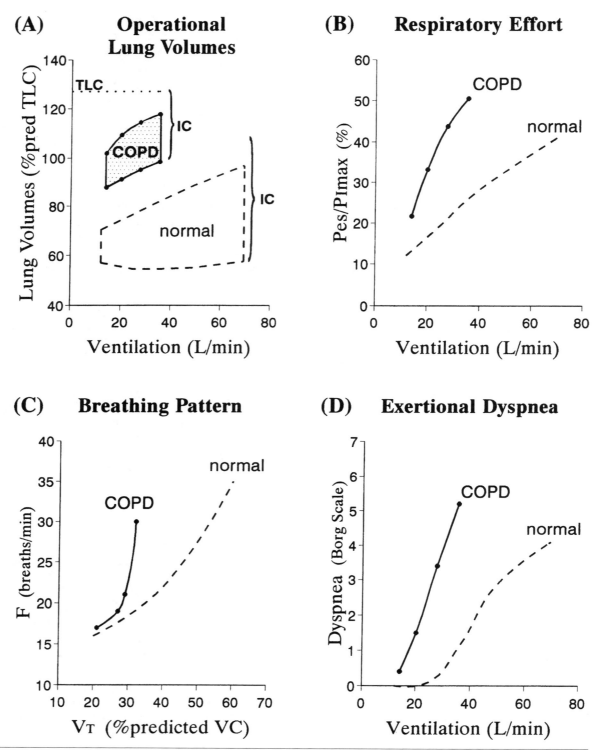

**Figure 11.2** Behaviour of (A) operational lung volumes, (B) respiratory effort (Pes/PI$_{max}$), and (D) exertional dyspnea as ventilation increases throughout exercise in normals and COPD. In COPD, tidal volume (V$_T$) takes up a larger proportion of the reduced inspiratory capacity (IC), and the inspiratory reserve volume (IRV) is decreased at any given ventilation—these mechanical constraints on tidal volume expansion are further compounded because of dynamic hyperinflation during exercise. (C) Due to a truncated V$_T$ response to exercise, patients with COPD must rely more on increasing breathing frequency (F) to generate increases in ventilation.

Data from DE O'Donnell et al., 1998, "Measurement of symptoms, lung hyperinflation and endurance during exercise in chronic obstructive pulmonary dieseaese," *American Journal of Respiratory and Critical Care Medicine* 158:1557-1565.

functional muscle strength is remarkably preserved in some patients with advanced chronic ventilatory insufficiency (21). Patients with acute-on-chronic hypercapnia during exercise have been shown to have no acute deterioration in maximal force generating capacity, and do not exhibit alteration in the pattern of ventilatory muscle recruitment compared with non-hypercapnic individuals matched for $FEV_{1.0}$ (22). The result of studies on the effects of specific inspiratory muscle training on exercise performance in COPD have been inconsistent (23). Nevertheless, the argument that acute inspiratory muscle weakness or fatigue contributes to ventilatory limitation in some individuals with COPD is supported by studies of acute VA during exercise (24-26). These studies will be reviewed in detail below.

## Expiratory Muscle Recruitment in COPD

In the presence of expiratory flow limitation, tidal expiratory flow rates are independent of expiratory transpulmonary pressures beyond a critical level (8). In fact, increasing expiratory effort beyond this level not only fails to increase expiratory flow, but results in dynamic airway compression of the airways downstream from the flow-limiting segment (8). Expiratory muscle recruitment appears to be highly variable in COPD during exercise (12,13,27). During constant-load exercise, some patients allow expiratory transpulmonary pressures to reach, but not exceed, the critical flow-limiting pressure, thus attenuating dynamic airway compression (27). Expiratory muscle recruitment may assist the inspiratory muscles by favourably altering diaphragmatic configuration or by the release of stored elastic energy at the onset of inspiration (12,13,22). Several studies have shown marked expiratory muscle activity at high work rates in COPD (12,13,22,20). This possibly maladaptive behaviour will not improve alveolar ventilation or operating lung volumes, and will aggravate dynamic airway compression which, in turn, likely contributes to increased exertional dyspnea (28,29). Excessive expiratory intrathoracic and abdominal pressures, with reduced velocity of shortening of the expiratory muscles, may also significantly impair cardiac function in exercising COPD patients (12). The net effect of intense expiratory muscle recruitment on exercise performance will vary among COPD patients; in many patients, the deleterious effects of vigorous expiratory muscle contraction on symptoms and cardiac performance may outweigh potential beneficial effects

on inspiratory muscle function.

## Increased Ventilatory Demand in COPD

The effects of the above-outlined mechanical derangements in COPD are often compounded by concomitant increases in ventilatory demand. Many studies have shown that $V_E$ at a given submaximal work rate is significantly increased compared with normal (30,31). Factors contributing to increased $V_E$ include high physiological deadspace, earlier lactate acidosis, hypoxemia, high metabolic demands, low arterial $CO_2$ set point, and other non-metabolic sources of ventilatory stimulation (i.e., anxiety, hyperventilation, etc.). For a given level of expiratory flow limitation, the extent of DH and its negative sensory consequences will vary with ventilatory demand. Those with the highest ventilation will develop limiting ventilatory constraints on flow and volume generation, and greater dyspnea early in exercise (31). There is abundant evidence that increased ventilatory demand contributes to dyspnea causation in COPD, and dyspnea intensity during exercise has been shown in several studies to correlate strongly with changes in $V_E$ or with $V_E$ expressed as a fraction of maximal breathing capacity (32-33). For a given $FEV_{1.0}$, patients who have greater ventilatory demands will have more severe chronic activity-related dyspnea (31). Moreover, exertional dyspnea relief following interventions such as exercise training (33), oxygen therapy (34), and opiates (35), has been shown to result, in part, from reduced submaximal ventilation.

## Dynamic Hyperinflation and Dyspnea

Dyspnea intensity during exercise has been shown to correlate strongly with measures of DH (10) and the consequent increased inspiratory effort/displacement ratio (14). This increased ratio ultimately reflects neuromechanical uncoupling of the respiratory system and may provide a neurophysiological explanation for perceived respiratory distress or some of its dominant qualitative dimensions.

Further evidence of the importance of DH in contributing to exertional dyspnea in COPD has come from a number of studies that have shown that dyspnea was effectively ameliorated by interventions that reduced operational lung volumes, either pharmacologically

(36-38) or surgically (39), or that counter-balanced the negative effects of DH on the respiratory muscle, i.e., continuous positive airway pressure (CPAP) (40,25).

## Dynamic Hyperinflation and Exercise Limitation in COPD

Accelerated DH during exercise hastens the onset of critical ventilatory limitation, which in turn leads to premature termination of exercise (figures 11.1 and 11.2). In flow-limited patients, the degree of resting lung hyperinflation, as reflected by reduced IC, is a powerful predictor of exercise capacity (41,42). In a recent study, the resting IC in conjunction with the $FEV_{1.0}$/FVC ratio together accounted for 72% of the variance in exercise capacity in a group (n = 52) of patients with COPD (42). Moreover, it has recently been shown that improvement in resting IC following bronchodilator therapy was the strongest correlate of improved exercise endurance in patients with severe COPD (43). The dynamic IC represents the true operational limits for $V_T$ expansion during exercise in COPD; when $V_T$ approximates the dynamic IC (minus a minimal IRV), further exercise is impossible. In COPD, symptom-limited peak $\dot{V}O_2$ correlates well with the peak $V_T$ achieved (figures 11.1 and 11.2).

## Ventilatory Assistance During Exercise: Overview of the Literature

It has become clear that the patient-ventilator interface during exercise in COPD is complex; VA likely affects multiple integrated physiological functions that are difficult to measure with precision. Thus, VA not only affects inspiratory muscle function and dyspnea, but also affects expiratory and accessory muscle function, cardiac performance, submaximal ventilation levels, breathing pattern, operational lung volumes, and perhaps even peripheral muscle blood flow and oxygen delivery in some circumstances. The ultimate effect of VA on exercise performance in a given individual will, therefore, depend on its net effect on these multiple integrated functions. In some cases, the salutary effects of VA may be negated by simultaneous perturbations of other physiological functions; for example, CPAP levels above the patient's ITL will lead to increased expiratory muscle recruitment which

may negate its positive effects on inspiratory muscle function (25).

The interpretation of available studies is confounded by small study sample sizes and variation in pathophysiological impairment at baseline. Most studies are not adequately controlled. In order to provide a true control for VA, nominal support, even when delivered in a blinded, randomized fashion does not adequately control for higher level pressure support. In addition, differences in technical factors between studies make direct comparisons difficult. These include: operating and response characteristics of the various ventilators (i.e., ability to keep pace with higher ventilation during exercise and phase delay between respired volume and pressure support); reduced trigger sensitivity, type of mask or oral appliance used, the propensity to compensate for air leaks, and other circuit design features such as minimization of circuit resistance and prevention of $CO_2$ rebreathing. In some studies, oxygen was added to the breathing circuit during VA making inter-study comparisons difficult. Also, VA pressure titration protocols have not been standardized and vary greatly, some titrating to patient comfort, others to breathing pattern or blood gas measurements, and others empirically based on suspected or measured mechanical abnormalities in a given patient. During exercise studies, there is great variation in the testing protocols used, in the mode of exercise, and in the approach to measurement of subjective and objective physiological variables. Despite all these methodological reservations, these studies have enhanced our understanding of the mechanisms of dyspnea and exercise intolerance in COPD and are outlined below. Most studies showed significant improvement in exercise endurance during VA (figure 11.3).

## CPAP—Counterbalancing the Effects of Dynamic Hyperinflation on the Inspiratory Muscles

The argument that DH, through its adverse effects on inspiratory muscle function, contributes importantly to exertional dyspnea and exercise curtailment in COPD, has been bolstered by the results of studies on the effects of applied CPAP in such patients. In five patients with COPD ($FEV_{1.0}$ 35% predicted), CPAP 4 to 5 cm $H_2O$ delivered during constant load, submaximal exercise (at approximately 50% of $\dot{V}O_2$max) significantly reduced breathlessness ratings (p < 0.025) and improved exercise endurance by an average of 48% (p < 0.01) compared with bracketing unassisted exercise runs (24) (figure 11.3). Insights into potential mechanisms of relief of breathlessness during CPAP were obtained from a second study that partitioned CPAP into its two components: inspiratory positive airway pressure (IPAP) and expiratory positive airway pressure (EPAP) (40). CPAP, IPAP and EPAP of equal magnitude (4 to 5 cm $H_2O$) were each administered in random order for brief intervals during steady state exercise in five patients with COPD, (mean $FEV_{1.0}$ of 40% predicted), and in five healthy subjects (40). Breathlessness was assessed by a bi-directional transition scale. CPAP and IPAP significantly reduced breathlessness, whereas EPAP had no significant effect in COPD patients (40). In normals, IPAP significantly improved breathing effort but both CPAP and EPAP made breathing more difficult. It was concluded that the beneficial effects of CPAP on exertional breathlessness occurred mainly as a result of the inspiratory assistance component (IPAP) and that EPAP's potential effect on expiratory airway splinting was less important. In that study, CPAP (4 to 5 cm $H_2O$) did not diminish volume-matched expiratory flow rates or result in increases in the EELV compared with unassisted control periods (40). These patients were, therefore, likely flow-limited throughout exercise. The potential beneficial effects of EPAP on airway splinting could have been negated since the applied pressure was terminated precisely at the end of expiration (i.e., onset of inspiration). EPAP did not, therefore, (unlike CPAP) counterbalance the ITL, which the patient had still to overcome.

Petrof et al. (25), studied ventilatory mechanics and breathlessness following CPAP (7.5 to 10 cm $H_2O$) during submaximal exercise (20 ± 4.8 watts) in eight patients with COPD ($FEV_{1.0}$ = 21 % predicted). CPAP relieved breathlessness in five of the eight subjects. Relief of breathlessness correlated with reduction in the pressure-time integral of esophageal pressure ($\backslash gS\backslash P_{es}.dt$) and was inversely related to the pressure-time integral of gastric pressure ($\backslash gS\backslash P_{ga}.dt$). It is clear from this study that the ameliorating effect of CPAP on breathlessness is a function of its ability to unload the inspiratory muscles, and that such effects can be negated by increased expiratory muscle recruitment which likely occurs when CPAP is not optimized to match the ITL.

In contrast to these studies, Keilty et al. (44) failed to show any significant improvement in submaximal treadmill endurance times when CPAP (6 cm $H_2O$) was delivered to eight patients with severe COPD ($FEV_{1.0}$ = 0.73 L) (figure 11.3). Dolmage et al (45) showed an average improvement of 20% in cycle endurance times during CPAP (5 cm $H_2O$) in ten patients with severe COPD ($FEV_{1.0}$ = 29% predicted) (figure 11.3). In 15 patients with stable hypercapnic COPD, Bianchi et al (46) showed significant improvements in cycle endurance time (at 80% of maximal work rate) by approximately 30% of control as well as improved dyspnea ratings.

The magnitude of response to CPAP varied considerably between subjects and between studies (figure 11.3). A minority of the study patients showed dramatic responses, while others showed little or no response. The difference in response likely reflects variability in baseline pathophysiology as well as differences in CPAP optimization protocols. As mentioned above, the pattern of DH varies substantially between patients; ideally, CPAP levels should be continuously adjusted to match the change in DH and the ITL throughout exercise. However, for practical purposes this is often impossible to achieve. There is marked variability in CPAP delivery methods: for best results, continuous pressure support should be provided throughout inspiration and expiration. Often there are wide phasic fluctuations with either an inspiratory or expiratory bias, which negates the physiological effects of CPAP. At this time it is impossible to predict, based on resting pathophysiological characteristics, which patient will benefit from ambulatory CPAP, but it is reasonable to assume that it would be most useful in patients in whom DH contributes importantly to exertional dyspnea.

## Pressure Support During Exercise in COPD

Given the difficulties in optimizing CPAP during exercise in COPD, Keilty et al. (44) have suggested that ventilatory assistance using pressure support (PS) may have wider application for this purpose. These investigators delivered PS (12 to 15 cm $H_2O$) to 8 men with severe COPD ($FEV_{1.0}$ = 0.75) during submaximal treadmill walking. PS increased walking distance by an average of 62% of the control value (i.e., sham circuit) (figure 11.3). Responses to PS varied greatly among this group, with one patient increasing walking distance by 533 metres while others showed a minimal response. Improved endurance was associated with a significant reduction of exertional dyspnea. Of interest, in this same patient group, CPAP (6 cm $H_2O$) increased walking

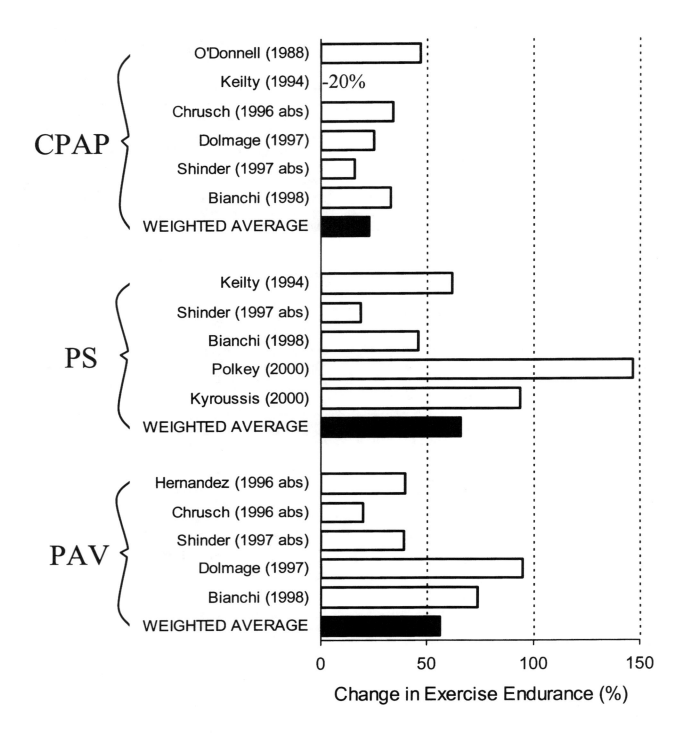

**Figure 11.3** From a number of controlled studies, changes in endurance during CPAP, PS and PAV assisted exercise tests are shown versus unassisted control or sham tests. Added oxygen was used during tests by Bianchi et al.(46) and Chrusch et al.(52); CPAP was used in combination with PAV in results reported from Chrusch et al.(52), Shinder et al.(53), and Dolmage et al.(45). The "weighted average" is the average change from the listed studies, after accounting for study sample sizes.

distance by an average of 20% of the control value, but this was not statistically significant.

Maltais et al. (47) delivered PS (11 – 15 cm $H_2O$) to 7 patients with severe COPD ($FEV_{1.0}$/FVC = 39% predicted) during constant load cycle exercise (at 50% maximal $\dot{V}O_2$). Five of the 7 patients received additional supplemental oxygen, which may have confounded the net physiological responses. PS reduced the $\Sigma P_{es}\cdot dt$ by an average of 32% and significantly reduced dyspnea ratings at isotime. The relief of dyspnea correlated well with measures of inspiratory muscle unloading. PS significantly stimulated ventilation, increased $\dot{V}CO_2$, and possibly improved alveolar ventilation. Stimulation of $V_E$ by 4 to 5 L/min at isotime would be expected to increase DH and result in earlier ventilatory limitation: under these circumstances, improvement in exercise endurance during PS is likely attributable to the simultaneous delay in the onset of intolerable exertional dyspnea.

To investigate the mechanisms by which PS reduced dyspnea, Polkey et al. (20) measured maximal sniff relaxation rates ($SnP_{es}MRR$) of inspiratory muscles during unassisted treadmill walking and compared these values with those obtained during PS (15 cm $H_2O$) in 6 patients with severe COPD ($FEV_{1.0}$ 22% predicted) at a comparable exercise level. Following unassisted walking there was a mean slowing of $SNP_{es}MRR$ by 41% indicating incipient inspiratory muscle fatigue. Following similar exercise assisted by PS, sniff esophageal MRR was delayed by a mean of 20% of baseline values, signifying effective inspiratory muscle unloading. The corollary of these findings is that inspiratory muscle loading, or its perception by the patient, contributes importantly to exercise intolerance in COPD.

Bianchi et al. (46) determined the effects of PS (12 to 16 cm $H_2O$), delivered by nasal mask in conjunction with oxygen (3 L/min), on dyspnea and exercise endurance in 15 patients with severe hypercapnic COPD ($FEV_{1.0}$ 32% predicted) and respiratory failure (figure 11.4). Endurance time improved by a mean of 46% from the control value and Borg dyspnea ratings fell significantly. In this study PS had minimal effects on ventilation and resulted in small, consistent effects on the $V_T$ (mean increase of 15%).

New insights into the effects of PS on respiratory muscle function during exercise in severe COPD were recently provided in a study by Kyroussos et al. (48). During unassisted walking in 12 patients with severe COPD ($FEV_{1.0}$ 27% predicted), the pressure time product of the inspiratory muscles rose rapidly at the onset of exercise, and then quickly plateaued despite increasing ventilation levels (figure 11.4). This behaviour may be explained by progressive DH which compromises inspiratory muscle function, while preserving or improving respirated flow rates. Consistent with other studies in severe COPD during unassisted breathing, patients recruited expiratory muscles increasingly throughout exercise, as measured by the expiratory gastric pressure time product, but with considerable variation in the range (figure 11.4). It is of interest that PS significantly reduced both the inspiratory and expiratory pressure time products throughout exercise, possibly indicating a reduced central drive to breathing related to mechanical unloading and reduced arterial $CO_2$ levels (figure 11.4). In 6 of the 12 patients, treadmill endurance times increased substantially in the setting of marked reductions in pressure time products of the inspiratory muscles. It is to be expected that reduced expiratory muscle activity during PS would have beneficial effects on cardiac function and this, of itself, may be an important contributor to the improved exercise performance and requires further study (12).

## Proportional Assist Ventilation

Proportional assist ventilation (PAV) provides positive airway pressure throughout the inspiratory cycle, in direct proportion to the patient's inspiratory effort (49). This proportionality can be amplified as desired. In other words, PAV directly augments the respiratory effort generated by the patient in synchrony with his or her spontaneous breathing pattern. When PAV provides pressure in proportion to the respired volume signal, volume assist (VA) or elastic unloading occurs; when pressure is in proportion to the respiratory flow, flow-assist (FA) resistive unloading is accomplished (49). Theoretically, PAV should enhance neuromechanical coupling and patient comfort to a greater degree than other pressure support modalities. However, preliminary results using PAV in the exercise setting of COPD have been mixed and its theoretical superiority remains conjectural.

Hernandez et al (50) compared the effects of unassisted breathing to PAV (VA = 2.8 cm $H_2O$/L, FA = 1.2 cm $H_2O$/L/sec) in five subjects with severe COPD ($FEV_{1.0}$ = 0.93+0.11 L) during incremental cycle exercise. With PAV, peak work rate improved from 48 to 53 watts, and exercise time increased by an average of 11%. Dyspnea ratings decreased

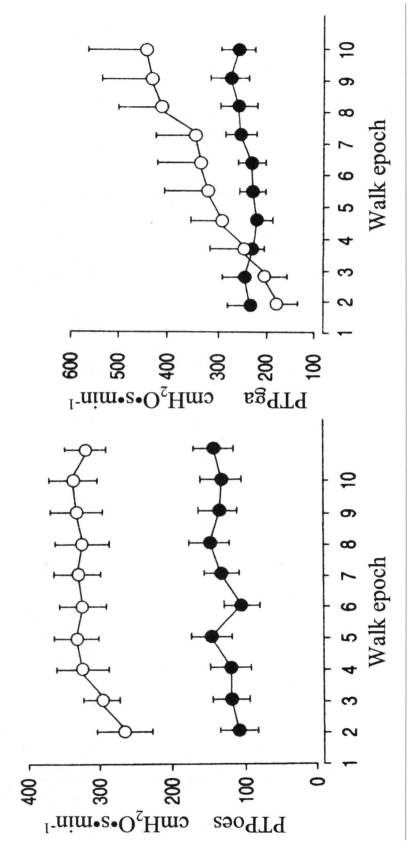

**Figure 11.4** (Left) Progression of mean pressure time product (PTP) of oesophageal pressure (O) and PTP of transdiaphragmatic pressure (Σ) by 10% epoch of walk duration for the free exhaustive walk (12 subjects). Data are presented as means ±SEM. (Right) Progression of pressure time product of gastric pressure ($PTP_{ga}$) by 10% epoch of walk duration during free (O) and equidistant positive pressure ventilation-assisted walking (Σ) (six subjects). Data are presented as mean ±SEM (from reference 48).

significantly and $V_T$ increased during PAV. A second study by the same authors compared higher levels of PAV (VA = 9.7 cm $H_2O$/L, FA = 3.4 cm $H_2O$/L/sec) using the Winnipeg ventilator and a mouthpiece. PAV improved exercise endurance (at 82% $\dot{V}O_2$max) by an average of 40% and significantly reduced Borg dyspnea ratings at isotime (51) (figure 11.3). In that study, PAV stimulated ventilation throughout exercise chiefly by increasing the $V_T$: compared with control $V_T$ was increased at isotime and peak exercise by 15% and 31%, respectively. These increases in $V_E$ have the potential to accelerate DH and its negative mechanical and cardiac consequences. However, in that study, regardless of these possible deleterious negative effects on ventilation, operational lung volumes, and ventilatory limitation, the onset of intolerable dyspnea during PAV was, nevertheless, delayed by 2 + minutes compared with the unassisted control.

Dolmage and Goldstein (45) examined the effects of PAV (VA = 6 cm $H_2O$/L, FA = 3 cm $H_2O$/L/sec) using the Winnipeg ventilator on dyspnea and exercise endurance during cycle exercise (at 60 to 70% of their pre-established peak work rate) in patients with severe COPD, and compared its effects with unassisted exercise. In that study, PAV alone had only small and insignificant effects on dyspnea and exercise endurance. In 10 hypercapnic COPD patients, Bianchi et al. (46) showed that PAV (VA = 8.6 cm $H_2O$/L, FA = 3.1 cm $H_2O$/L/sec) delivered by a portable ventilator (Respironics) and nasal mask, showed an increase in endurance (at 80% of their maximal work rate) by 66% of the unassisted control value (figure 11.3). In that study, PAV increased $V_T$ significantly at isotime while decreasing end-tidal $CO_2$, and dyspnea ratings were similarly decreased. In this, as in other studies, the responses varied considerably within the group with a few subjects showing marked improvements. In this study by Bianchi et al. (46), supplemental oxygen was added to PAV and may have had independent effects on exercise performance.

## Combined Ventilatory Assist Modalities During Exercise

The combination of CPAP, to counter the inspiratory threshold load, and additional inspiratory assist with PS or PAV should, theoretically, provide more effective unloading than either alone and this should, therefore, translate into greater improvements in dyspnea and exercise performance. There is some evidence to support this claim. Dolmage and Goldstein (45) showed that combined PAV (VA = 6 cm $H_2O$, FA = 3 cm $H_2O$/L/sec) + CPAP (5 cm $H_2O$) had a significantly greater effect on exercise endurance and dyspnea than either modality alone (Figure 4). By contrast, Chrush et al. (52), in a preliminary study found that the addition of PAV (VA 2.3 cm $H_2O$/L, FA = 1.4 cm $H_2O$/L/sec) to oxygen (fractional concentration of $O_2$ = 0.35) and CPAP (5.4 cm $H_2O$) did not result in further increases in endurance times or dyspnea ratings when compared with CPAP plus $O_2$ alone (figure 11.3). Similarly, Shinder et al. (53) showed that the addition of PAV (VA = 2 cm $H_2O$/L, FA = 1 cm $H_2O$/L/sec) to CPAP (4 cm $H_2O$) did not improve exercise endurance or dyspnea over that provided by CPAP alone. In the study of Bianchi et al. (46), which compared PAV and PS, PAV showed significantly greater improvements in dyspnea and exercise endurance. However, the authors conceded that these difference could reflect differences in optimization schedules for the two ventilatory assist modalities rather than any technical superiority of PAV.

It would appear that the magnitude of PAV that can be tolerated varies considerably depending on which commercial ventilator is used for delivery: it was possible to deliver greater levels of unloading with the original Winnipeg ventilator than with the Respironics portable ventilator and this may account for the greater success of the former.

## Clinical Experience With Ventilatory Assistance during Exercise

A few generalizations can be made from the existing sparse literature on VA during exercise in COPD. (1) VA can be administered safely to patients with severe stable COPD during exercise. (2) VA can sufficiently unload the overburdened muscles of breathing. (3) VA can effectively ameliorate dyspnea and improve exercise tolerance. (4) Responses to VA are highly variable, but some patients show remarkable, acute improvements in both dyspnea and exercise performance.

Some further observations can be made with respect to the effects of VA on exertional dyspnea. Subjective responses to various VA modalities may vary in a given individual—for example, CPAP may be very effective in relieving dyspnea while PS at a level which provides greater muscle unloading, may be relatively ineffective, and vice versa. A common observation, at least in some patients, is that while VA effectively reduced tidal esophageal pressure swings during exercise, it simultaneously failed to influence dyspnea. The relationship between muscle unloading and dyspnea relief is not often reflected as a linear dose-response relation. For many patients, there appears to be a critical level of unloading where dyspnea relief is maximal: levels below or beyond this point are often not as beneficial. A lack of symptomatic recovery during VA suggests the existence of alternative sources of unpleasant respiratory sensations to muscle loading per se, i.e., increased chemical drive, excessive ventilatory demand, or severe mechanical restriction (dynamic IC < 1 L), which are not specifically addressed by the particular VA modality. Finally, VA may improve some qualitative aspects of breathing difficulty without sufficiently diminishing the overall intensity of respiratory discomfort. VA remains an important research tool for the study of the mechanisms of exertional dyspnea in COPD. A comparison of the effects of the different VA modalities in the same patient allows a determination of the role of various mechanical perturbations in dyspnea causation, in relative isolation.

## Future Clinical Utility of Ventilatory Assistance

There is currently considerable interest in the question of whether VA could be employed as an adjunct to exercise training in patients with advanced COPD. During VA, dyspnea may be displaced by leg discomfort as the main exercise limiting symptom, thus indicating a shift in the locus of sensory limitation. VA could, theoretically, permit such patients to exercise for a longer duration and with a greater intensity that during unassisted breathing. This would allow them to reach the hitherto, unattainable threshold where cardiovascular, metabolic, and peripheral muscle training effects could be achieved. VA training could improve aerobic capacity and this in turn, may lead to reduced submaximal ventilation and delay the attainment of ventilatory limitation and intolerable dyspnea in these patients during unassisted breathing. This hypothesis, however, remains to be tested. It is clear that in some patients, ventilatory limitation will remain the proximate limitation to exercise, despite improved peripheral muscle function as a result of adjunct VA training.

In general, the acute effects of VA on exercise endurance are modest in the majority of patients, and comparable in magnitude to that achieved using supplemental ambulatory oxygen alone. Supplemental oxygen may be a more convenient form of enhancing exercise training responses than the more cumbersome VA, but this question requires systematic study. Given the pathophysiological heterogeneity of COPD, the challenging technical difficulties involved in optimizing VA during exercise, and the complex effects of VA on integrated physiological functions, definitive conclusions about its eventual utility in pulmonary rehabilitation will require large randomized control trials.

## References

1. Hamilton AL, Killian KJ, Summers E, Jones NL. Muscle strength, symptom intensity, and exercise capacity in patients with cardiorespiratory disorders. *Am J Respir Crit Care Med* 1995;152:2021-2031.
2. Grassino A, Gross D, Macklem PT, Roussos C, Zagelbaum G. Inspiratory muscle fatigue as a factor limiting exercise. *Bull Europ Pathophysiol Respir* 1979;15:105-111.
3. Montes de Oca M, Rassulo J, Celli BR. Respiratory muscle and cardiopulmonary function during exercise in very severe COPD. *Am Rev Respir Dis* 1996;154:1284-1289.
4. Bauerle O, Chrusch CA, Younes M. Mechanisms by which COPD affects exercise tolerance. *Am J Respir Crit Care Med* 1998;157:67-68.
5. Neder JA, Jones PW, Nery LE, Whipp BJ. Determinants of the exercise endurance capacity in patients with chronic obstructive pulmonary disease. *Am J Respir Crit Care Med* 2000;162:497-504.
6. Gosselink R, Troosters T, Decramer M. Peripheral muscle weakness contributes to exercise limitation in COPD. *Am J Resp Crit Care Med* 1996;153:976-980.
7. Pride NB, Macklem PT. Lung mechanics in disease. In: AP Fishman, editor. Handbook of Physiology, Section 3, Vol. III, Part 2: The Respiratory System. Bethesda MD: American Physiological Society: 1986. P. 659-692.
8. Hyatt RE. Expiratory flow limitation. *J Appl Physiol* 1983;55:1-8.
9. Henke KG, Sharatt M, Pegelow DF, Dempsey JA. Regulation of end-expiratory lung volume during exercise. *J Appl Physiol* 1988;64:135-146.
10. O'Donnell DE, Webb KA. Exertional breathlessness in patients with chronic airflow limitation:

the role of lung hyperinflation. *Am Rev Respir Dis* 1993;148:1351-1357.

11. Grimby G, Bunn J, Mead J. Relative contribution of rib cage and abdomen to ventilation during exercise. *J Appl Physiol* 1968;24:159-166.

12. Potter WA, Olafson S, Hyatt RE. Ventilatory mechanics and expiratory flow limitation during exercise in patients with obstructive lung disease. *J Clin Invest* 1971;50:910-919.

13. Dodd DS, Brancatisano T, Engel LA. Chest wall mechanics during exercise in patients with severe chronic airway obstruction. *Am Rev Respir Dis* 1984;129:33-38.

14. O'Donnell DE, Chau LKL, Bertley JC, Webb KA. Qualitative aspects of exertional breathlessness in chronic airflow limitation: pathophysiologic mechanisms. *Am J Respir Crit Care Med* 1997;155:109-115.

15. Levison H, Cherniack RM. Ventilatory cost of exercise in chronic obstructive pulmonary disease. *J Appl Physiol* 1968;25:21-27.

16. Bye PT, Esau SA, Levy RD, et al. Ventilatory muscle function during exercise in air and oxygen in patients with chronic airflow limitation. *Am Rev Respir Dis* 1985;132:236-240.

17. Grassino A, Gross D, Macklem PT, Roussos C, Zagelbaum. Inspiratory muscle fatigue as a factor limiting exercise. *Bull Europ Pathophysiol Respir* 1979;15:105-111.

18. Kyroussis D, Polkey MI, Keilty SEJ, et al. Exhaustive exercise slows inspiratory muscle relaxation rate in chronic obstructive pulmonary disease. *Am J Respir Crit Care Med* 1996;153:787-793.

19. Kryoussis D, Polkey MI, Hammegard G-H, Mills GH, Green M, Moxham J. Respiratory muscle activity in patients with COPD walking to exhaustion with and without pressure support. *Eur Respir J* 2000;15:649-655.

21. Polkey MI, Hawkins P, Kyroussis D, Ellum SG, Sherwood R, Moxham J. Inspiratory pressure support prolongs exercise induced lactataemia in severe COPD. *Thorax* 2000;55:547-549.

22. Similowski T, Yan S, Gauthier AP, Macklem PT, Bellemere F. Contractile properties of the human diaphragm during chronic hyperinflation. *N Engl J Med* 1991;325:917-923.

24. Montes de Oca M, Celli BR. Respiratory muscle recruitment and exercise performance in eucapnic and hypercapnic severe chronic obstructive pulmonary disease. *Am J Respir Crit Care Med* 2000;161:880-885.

25. Smith K, Cook D, Guyatt GH, Madhoven J, Oxman AD Respiratory muscle training in chronic airflow obstruction. *Am Rev Respir Dis* 1992;145:533-539.

26. O'Donnell DE, Sanii R, Younes M. Improvement in exercise endurance in patients with chronic airflow limitation using CPAP. *Am Rev Respir Dis* 1988;138:1510-1514.

27. Petrof BJ, Calderini E, Gottfried SB. Effect of CPAP on respiratory effort and dyspnea during exercise in severe COPD. *J Appl Physiol* 1990;69:178-188.

28. Polkey MI, Kyroussis D, Mills GH, et al. Inspiratory pressure support reduces slowing of inspiratory muscle relaxation rate during exhaustive treadmill walking in severe COPD. *Am J Respir Crit Care Med* 1996;154:1146-1150.

29. Leaver DG, Pride NB. Flow volume curves and expiratory pressures during exercise in patients with chronic airflow obstruction. *Scand J Respir Dis* 1971;42(Suppl 1):23-27.

30. O'Donnell DE, Sanii R, Antonisen NR, Younes M. Effect of dynamic airway compression on breathing pattern and respiratory sensation in severe chronic obstructive pulmonary disease. *Am Rev Respir Dis* 1987;135:912-918.

31. O'Donnell DE, Sanii R, Antonisen NR, Younes M. Expiratory resistive loading in patients with severe chronic airflow limitation: an evaluation of ventilatory mechanics and compensatory responses. *Am Rev Respir Dis* 1987;136:102-107.

32. Dillard TA, Piantadosi S, Rajagopal KR. Prediction of ventilation at maximal exercise in chronic airflow obstruction. *Am Rev Respir Dis* 1985;132:230-235.

33. O'Donnell DE, Webb KA. Breathlessness in patients with severe chronic airflow limitation: physiologic correlates. *Chest* 1992;102:824-831.

34. Leblanc P, Bowie DM, Summers E, Jones NL, Killian KJ. Breathlessness and exercise in patients with cardio-respiratory disease. *Am Rev Respir Dis* 1986;133:21-25.

35. O'Donnell DE, McGuire M, Samis L, Webb KA. The impact of exercise reconditioning on breathlessness in severe chronic airflow limitation. *Am J Respir Crit Care Med* 1995;152:2005-2013.

36. O'Donnell DE, D'Arsigny C, Hollingworth EN, Webb KA. Oxygen reduces dynamic hyperinflation and improves exercise performance in hypoxic patients with COPD. *Am J Respir Crit Care Med* 2000;161:A753.

37. Light RW, Muro JR, Sato RI, Stansbury DW, Fischer CE, Brown SE. Effects of oral morphine on breathlessness and exercise tolerance in patients with chronic obstructive pulmonary disease. *Am Rev Respir Dis* 1989;139:126-133.

38. O'Donnell DE, Lam M, Webb KA. Measurement of symptoms, lung hyperinflation and endurance during exercise in chronic obstructive pulmonary disease. *Am J Respir Crit Care Med* 1998;158:1557-1565.

39. Chrystyn H, Mulley BA, Peak MD. Dose response relation to oral theophylline in severe chronic obstructive airways disease. *Br Med J* 1988;297:1506-1510.

40. Belman MJ, Botnick WC, Shin JW. Inhaled bronchodilators reduce dynamic hyperinflation during exercise in patients with chronic obstructive pulmonary disease. *Am J Respir Crit Care Med* 1996;153:967-975.

41. Martinez FJ, Montes de Oca M, Whyte RI, Stetz J, Gay SE, Celli BR. Lung-volume reduction improves dyspnea, dynamic hyperinflation and respiratory muscle function. *Am J Respir Crit Care Med* 1997;155:1984-1990.

42. O'Donnell DE, Sanni R, Giesbrecht G, Younes M. Effect of continuous positive airway pressure on respiratory sensation in patients with chronic obstructive pulmonary disease during submaximal exercise. *Am Rev Respir Dis* 1988;138:1185-1191.

43. Milic-Emili J. Inspiratory capacity and exercise tolerance in chronic obstructive pulmonary disease. *Can Respir J* 2000;7:282-285.

44. Diaz O, Villafranco C, Ghezzo H, Borzone G, Leiva A, Milic-Emil J, Lisboa C. Exercise tolerance in COPD patients with and without tidal expiratory flow limitation at rest. *Eur Respir J* 2000;16:269-275.

45. O'Donnell DE, Lam M, Webb KA. Spirometric correlates of improvement in exercise performance after anticholinergic therapy in COPD. *Am J Respir Crit Care Med* 1999;160:524-549.

46. Keilty SJ, Ponte J, Fleming TA. Effect of inspiratory pressure support on exercise tolerance and breathlessness in patients with severe stable chronic obstructive pulmonary disease. *Thorax* 1994;49:990-994.

47. Dolmage TE, Goldstein RS. Proportional assist ventilation and exercise tolerance in subjects with COPD. *Chest* 1997;111:948-954.

48. Bianchi L, Foglio K, Pagoni M, Vitacca M, Rossi A, Amgrosino N. Effect of proportional assist ventilation on exercise tolerance in COPD patients with chronic hypercapnia. *Eur Respir J* 1998;11:422-427.

49. Maltais F, Reissmann H, Gottfried SB. Pressure support reduces inspiratory effort and dyspnea during exercise in chronic airflow obstruction. *Am J Respir Crit Care Med* 1995;151:1027-1033.

50. Kyroussis D, Polkey MI, Hammegard G-H, Mills GH, Green M, Moxham J. Respiratory muscle activity in patients with COPD walking to exhaustion with and without pressure support. *Eur Respir J* 2000;15:649-655.

51. Younes M. Proportional assist ventilation. A new approach to ventilatory support: theory. *Am Rev Respir Dis* 1992;145:114-120.

52. Hernandez P, Maltais F, Gursahaney A. Proportional assist ventilation improves exercise performance in severe COPD. *Am J Respir Crit Care Med* 1996;153:A172.

53. Hernandez P, Maltais F, Gursahaney A, LeBlanc P, Navalesi P, Gottfried SB. Proportional assist ventilation (PAV) improves exercise performance in severe COPD. *Am J Respir Crit Care Med* 1996;153:A172.

54. Chrusch C, Baurele O, Younes M. The effect of proportional assist ventilation (PAV) on exercise endurance in COPD. *Am J Respir Crit Care Med* 1996;153:A171.

55. Shinder N, Webb KA, O'Donnell DE. Relief of exertional dyspnea during different modes of non-invasive ventilation in severe COPD. *Am Rev Respir Crit Care Med* 1997;155:A912.

# Chapter 12

# Oxygen in COPD Rehabilitation

Roger S. Goldstein, MD, Canada

Oxygen therapy is part of the continuum of care for the patient with COPD. Other components include: cessation of smoking, optimal pharmacological therapy, appropriate vaccinations, prompt attention to infectious exacerbations, supervised rehabilitation, education and psychosocial support as well as surgery for highly selected individuals. Compliance with oxygen therapy will be enhanced by psychosocial factors such as good coping skills, motivation, optimism and flexibility as well as the involvement of a supportive family. Patient and family education improves the understanding of the technical aspects of oxygen delivery and facilitates setting realistic goals and expectations (1). This article addresses the role of oxygen therapy in the rehabilitation of the patient with COPD.

## Life Saving Effects of Oxygen Therapy

In a study reported by the Nocturnal Oxygen Therapy Trial Group (2), 203 subjects were randomly allocated to continuous oxygen therapy (21-24 hours) or to nocturnal oxygen therapy (12 hours). Oxygen was administered to maintain the resting $PaO_2 > 60$ mmHg. The flow rate was increased by 1 litre/minute during exercise and sleep. The average patient was 66 years of age and had severe airflow limitation ($FEV_1 < 30\%$ predicted), a limited maximal exercise capacity (37 watts) and moderate pulmonary hypertension (mean pulmonary artery pressure 29 mmHg). The resting $PaO_2$ was 45 mmHg. After 12 months, 64 patients had died, 41 in the nocturnal oxygen therapy group and 23 in the continuous oxygen therapy group. Thus, the 12 month mortality was 21% for nocturnal oxygen therapy and 12% for continuous oxygen use. Several measures of quality of life and neuropsychological functioning improved in both treatment groups. In a second study, the British Medical Research Council (3), reported the results of a randomized controlled trial in which oxygen was given to hypoxemic patients for 15 hours a day. A randomly assigned control group received no oxygen. In 87 subjects with severe airway obstruction, pulmonary hypertension (mean pulmonary artery pressure 34 mmHg) and hypercapnia (mean $PaCO_2$ 51 mmHg), the between group mortality differed. In the treatment group 19 of the 42 patients died and in the control group, 30 of the 45 patients died.

These studies (figure 12.1 [4]) have provided evidence that sustained hypoxemia resulted in an increased morbidity and mortality presumably from target organ damage (erythrocytosis, pulmonary hypertension, cardiac and neuro-cognitive dysfunction). These effects were reversed by long term oxygen therapy with an attendant reduction in morbidity and mortality. As a result of these studies, oxygen therapy has been recommended by several professional societies and many countries have programs for providing domiciliary oxygen. Entry criteria usually include resting hypoxemia ($PaO_2 < 55$ mmHg and $SaO_2 < 88\%$) or $PaO_2$ 56-60 mmHg plus cor pulmonale, pulmonary hypertension or persistent erythrocytosis.

## Transient Exercise Hypoxemia in COPD—Should Oxygen be Prescribed for Rehabilitation?

A number of studies have demonstrated that many patients with a resting $SaO_2 > 90\%$ will exhibit transient exercise desaturation (5). These decreases in $SaO_2$ have been noted during physical activity levels

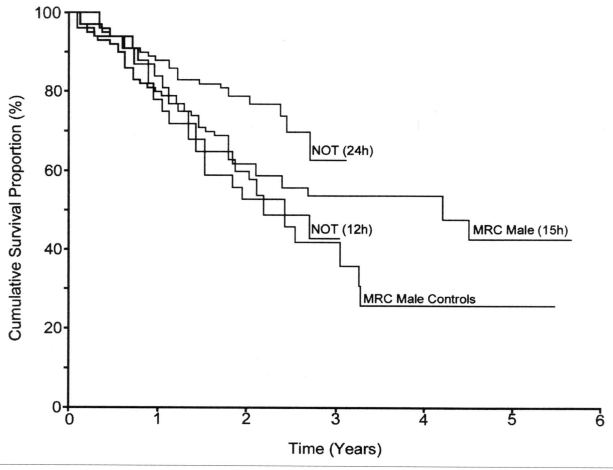

**Figure 12.1**    Combined data from the Nocturnal Oxygen Therapy (NOT) trial and the Medical Research Council (MRC) trial showing the improvement in survival proportional to the duration of oxygen therapy (h).
Reprinted, by permission, from CB Cooper, 1993, Long term oxygen therapy. In *Principles and practice of pulmonary rehabilitation*, edited by Casaburi and Petty (WB Saunders Company), 183-203.

comparable to those often encountered during activities of daily living (6). In a recent study by Garrod (7), 14 patients with COPD (FEV$_1$ 0.83 ± 0.28, PaO$_2$ 62 ± 9.2 mmHg), PaCO$_2$ 44 ± 6.4 mmHg) were randomized to a shuttle walk test while breathing room air or oxygen at 2 litres/minute. Walking saturation fell to 79.2 ± 8.6% with subjects breathing room air but with pulsed oxygen, the saturation fell to only 86 ± 7.4%. Subjects walked 189 ± 110 metres on room air and 208 ± 110 metres (p < 0.05) on oxygen. The dyspnea score did not change with oxygen. This study and a number of others addressed the benefits of acute oxygen therapy for patients with mild hypoxemia (8, 9, 10, 11).

One study (12) evaluated the factors contributing to the relief of exertional dyspnea during hyperoxia in COPD. Eleven subjects (FEV$_1$ 39% predicted, resting PaO$_2$ 74 ± 3 mmHg) exercised at 50%

$\dot{V}O_2$max while breathing room air or 60% oxygen. Oxygen was noted to improve saturation, decrease ventilation and decrease lactate levels. Oxygen was associated with reduced dyspnea and reduced leg effort at comparable exercise times. The decreased exertional symptoms and improved exercise endurance was noted to be in proportion to the decreased ventilation consequent upon improved peripheral muscle aerobic metabolism (12). Oxygen enabled some patients to achieve a level of exercise that has been associated with physiological training.

Many rehabilitation programs test patients with COPD for transient exercise desaturation. The patient exercises while breathing room air or oxygen in a randomized, single blind test. Saturation, heart rate, dyspnea, leg effort and endurance time are monitored.

# Training with Oxygen in COPD

Two recent studies have evaluated the influence of supplemental oxygen administered to COPD patients with hypoxemia during exercise. Rooyackers (13) asked whether supplemental oxygen during training advanced the effect of training. Twenty-four subjects (FEV$_1$ 29 – 31%, resting PaO$_2$ 75 – 78 mmHg, exercise saturation < 90%) undergoing inpatient rehabilitation (5 days a week for 10 weeks), were randomized to exercise on room air or supplemental oxygen at 4 litres/minute. Maximum workload, 6 minute walk test and quality of life improved in both groups (table 12.1). Training on oxygen did not confer additional benefit over training on room air.

Garrod (14) randomized 25 subjects (FEV$_1$ 0.76 ± 0.29, PaO$_2$ 63 ± 9 mmHg, PaCO$_2$ 47 ± 8 mmHg, exercise SaO$_2$ 82 ± 10.4%) to 6 weeks of exercise on 4L/min air (12 subjects) or oxygen (13 subjects). Oxygen improved the baseline shuttle walk test by 27.3 metres (14.7 – 39.8) and the dyspnea score fell –0.69 (-1.05 to -0.31). Post rehabilitation, dyspnea was reduced in the oxygen trained group (difference in Borg score –1.46 (-2.72 to -0.19)). However there was no difference between the groups in the shuttle walk test or in measures of quality of life (Chronic Respiratory Disease Index, the Hospital Anxiety Depression Scale and a locally developed Activities of Daily Living Scale). Supplemental oxygen during exercise training did little to enhance exercise tolerance although there was a small reduction in dyspnea in the group trained with oxygen.

# Home Oxygen for Dyspnea in COPD

In both of the above studies subjects underwent pulmonary rehabilitation with or without supplemental oxygen. A third study (15) evaluated the influence of oxygen or air given at home during activities that resulted in dyspnea. The authors wished to know whether the short-term benefits of supplemental oxygen during exercise could translate into improved health related quality of life. Twenty-six subjects (aged 73 ± 6 years, FEV$_1$ of 0.9 ± 0.4 L, PaO$_2$ 69 ± 9 mmHg, PaCO$_2$ 41 ± 3 mmHg) with exertional dyspnea, participated in a 12 week, double-blind, randomized cross-over assessment of air (6 weeks) versus oxygen (6 weeks) during activities (figure 12.2). At the end of the air phase and the oxygen phase, subjects demonstrated the acute effects of oxygen on the 6 minute walk distance. However, neither the 6 minute walk nor the Borg dyspnea score differed between the air and the oxygen groups. Health related quality of life did improve during the oxygen phase (compared with baseline), but this improvement did not reach statistical significance when compared with the air phase. Despite small acute benefits in exercise performance with oxygen, there were no longer term benefits in exercise tolerance, quality of life or respiratory symptoms after 6 weeks of oxygen used during activities (table 12.1). When asked which period they preferred, 50% of subjects chose the 6 week period on oxygen and the other 50% chose the 6 week period on air, or had no preference.

Consistent with the above, a recent study confirmed that patient preference was not a reliable

**Table 12.1   Single Stage Exercise Test and Activities of Daily Life Breathing Room Air Before and After Pulmonary Rehabilitation**

|  | Air training | | Oxygen training | |
| --- | --- | --- | --- | --- |
|  | Before | After | Before | After |
| Dyspnea | 15 ± 6 | 22 ± 5* | 16 ± 5 | 22 ± 6* |
| Fatigue | 17 ± 5 | 20 ± 5 | 16 ± 4 | 19 ± 4 |
| Emotional function | 32 ± 7 | 35 ± 9 | 30 ± 7 | 35 ± 6* |
| Mastery | 20 ± 4 | 23 ± 4* | 18 ± 6 | 22 ± 3* |
| Total score | 85 ± 16 | 100 ± 17* | 79 ± 18 | 98 ± 16* |

*p<0.01 within-group comparison before versus after rehabilitation

Reprinted, by permission, from JM Rooyackers et al., 1997, "Training with supplemental oxygen in patients with COPD and hypoxemia at peak exercise," *European Respiratory Journal* 10:1278-1284.

## Exertional Oxygen in COPD

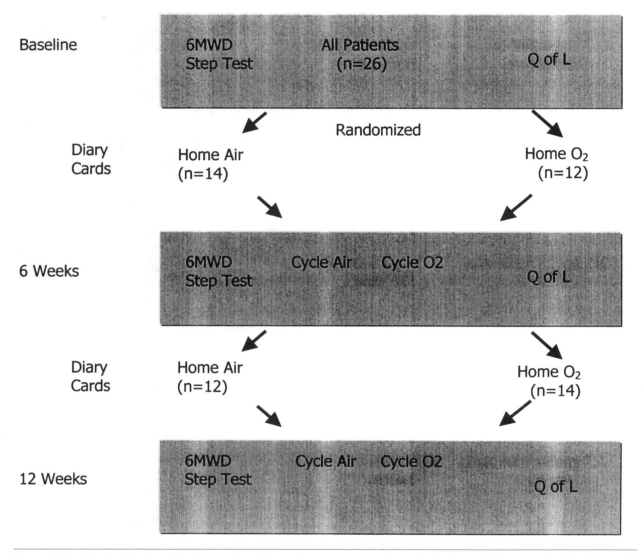

**Figure 12.2**  Study plan for 6 week periods of domiciliary oxygen or air used during activities associated with dyspnea. Cyl Air = Cylinder Air, Cyl O$_2$ = Cylinder O$_2$, QoL = Quality of Life.
CR McDonald et al., 1995, "Exertional oxygen of limited benefit in patients with chronic obstructive pulmonary disease and mild hypoxiemia," *American Journal of Respiratory and Critical Care Medicine* 152: 1616-1619. Official Journal of the American Thoracic Society © American Lung Association.

guide as to who might meet criteria for domiciliary oxygen. In an audit of a provincial domiciliary oxygen program (16) only 59% of 237 patients audited met accepted provincial criteria for long term oxygen therapy. The remaining 41% of patients receiving long term oxygen therapy did not have an accepted indication for it at the time of the audit. When patients were asked to comment on the sub-

jective benefits of home oxygen, the comments of those who met criteria could not be distinguished from the comments of those who did not. The results were as follows; very beneficial 82% vs 88%, moderately beneficial 16% vs 8%, slightly beneficial 2% vs 3%, no benefit 0% vs 1%. Thus, individuals experienced oxygen as beneficial irrespective of whether or not they met criteria.

**Table 12.2   Quality of Life With Oxygen or Air Used for Activities (6 Week Periods)**

|  | Dyspnea | Fatigue | Emotional function | Mastery |
|---|---|---|---|---|
| Baseline | 14 ± 5 | 13 ± 4 | 33 ± 9 | 17 ± 6 |
| Home air | 17 ± 6 | 15 ± 4 | 35 ± 9 | 19 ± 5† |
| Home O$_2$ | 19 ± 6* | 16 ± 4* | 36 ± 8* | 20 ± 6* |
| Maximum score | 35 | 28 | 49 | 28 |

*Home O$_2$ compared with baseline (p<0.02).

†Mastery improved with home air compared with baseline (p<0.03). There was no significant difference between oxygen and air.

CR McDonald et al., 1995, "Exertional oxygen of limited benefit in patients with chronic obstructive pulmonary disease and mild hypoxiemia," *American Journal of Respiratory and Critical Care Medicine* 152: 1616-1619. Official Journal of the American Thoracic Society © American Lung Association.

## Survival With Oxygen in Patients With COPD and Mild Hypoxemia

Another way of looking at the influence of oxygen for patients with mild hypoxemia is to evaluate its impact on survival. Góreka (17) reported the three year follow-up of 68 subjects who received long term oxygen therapy in whom the resting PaO$_2$ was 55 mmHg at the time of prescription. These subjects were compared with 67 control subjects with COPD who had similar lung mechanics but higher oxygen levels at rest (PaO$_2$ > 55 mmHg) and who therefore did not receive supplemental oxygen. There were 32 deaths among the control subjects and 38 deaths among those receiving oxygen. Survival was predicted by age, FEV$_1$ and body mass.

The characteristics of patients prescribed long term oxygen therapy outside of prescription guidelines between 1984 and 1995 (18) were reviewed by the Association Nationale pour le Traitement à Domicile de l'Insuffisance Respiratoire (ANTADIR). It

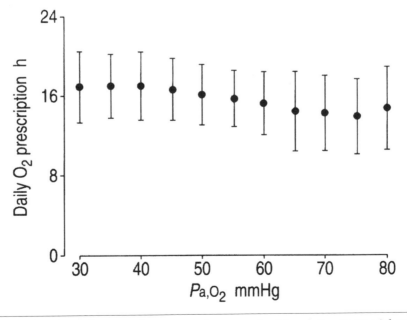

**Figure 12.3**   Variation in duration of oxygen therapy per day prescribed in relation to arterial oxygen tension (PaO²) (mean ± SD). (1 mmHg = 0.133 kPa). Note that the duration of therapy has no association with the resting oxygen tension.
Reprinted, by permission, from D Veale, E Chailleus, and A Taytard, 1998, "Characteristics and survival of patients prescribed long term oxygen therapy outside prescription guidelines," *European Respiratory Journal* 12: 780-784.

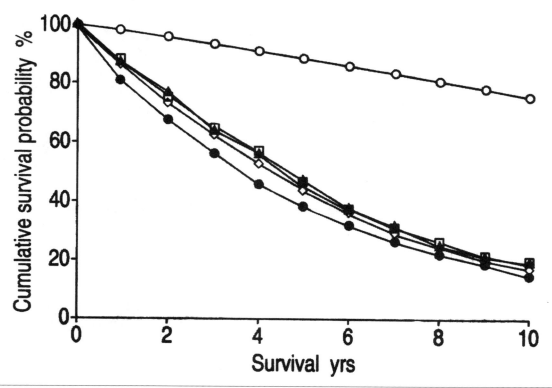

**Figure 12.4**   Cumulative probability of survival (yrs) at four different levels of arterial oxygen tensions (PaO²) at the time of prescription of long term oxygen therapy. Patients with PaO² < 50 mmHg had worse survival (p<0.001) than the other groups. ○: expected survival; □: PaO² 60 mmHg (8 kPa); ▲: PaO² 55-59 mmHg (7.3-7.9 kPa); (◊: PaO² 50-54 mmHg (6.7-7.2 kPa); ●: PaO² < 50 mmHg (6.6 kPa). (0.133 kPa =1 mmHg).
Reprinted, by permission, from D Veale, E Chailleus, and A Taytard, 1998, "Characteristics and survival of patients prescribed long term oxygen therapy outside prescription guidelines," *European Respiratory Journal* 12: 780-784.

was noted that patients with a resting $PaO_2$ > 60 mmHg at the time of prescription differed little from those with a $PaO_2$ < 60 mmHg. In fact, 18.5% of 7,700 patients on long term oxygen therapy had a $PaO_2$ > 60 mmHg at the time of prescription. The two groups were of similar age and lung function. Those with a $PaO_2$ < 60 mmHg had a slightly lower $PaCO_2$. Their oxygen prescription characteristics were similar, with most subjects being prescribed oxygen for just over 16 hours a day. Survival was similar between those with a $PaO_2$ > 60 mmHg and those with a $PaO_2$ of 55 – 59 mmHg. Survival only differed for the group with a resting $PaO_2$ < 50 mmHg.

## Summary

In summary, oxygen is known to be life prolonging for patients with COPD who have resting hypoxemia. Morbidity and mortality was reduced, presumably by reversing target organ damage especially to the heart and the pulmonary vasculature.

For patients with a resting $SaO_2$ > 90% who exhibited transient exercise hypoxemia, oxygen acutely reduced dyspnea and improved exercise tolerance. However, training with supplemental oxygen did not improve exercise duration or health related quality of life when compared with room air. Oxygen at home, used for activities that resulted in dyspnea did not improve exercise or quality of life. Retrospective studies of oxygen in mild hypoxemia, have not provided evidence of a survival benefit. The patient's subjective evaluation of the beneficial effects of oxygen was not a useful guide for identifying those who met evidence based criteria for the life prolonging effects of domiciliary oxygen therapy.

## References

1. Goldstein RS. "Supplemental oxygen in chronic respiratory disease." Pulmonary Rehabilitation: The Obstructive and Paralytic Conditions. Bach JR (Ed). Hanley and Belfus Inc. 1996;6:65-83.

2. Nocturnal Oxygen Therapy Trial Group. Continuous or nocturnal oxygen therapy in hypoxemic chronic obstructive lung disease. Annals of Internal Medicine 1980;93:391-398.

3. Report of the British Medical Research Council Working Party: Long term domiciliary oxygen therapy in chronic hypoxic cor pulmonale complicating chronic bronchitis and emphysema. Lancet 1981;1:681-686.

4. Cooper CB, Howard P. "Long term oxygen therapy" Principles and Practice of Pulmonary Rehabilitation. Casaburi R & Petty T (Eds). WB Saunders Company. 1993;15:183-203.

5. D'Urzo, AD, Mateika J. Bradley TD, et al: Correlates of arterial oxygenation during exercise in severe chronic obstructive pulmonary disease. Chest 1989;95:13-17.

6. Mak VHF, Bugler JR,. Roberts CM, et al. Effect of arterial oxygen desaturation on six minute walk distance, perceived effort and perceived breathlessness in patients with airflow limitation. Thorax 1993;48:33-38.

7. Garrod R, Bestall JC, Paul E, et al. Evaluation of a pulsed dose oxygen delivery during exercise in patients with severe chronic obstructive pulmonary disease. Thorax 1999;54:242-244.

8. Woodcock AA, Gross ER, Geddes DM. Oxygen relieves breathlessness in "Pink Puffers". Lancet 1981;1:907-909.

9. Davidson AC, Leach R, George RJD, et al. Supplemental oxygen and exercise ability in chronic obstructive airways disease. Thorax 1988;43:965-971.

10. Dean NC, Brown JK, Himelman RG, et al. Oxygen may improve dyspnea and endurance in patients with chronic obstructive pulmonary disease and only mild hypoxemia. Am Rev Respir Dis 1992;146:941-945.

11. Leach RM, Davidson AC, Chinn S, et al. Portable liquid oxygen and exercise ability in severe respiratory disability. Thorax 1992;47:781-789.

12. O'Donnell DE, Bain, DJ, Webb KA. Factors contributing to the relief of exertional breathlessness during hyperoxia in chronic airflow limitation. AJRCCM 1997;155:530-535.

13. Rooyackers JM, Dekhuijzen PNR, Van Herwaarden CLA, et al. Training with supplemental oxygen in patients with COPD and hypoxemia at peak exercise. ERJ 1997;10:1278-1284.

14. Garrod R, Paul EA, Wedzicha JA. Supplemental oxygen during pulmonary rehabilitation in patients with COPD with exercise hypoxemia. Thorax 2000;55:539-543.

15. McDonald CF, Blyth CM, Lazarus MD, et al. Exertional oxygen of limited benefit in patients with chronic obstructive pulmonary disease and mild hypoxemia. AJRCCM 1995;152:1616-1619.

16. Guyatt GH, McKim D, Austin P, et al. Appropriateness of domiciliary oxygen delivery. Chest 2000;118:1303-1308.

17. Góreka D, Gorzelak K, Sliwinski P, et al. Effect of long term oxygen therapy on survival in patients with chronic obstructive pulmonary disease with moderate hypoxemia. Thorax 1997;52:674-679.

18. Veale D, Chailleux E, Taytard A, et al. Characteristics and survival of patients prescribed long term oxygen therapy outside prescription guidelines. ERJ 1998;12:780-784.

PART V

# Home Rehabilitation Programs

# Chapter 13

# Case Management: Making Cardiovascular Risk Reduction Work In a Variety of Practice Settings

Kathy Berra, MSN, ANP, USA

## Introduction

Cardiovascular risk reduction involves the integration of medical and psychosocial therapies and lifestyle changes. The past 40 years have provided us with landmark scientific research defining the pathophysiology and management of diseases of the vascular system. Vascular biology, percutaneous interventions, innovative surgeries, new and more effective medications, advances in understanding the role of genetics, improved noninvasive assessment techniques and more effective lifestyle interventions have led the way in the reduction of death and disability from coronary heart disease (CHD) and stroke. It is through the systematic application of these advances and through continued scientific research that " evidence based practice guidelines" have been developed. The future of CHD and stroke prevention and treatment lies in the effective implementation of these guidelines. Effective implementation relies heavily on a systematic approach to risk reduction. Medical care systems such as employee wellness programs, health maintenance organizations, group practice settings, individual physician associations, cardiac rehabilitation programs and hospital-based clinics can provide such systems. Disease management is the term often used to describe such systems. Case management provides a fundamental approach to patient care in a disease management system.

Case management is the cornerstone of multiple risk reduction and provides an excellent model for vascular disease management (fig. 13.1). The vascular risk factors demand an integrated approach to medical and lifestyle management. Lifestyle skills will always remain the foundation of risk factor interventions, providing both important metabolic and psychosocial benefits (1).

## The Case for Case Management

Research is filled with successful models of case management. As early as the 1970's, case management was shown to be effective when compared to usual care. Case management for the treatment of vascular diseases is based on the following:

1. Population screening to identify persons at risk for disease
2. Risk stratification and triage of those identified
3. Institution of intensive risk reduction interventions based on clinical practice guidelines
4. Surveillance of safety, efficacy and adherence to risk reduction efforts
5. Measurement of medical outcomes and patient satisfaction
6. Systematic follow-up and institution of change in therapies as indicated

Usual care in the 21st century has been further complicated by reimbursement issues, lack of continuity in medical care resulting from an ever changing health care system, lack of continuity of health care providers, limited time with health care providers, and a focus on isolated "chief complaint" physician office visits. Thus effective disease management must rely on integrated approaches. Case management provides a model for vascular disease management by integrating patent, family, environment, lifestyle and community. Sueta et al. evaluated the degree of treatment of hyperlipidemia and congestive heart failure in patients with coronary artery disease (CAD) (2). This study reviewed patient billing records and audited medical charts in 140 predominately cardiovascular practices in the United States. A total of 58,890 outpatient records

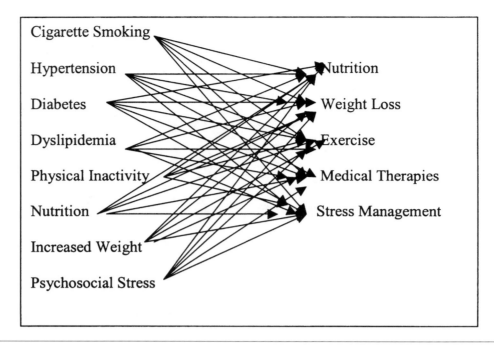

**Figure 13.1**   Relationships of the modifiable vascular disease risk factors.

were reviewed - 83% or patients had CAD, 28% had CHF and 10% had both CAD and CHF. All patients reviewed had at least two office visits recorded in a 12 month period between Jul 1, 1994 and October 1996. The findings are described in tables 13.1 and 13.2. It is important to note that this study revealed a large identification gap with 56% of patients not having a recent low density lipoprotein cholesterol (LDL-C) documented, 61% of patients not receiving lipid lowering therapy and only 25% of patients were at the NCEP II goal of < 100 mg/dL. In addition, patients with a documented LDL-C in their charts were 4 times more likely to receive therapy.

**Table 13.1   Aggregate Data (From Sueta et al., Ref 1)**

Total of 58,890 outpatient records reviewed

80% from cardiology-only practices

48,586 with CAD (83%)

16,603 with Heart Failure (28%)

10% of patients had both CAD and CHF

Minimum of 2 office visits within a 12-month period (last visit between July 1, 1994 and October 1, 1996)

**Table 13.2   CAD Summary (From Sueta et al., Ref 1)**

Large identification gap

56% of CAD patients did not have a recent LDL-C documented in their chart

Large treatment gap

61% of CAD patients were not receiving lipid-lowering therapy

LDL-C documentation

Patients with a documented LDL-C in their chart were 4 × more likely to receive therapy

Large treatment gap

Only 25% of CAD patients were at NCEP goal of <100 mg/dL

65% of CAD patients on statin therapy starting dose

The Lipid Treatment Assessment Project (L-TAP) evaluated the percentages of dyslipidemic patients receiving lipid-lowering therapy and achieving low density lipoprotein cholesterol (LDL-C) goals (3). In this study, Pearson et al. targeted primary care physician offices where patients with dyslipidemia were regularly seen. Participating physicians completed a survey regarding their demographic status, professional characteristics and practice profiles. Awareness and adherence to NCEP II guidelines was also assessed. In L-TAP, the primary outcome measured was the success rate of appropriately screened and stratified patients reaching NCEP II LDL-C levels. The results of this study are seen in tables 13.3 and 13.4. These results demonstrate that in primary care, as in specialty practices, a large gap exists in the achievement of LDL-C goals. These studies are pivotal in that they demonstrate clearly the need for improved models for health care delivery.

**Table 13.3   L-TAP (From Pearson et al., Ref 2)**

Approximately 95% of investigators indicated that they were aware of the NCEP guidelines and follow them in practice.

Furthermore, these investigators believe that LDL-C levels influence risk of CHD.

Nevertheless, only small proportions of patients are actually reaching LDL-C levels that the investigators consider desirable.

Therefore, the results of this survey suggest that factors other than knowledge of and attitude toward NCEP guidelines account for the low success rates.

**Table 13.4   L-TAP ~ Conclusion (From Pearson et al., Ref 2)**

The NCEP guidelines were originally formulated to reduce the risk of CHD as both primary and secondary prevention.

Landmark trials (4S, WOS, AFCAPS/TexCAPS) have reaffirmed the validity of these guidelines.

The L-TAP survey demonstrates that only 38% of patients being treated in community practice are achieving their LDL-C goals.

More aggressive treatment will be required if the NCEP treatment goals are to be achieved. This includes:

More use of drug therapy after failure of diet

More use of statins (relative to other lipid-lowering drugs)

Greater use of higher doses of drugs

What about studies that evaluate the benefits of case management? Aubert et al evaluated the difference between special intervention (nurse case management) and usual care over 12 months in primary care clinics in Jacksonville Florida (4). The case managers saw patients 4 times over 12 months and utilized biweekly phone follow-up regarding blood glucose control, medications, weight, exercise and nutrition. Primary care providers followed usual care patients. table 13.5 shows the benefit to both HgA1c as well as blood glucose control for the case managed patients.

Additional support for case management comes from the Butterworth Health System following an assessment of their revamped cardiac rehabilitation program (5). They focused on the integration of case management by using referral pathways, education sessions and intervention by social workers as indicated. In addition, they added regular phone call follow-up to assess the effectiveness of the risk reduction interventions. At one year, the case management group showed excellent risk reduction results. Seventy-seven percent were on lipid lowering medications, 78% reported exercising at least 3 days per week and 66% reported smoking cessation. Although these results are based on self-report, the case management model of care seems to support the benefit of this approach. Shaffer et al compared diet and medication management for patients with dyslipidemia managed by a specialized team versus those seen in Internal Medicine Clinics (6). Patients were seen by a special team of nurse case managers, pharmacists, nutritionists, psychologists and physicians versus usual care. At the end of the study period, changes in Total Cholesterol (TC) and LDL-C were improved in intervention versus usual care.

Two key studies the MUTIFIT Study and the Stanford Coronary Risk Reduction Project (SCRIP)

**Table 13.5   Nurse Case Management in Diabetic Patients (Aubert et al., Ref 5)**

|  | Intervention (N = 71) | UC (N = 67) | p |
|---|---|---|---|
| Change in HgA1c | -1.7 (9.0 → 7.3) | -0.6 (8.9 → 8.3) | <0.001 |
| Change in fasting BG | -48.3 (194 → 146) | -14.5 (191 → 176) | 0.003 |

also demonstrated the powerful effect of case management (7,8). MULTIFIT, is a randomized controlled trial of both men and women hospitalized for Acute Myocardial Infarction in Northern California. This study randomized patients to special risk reduction intervention (SI) by nurse case managers versus usual care (UC). The SI patients received education and counseling regarding smoking cessation, regular physical activity and nutrition. Medical management was instituted as indicated for risk factors not controlled by lifestyle change. Much of the intervention was mediated via phone and mail contact. Outcomes were measured at 6 months and one year and revealed what you might expect. The SI group had significant changes in functional capacity, smoking cessation and changes in LDL-C. This important case management study set the stage for the inclusion of case management into the Kaiser Permanente Health Care System, one of the largest Health Care Organizations in the Western States. At about the same time, the Stanford Coronary Artery Intervention Project (SCRIP) was funded by the National Institutes of Health to evaluate the efficacy of multifactor risk intervention, in men and women, as defined by quantitative coronary arteriography. This study utilized nurse case managers who supervised and coordinated the care. The case managers worked with a team of nutritionists, psychologists and physicians to provide clinical and lifestyle interventions, which brought participants to nationally, recognized goals for CVD risk factor reduction. The study was conducted over 4 years and was able to demonstrate angiographic benefit as measured by less progression and greater stabilization of plaque in the Special Intervention group compared to the Usual Care group. More striking, however, was the 46% benefit seen in the reduction of clinical coronary events in the SI group.

Fonarow et al recently published the results of the Cardiac Hospitalization Atherosclerosis Management Program (CHAMP) (9). In this study, the investigators attempted to evaluate the efficacy of a case management approach to discharge planning for persons admitted to the University of California at Los Angeles Medical Center with a diagnosis of CAD or other vascular diseases. The study was initiated in 1994 and followed a case management approach emphasizing the appropriate us of aspirin, cholesterol lowering, beta blockers and angiotensin converting enzyme inhibitors (ACEI). These interventions were applied in conjunction with exercise, nutrition and smoking cessation counseling. At the end of the study, medication utilization (table 6) was

analyzed for beta blockers, ACEI, Aspirin, Lipid lowering, antianginal therapies, and calcium channel blockers. Physiologic measures of efficacy for LDL-C were also measured. As can be seen from the results, appropriate risk factor modification can be integrated into existing hospital heath care systems. This data supports the potential for greater application of national guidelines in the acute care system which has the potential of improving outcomes and influencing long term adherence to risk reduction efforts.

An important model based on the case management model has been developed to disseminate aggressive CVD risk reduction programs. The HEAR$^2$T Program (Health Education and Risk Reduction Training Program) is based on the successes of the case management research of the 1980's and 1990's. The HEAR$^2$T model can be implemented at the worksite, within an existing health care organization, in a private medical practice, in a cardiac rehabilitation program and in other models of health care delivery. The HEAR$^2$T program is based upon the premise that CVD risk reduction is synergistic—and that greater benefit to atherosclerosis management will occur by reducing all of the lifestyle risk factors while integrating appropriate medical therapies.

The goals of the HEAR$^2$T program are to:

- Identify high risk persons for CHD and stroke within a care system.
- Implement risk reduction programs for those identified at high risk in a variety of settings.
- Utilize case management as the key method of applying risk reduction efforts.
- Provide effective therapies to reduce coronary risk factors through case management.
- Reduce death and disability from CAD and stroke through risk reduction efforts.
- Show measurable effects in health care utilization as a result risk reduction efforts.
- Have a high level of acceptance by participants and their health care providers.

The HEAR$^2$T Program has been successfully implemented in three demonstration projects. They included a worksite, an individual physician association and a large county employer. All three of these demonstration projects were successful in identifying the highest risk participants and involve them in a case management program lasting one year. In all three settings, the overall risk status of the individual participants were successfully reduced towards national goals.

**Table 13.6    CHAMP ~ Medical Regimen for Patients With Atherosclerosis (From Fonarow et al., Ref 8)**

Aspirin

Patients should continue on 81-325 mg aspirin/day indefinitely after discharge.

Cholesterol-lowering medications

Patients with CAD should be started on an HMG-CoA reductase inhibitor to lower cholesterol and treat the underlying atherosclerosis disease process. Starting dose should be the dose estimated to achieve and LDL < 100 mg/dL based on the lipid panel.

Beta blockers

These agents should be considered in all patients with CAD, because they reduce the risk of MI and make it more likely that a patient will survive an infarction. Use target doses as clinically tolerated.

ACE inhibitors

These agents have potent vascular and cardiac protective effects. These agents are potentially indicated in all patients with atherosclerosis. All patients with myocardial infarction without contraindications should be started on ACEIs within 24 hours and treated long term. Use target doses.

Nitrates

These agents should be considered second-line agents after b-blockers for the symptomatic control or angina. There is no long term data showing that nitrates improve prognosis in patients with CAD, so their use is simply for symptom relief.

Calcium antagonists

These agents decrease chest pain but do not decrease the risk of a cardiac event or improve survival. They should, in general, not be prescribed to patients with known CAD.

Antiarrhythmic agents

Type I antiarrhythmic agents increase the risk of sudden death in patients with CAD. These agents should be avoided in all patients with CAD except those with implantable cardioverter defibrillators or in whom the risk/benefit ratio has been carefully considered. Amiodarone should be considered the only safe antiarrhythmic agent in patients with CAD.

The HEAR²T Program was designed and implemented at the Stanford Center for Research in Disease Prevention. More information about this multiple risk reduction program can be found on the website at **www. stanfordheart.net**.

## Summary

Extensive data exists to support the importance of multiple risk reduction utilizing a case management approach. Systematic approaches involving case management will greatly aid in the:

- Identification of high risk persons for CHD and stroke
- Implementation of effective methods of multiple risk reduction
- Achievement of national goals for risk reduction therapies
- Reduction of morbidity and mortality from CHD and Stroke

Extensive research exists to support the safe and effective use of case management in the primary and secondary prevention of CHD and stroke. Models of care involve a team approach utilizing written, trans-telephonic and electronic education. Face to face medical visits can be streamlined to allow for individualized care as well as to assess compliance to interventions and plans for follow-up. Medical management should be based on nationally established goals for coronary risk reduction and stroke prevention. The lifestyle interventions for CHD and stroke prevention reach across all of the risk factors. Case management is ideally suited to deliver important lifestyle interventions both successfully and cost effectively.

# References

1. Ades P, Balady G, Berra K. Transforming Exercise-based Cardiac Rehabilitation Programs Into Secondary prevention centers: A national imperative. *J Cardiopulm Rehabil* 2001;21(5):263-272

2. Sueta CA, Chowlhury M, Boccuzzi SJ, Smith S, Alexander CM, Londle A, Lulla A, Simpson RJ. Analysis of the degree of undertreatment of hyperlipidemia and congestive heart failure secondary to coronary artery disease. *Am J Cardiol* 1999:83:1303-07.

3. Pearson TA, Laurora I, Chu H, Kafonek S. The lipid treatment assessment project (L-TAP): A multicenter survey to evaluate the percentages of dyslipidemic patients receiving lipid-lowering therapy and achieving low-density lipoprotein cholesterol goals. *Arch Intern Med* 2000. 28;160 (4):459-67.

4. Aubert RE, Herman WH, Waters J, Moore W, Sutton D, Peterson BL, Bailey CM, Koplan JP. Nurse case management to improve glycemic control in diabetic patients in a health maintenance organization. A randomized, controlled trial. *Ann Intern Med* 1998 Oct 15;129(8):605-12.

5. Levknecht L, Schrieffer J, Maconis B. Combining case management, pathways and report cards for secondary prevention. *Joint Commission Journal for Quality Improvement.* 1997;162-174.

6. Shaffer J, Wexler L. Reducing low-density lipoprotein cholesterol levels in an ambulatory care system. Results of a multidisciplinary collaborative practice lipid clinic compared with traditional physician-based care. *Arch Inter Med* 1995 Nov 27;155(21):2330-5.

7. DeBusk RF, Miller NH, Superko HR, Dennis CA, Thomas RJ, Lew HT, Berger WE 3rd, Heller RS, Rompf J, Gee D, et al. A case-management system for coronary risk factor modification after acute myocardial infarction. *Ann Intern Med* 1994;May 1;120(9):721-9.

8. Haskell WL, Alderman EL, Fair JM, Maron DJ, Mackey SF, Superko HR, Williams PT, Johnstone IM, Champagne MA, Krauss RM, et al. Effects of intensive multiple risk factor reduction on coronary atherosclerosis and clinical cardiac events in men and women with coronary artery disease. The Stanford Coronary Risk Intervention Project (SCRIP). *Circulation* 1994 Mar;89(3):975-90.

9. Fonarow GC, Gawlinski A. Rationale and Design of the Cardiac Hospitalization Atherosclerosis Management Program (CHAMP) University of California Los Angeles. *Am J Cardiol* 2000;85:10A-17A.

# Chapter 14

# COPD Rehabilitation:
# Maintenance on the Long Term

Jean-Marie Grosbois, MD, France

It is now well documented that the rehabilitation of patients suffering from chronic obstructive pulmonary disease (COPD) improves their exercise tolerance, dyspnea, and quality of life (1,2). Although these benefits are obvious at the beginning, it is important that patients be motivated to maintain these programs in order to consolidate or even improve the benefits acquired early on. This long term global care must be supervised by a multidisciplinary team and is currently the most important challenge of pulmonary rehabilitation. Ideally, this team should be coordinated by a respirologist, and include nurses, kinesitherapists, physical educators-exercise rehabilitation specialists, psychologists, nutritionists, patient associations, and recreational organizations. All aspects of rehabilitation such as exercise training, respiratory therapy, education, and psychosocial support, must be continued at home or in the community.

One possible limiting factor for the long term use of adapted physical activities without medical supervision is the risk of accidents or medical incidents. To lower this risk and identify possible contraindications such as myocardial ischemia, arrhythmias or hypertension, patients must have an exercise test with measurements of some cardiovascular and pulmonary parameters before even starting rehabilitation. Based on the results, the medical prescription of adapted physical activities can be personalized and adapted to the patient's characteristics with regard to targeted heart rates (at ventilatory threshold or 50-60% of $\dot{V}O_2$max) and / or to onset of dyspnea. To increase the likelihood of long term maintenance, activities must also be diversified and playful, and they must take into account patient's preferences and on site possibilities. These activities can be done under the supervision of trained personnel, or even in a completely non-medical environment for less severely ill patients.

One of the most important aspect of patient education is to provide her or him with a better perception of its own limitations so that he or she can suspend exercise training in the presence or even fear of clinical instability (chest pain, fever, infection, uneasiness . . .). One other important question yet to be answered concerns the safety and efficiency of home rehabilitation versus rehabilitation supervised in in- or out-patient facilities.

Walking is one of the easiest forms of activity because it can be done at home, it is cheap, and it does no require any special learning skill. In several studies, walking has been suggested as the main activity for short term home rehabilitation. In four of those studies (3-6), patients were aged 61 to 73, they had a $FEV_1$ of about 40% of predicted, and the exercise sessions lasted 20 to 60 minutes, for 10 to 12 weeks. Supervision to monitor and if necessary to readjust training intensity, motivate patients, or modulate self management was done through weekly or biweekly visits to the center. Exercise intensity was determined by the patient's tolerance (3,4) at 70% of maximal level reached in the shuttle run test (5) or at a walking speed of 3-4 km · hr⁻¹ (2-2.5 mph) with a pedometer. (6) No accidents nor incidents were reported and compliance to the training regimen was reported as being be very good. Efficiency was evidenced by increased distances on the 6 minute walking test (3) or shuttle run rest (4), increased power output on the clinical exercise test (3, 6), increased endurance time (5), and improved dyspnea (5,6) and quality of life. (4-6) In one study, Wedzicha et al. were unable to document improvements in exercise tolerance or quality of life in the most dyspneic of their patients (MRC: 5) (4), probably because the training intensity was too low.

Currently, the cycle ergometer is the most commonly suggested mode of exercise because it allows for a precise personalized exercise prescription. The

119

cycle is however expensive to buy and on the long run, this form of exercise may not be so attractive to patients. In the six studies where it was proposed for home exercise (7-12), patients were aged 60 to 66 and had a $FEV_1$ ranging from 30 to 66% of predicted. The duration of exercise was 20 to 45 min. and the sessions were done 2 to 7 times a week for 10 to 12 weeks. The initial exercise intensity was 50-60 percent of the maximal power output as determined by the clinical exercise test and supervision was done by kinesitherapists (10), nurses (11), kinesitherapists and nurses (7-9), or simply through the phone (12). The efficiency of exercise was documented by improved walking distance on the 6 minute walking test (10,12), increased maximal power output (9,12) or $\dot{V}O_2$max (9,11,12) improved dyspnea (9-11), and quality of life (7,10). Again, no accident nor incident were reported and it is worth noting that the sickest patients (24 individuals with mean $FEV_1$ of 30% predicted, referred for lung reduction surgery) were only supervised by phone once a week (12). In general, exercise was started after 2 to 3 days of hospitalization where, in addition to clinical and para-clinical evaluation, teaching of exercise training techniques and education were provided.

Skeletal muscle strengthening can also be done fairly easily by most patients. In 1996, Clark et al. showed that this type of training improves muscle strength and endurance as well as ventilation at submaximal work loads (13). They used 10 simple exercises designed for upper and lower limbs and each exercise was repeated, as many times as possible over 30 to 60 seconds for a period of 12 weeks. In several studies, skeletal muscle strengthening was associated to exercise training on a cycle ergometer or to walking, so that the exact type of activity being studied is not clear (4,12,14).

When adjusted for COPD patients and personalized in terms of frequency, intensity and duration, all of these activities produce, initially at least, some improvement in exercise tolerance, dyspnea and quality of life. It therefore seems reasonable to enroll patients with moderately severe to severe COPD, in home based rehabilitation programs that are likely to be efficient while being at low risk providing the patient is stable and has previously benefited from preparation in a specialized center. Excluding safety considerations, would such a program still be efficient on the long run?

It is well documented that irrespective of age (15), aerobic capacity correlates well with daily physical activity and that any stoppage of physical activity even for a few weeks may bring about a decrease in work capacity (16,17). These findings emphasize the importance of maintaining regular physical activities for long periods of time specially for patients who have adopted a sedentary life style for many years, or for those who experience regularly respiratory difficulties that may keep them in bed for several days at the time.

Several studies have looked at the long term evolution of benefits acquired after community based (14,18,19,21,22) or home based (7,9,20), pulmonary rehabilitation programs. In these studies, patients were aged 60 to 68, their $FEV_1$ varied from 32 to 40% of predicted, and the follow up period was between 12 to 18 months. Supervision was done as usual or through specialized consultations, 2 to 3 times a year. In some cases, the patient was on its own most of the time (14,18,19,21), while at other times there were weekly (7,8,18,22) or monthly (7,8,14) feedbacks by a kinesitherapist and/or a nurse. The purposes of these latter interventions were to stimulate patient motivation and education as well as making sure that all patients had a personalized program. Overall, the results show improved exercise tolerance but irrespective of the type of test used (walking test, clinical exercise test (power output and/or $\dot{V}O_2$max), endurance test), the values are lower than those recorded at the end of the inpatient program (7-9,14,18,19,21,22). Further, the values are also lower than what they were at the time of the initial evaluation of control patients (7-9,14,19,22) or of those patients who stopped exercising after an outpatient program (18). Independent of the questionnaire used (Saint-George or CRDQ) the overall results show a significant improvement after outpatient rehabilitation, and this improvement is still significant at 12 and 18 months (8,14,19,21,22). The level of dyspnea also improved (7,9,18,22) but well being, anxiety, and depression (HAD, Hospital Anxiety Depression) did not (14).

The review of economic data also indicates that there are significant decreases in the number of visits to the physician (19) or to emergency rooms (20), in exacerbations (20-22), and in days of hospitalization (19-21) when compared to what it had been previously (21) or to control groups (19,20,22). Some investigators have also reported that a decrease in the number of days in hospital (14,22-24) was an important factor in lowering the long term costs of treating COPD patients. What may be more important is the fact that the calculated ratio cost/benefit makes these inpatient programs attractive because overall costs are lower and benefits higher than they would be if there was no rehabilitation at all. Considering these results, the next question to be asked is what type of program should be recommended to maintain the benefits acquired during the initial intervention?

Although it is difficult to compare different types of interventions, there appears to be no significant difference at 18 months in either exercise tolerance as measured by the 6 minute walking test and quality of life between patients having been supervised once a week or once a month (7,8) In 1996, Strijbos et al. reported however that patients who initially participated in a home program had better results at 18 months than those registered in an outpatient program (9). In a nonrandomized prospective study, we also showed that patients who elected to come back once a week in our community based program still maintained at 18 months better values for $\dot{V}O_2$max and power output (watts) than what they were at the end of the inpatient program. Patients who choose to come twice a week had similar results. By contrast, patients who stopped all regular physical activities had values that were lower than those recorded at the initial time of evaluation (18). Wijkstra et al (7) and Strijbos et al (9) hypothesized that patients for whom physical activities are initiated at home may be more motivated to maintain a certain level of activity than those where the same activities have been initiated in the hospital. These patients are also more likely to benefit from positive family involvement. We finally believe that the motivation of patients choosing their autonomy or of those who visit us once or twice a week is an important determinant of their continued adherence to physical activity and therapeutic compliance. Patients coming back twice a week have been found to be very dependent on the professional team.

Patient and team's motivation, and frequency of follow up visits are not the only predictors of good long term results. Indeed, there is some evidence to suggest that lack of compliance with pulmonary rehabilitation may not be solely related to clinical parameters, but also to socio-economical factors. Patients that are divorced, or are living alone, smokers, patients not taking inhaled corticoids, or patients not satisfied with medical services, are less inclined to start or maintain for some time this type of intervention (25). Similar predictors for home compliance to respiratory therapy include perceived therapeutic efficiency, dyspnea, and severe obstructive ventilatory disorders (26).

We think that patient education and psychosocial support are paramount to improve long term quality of life. This can be done by compliance with medical treatment and daily physical activities, and by a return to social and leisure activities that may

have been abandoned over the years. This type of multidisciplinary and multifactorial approach has proven to be beneficial in other chronic illnesses such as diabetes and asthma but to our knowledge, such extensive interventions have not been done in COPD patients. This is why the multicenter program of Bourbeau et al (20) should be considered a landmark. In that program, the educational interventions were made of 7 learning modules, which were taught at home by a team especially trained on pedagogical techniques. That program also provided counseling as how to go back to daily physical activities. At one year follow-up, patients in the intervention group improved their quality of life, and lowered the number of days in hospital, and number of emergency room visits when compared to a control group receiving the usual care. Thus interventions based on patient education can lead to better quality of life and less hospitalizations. Further, personalized physical activity programs are likely to also improve exercise tolerance.

It is now well documented that return to daily physical activities initially improves exercise tolerance, dyspnea, and quality of life, and that these benefits can be maintained for at least 12-18 months. Like many other investigators (4,12,20), we are convinced that a global approach centered on the patient, its education and appropriate psychosocial support, will prolong and likely further improve the benefits obtained through short duration interventions.

It can be stated, in conclusion, that management of chronic diseases is different than that of acute illnesses and that specific training must be offered to health care professionals involved in long term management of COPD patients. Further studies will however be needed to identify the best possible follow up procedures based on the severity of disease and associated illnesses. These procedures must also be adjusted to the patient's personal situation.

# References

1. Lacasse Y, Wong E, Guyatt G; King D, Cook D, Goldstein R: Meta-analysis of respiratory rehabilitation in chronic obstructive pulmonary disease. *Lancet* 1996; 26: 1115-1119.
2. A.T.S. Pulmonary Rehabilitation. Medical section of the american lung association. *Am J Respir Crit Care Med* 1999; 159: 1666-1682.
3. Mc Gavin, Gupta SP, Lloyd EL, Mc Hardy GJR: Physical rehabilitation for the chronic bronchitis:

results of a controlled trial of exercises in the home. *Thorax* 1977; 32: 307-311.

4. Wedzicha JA, Bestall JC, Garrod R, Garnham R, Paul EA, Jones PW: Randomized controlled trial of pulmonary rehabilitation in severe chronic obstructive pulmonary disease patients, stratified with the MRC dyspnoea scale. *Eur Respir J* 1998; 12: 363-369.

5. Hernandez MTE, Rubio TM, Ruiz FO, Riera HS, GIL RS, Gomez JC: Results of home based training program for patients with COPD. *Chest* 2000; 118: 106-114.

6. Puente-Maestu L, Sanz ML, Sanz P, Cubillo JM, Mayol J, Casaburi R: Comparison of effects of supervised versus self monitored training programmes in patients with chronic obstructive pulmonary disease. *Eur Respir J* 2000; 15: 517-525

7. Wijkstra PJ, Ten Vergert E.M., Van Altena R. et al. Long term benefits of rehabilitation at home on quality of life and exercise tolerance in patients with COPD. *Thorax* 1995; 50: 824-828.

8. Wijkstra PJ, Van Der Mark TW, Kraan J, Van Altena R, Koeter GH, Postma DS. Long term effects of home rehabilitation on physical performance in chronic obstructive pulmonary disease. *Am J Respir Crit Care Med* 1996; 153: 1234-1241.

9. Strijbos JH, Postma DS, Van Altena R, Gimeno F, Koeter GH: A comparison between an outpatient hospital based pulmonary rehabilitation program and a home care pulmonary rehabilitation program in patients with COPD. A follow-up of 18 months. *Chest* 1996; 109: 366-372.

10. Cambach W, Chadwick-Straver RVM, Wagenaar RC, Van Keimpema ARJ, Kemper HCG: The effects of a community-based pulmonary rehabilitation programme on exercise tolerance and quality of life: a randomised controlled trial. *Eur Respir J* 1997; 10: 104-113.

11. Larson JL, Covey MK, Wirtz SE, et al.: Cycle ergometer and inspiratory muscle training in chronic obstructive pulmonary disease. *Am J Respir Crit Care Med* 1999; 160: 500-507.

12. Debigaré R, Maltais F, Whittom F, Deslauriers J, Leblanc P: Feasibility and efficacy of home exercise training before lung volume resection. *J Cardiopulmonary Rehab* 1999; 19: 235-241.

13. Clark CJ, Cochrane L, Mackay E: Low intensity peripheral muscle conditioning improves exercise tolerance and breathlessness in COPD. *Eur Respir J* 1996; 9: 2590-2596.

14. Ries AL, Kaplan RM, Limberg TM, Prewitt LM: Effects of pulmonary rehabilitation on physiologic and psychosocial outcomes in patients with chronic obstructive pulmonary disease. *Ann Inter Med* 1995, 122: 823-832.

15. Berthouze S, Minaire P, Castells J, Busso T, Vico L, Lacour JR: Relationship between mean habitual daily energy expenditure and maximal oxygen uptake. *Med Sci Sports Exerc* 1995; 2:1170-1179.

16. Saltin B, Blomqvist G, Mitchell JH et al.: Response to exercise after bed rest and after training. *Circulation* 1968; 38 (Suppl 7):1-78.

17. Coyle EF, Martin WH, Sinacore DR, Joyner MJ, Hagberg JM, Holloszy JO: Time course of loss of adaptations after stopping prolonged intense endurance training. *J Appl Physiol* 1984; 57: 1857-1864.

18. Grosbois JM, lamblin C, Lemaire B et al.: Long term benefits of exercise maintenance after out patient rehabilitation program in patients with chronic obstructive pulmonary disease. *J Cardiopulm Rehabil* 1999; 19: 216-225.

19. Griffiths TL, Burr ML, Campbell IA, et al.: Results at 1 year of outpatient multidisciplinary pulmonary rehabilitation: a randomised controlled trial. *Lancet* 2000; 355: 362-368.

20. Bourbeau J et al.: Integrating rehabilitative elements into a COPD self management program reduces exacerbations: A randomized clinical trial. *Am J Respir Crit Care Med* 2000; 161(3): A254.

21. Foglio K, Bianchi L, Bruletti G, Battista L, Pagani M, Ambrosino N: Long term effectiveness of pulmonary rehabilitation in patients with chronic airway obstruction. *Eur respir J* 1999; 13: 125-132.

22. Guell R, Casan P, Belda J, et al.: Long term effects of outpatient rehabilitation of COPD. A randomised trial. *Chest* 2000; 117: 976-98.

23. Sneider R, O'Malley JA, Kahn M: Trends in pulmonary rehabilitation at Eisenhower Medical Center: An 11-years' experience. *J Cardiopulmonary Rehabil* 1988; 11: 453-461.

24. Hodgkin JE: Benefits and the future of pulmonary rehabilitation. In Hodgkin JE, Celli BR, Connors GL, eds. Pulmonary rehabilitation: Guidelines to success. Lippincott Williams Wilkins, 2000: 693-710.

25. Young P, Dewse M, Fergusson W, Kolbe J: Respiratory rehabilitation in chronic obstructive pulmonary disease: Predictors of nonadherence. *Eur respir J* 1999; 13: 855-859.

26. Turner J, Wright E, Mendella L, Anthonisen N, and the IPPB Study Group: Predictors of patients adherence to long term home nebulizer therapy for COPD. *Chest* 1995; 108: 394-400.

# PART VI

# Cardiopulmonary Rehabilitation and Cardiac and Thoracic Surgery

# Chapter 15

# Rehabilitation in Thoracic Surgery

Jean Deslauriers, MD, Canada

In the 1960's, many centers across North America and Europe began to include rehabilitation as an integral part of the management of patients with chronic obstructive pulmonary disease (COPD). Striking improvements were noted after exercise training and it soon became clear that exercise tolerance and quality of life (QL) could be optimized through formal rehabilitation. In addition, rehabilitation programs could integrate a comprehensive approach to management that included patient education, energy conservation, relaxation, nutrition, and psychosocial counseling.

As a result, patients undergoing surgical procedures for emphysema whether lung volume reduction surgery (LVRS) or lung transplantation have also been asked to participate in formal rehabilitation programs. Indeed, several institutions will not operate on a patient without his active participation in programs where the focus is on the teaching of proper breathing exercises, pulmonary toilet, upper body strengthening, and nutritional repletion. In most of these centers, formal pulmonary rehabilitation is continued postoperatively where it is used to improve exercise tolerance and chest wall mechanics.

Rehabilitation of patients with COPD who are to undergo pulmonary resection for lung cancer is based on similar objectives but is currently done in very few centers across North America. The ultimate goal of these programs is to improve patient's endurance and likelihood of normal postoperative recovery.

This paper will review the principles of rehabilitation as they apply to patients scheduled to undergo a major thoracic surgical procedure.

## Objectives of Pulmonary Rehabilitation

The goals of pulmonary rehabilitation, according to the American Thoracic Society (1), are to lessen airflow limitation, to prevent and treat secondary medical complications such as hypoxemia and infections, and to decrease respiratory symptoms and improve quality of life. With the advent of physiological operations designed for patients with end-stage COPD as well as an increase in the number of lung cancer resections done in patients with severe pulmonary dysfunction, the role of pulmonary rehabilitation undertakes a fourth major objective not addressed in the American Thoracic Society statement (2). Its goal prior to thoracic surgical intervention is to improve patient's endurance and emotional health in the hope that these improvements will translate into greater likelihood of normal postoperative period. Stated differently, the assumption is that if the patient is in better physical condition preoperatively, it is less likely that he will suffer from major postoperative complications.

After LVRS, pulmonary rehabilitation is deemed necessary so that patients can relearn how to breathe efficiently and use atrophied respiratory muscles again. For these individuals, the functional gains after surgery are fewer without rehabilitation regardless of any improvement seen in pulmonary function studies. These patients are expected to maintain their pulmonary fitness for the rest of their lives.

# Rehabilitation Prior to Lung Cancer Surgery

## Background

Lung cancer is currently the most common malignancy in men and women and approximately 175,000 new cases are diagnosed each year in the US (3). Of these, 70,000 are limited to the chest and therefore potentially operable. Since most of these patients are smokers, Olsen (4) has estimated that 80 to 90% of them have COPD and that 20 to 30% have severe disease. In numerous studies, COPD patients have been found to be at higher risk for postoperative morbidity and death.

## Approaching the High Risk Patient

In approaching the high risk patient, judgement and experience are paramount in assessing the risks of operation versus its benefits. Unfortunately, the numbers tell only part of the story. A carefully obtained clinical history and physical examination with particular detail to the patient's overall activity level, stamina, and motivation are important.

Over the years, many combinations of parameters such as forced expiratory volume in one second ($FEV_1$), forced vital capacity (FVC), and diffusion capacity (DLCO) have been used to assess patients. Unfortunately, these traditionally used criteria only have a modest ability to predict risk. In addition, there has never been unanimity as regards to which of there values are absolute contraindications to resection. In some situations where the tumor is located in an emphysematous lobe, for instance, a combination of cancer resection and LVRS may result in an appropriate cancer operation and improved pulmonary function.

Exercise testing has also become increasingly popular to assess operative risk. The implication being that if the results of the test correlate well with morbidity, the risks of postoperative complications may be reduced if exercise tolerance is maximized preoperatively.

One of the first publications on the role of exercise testing in the preresectional evaluation of risk from pneumonectomy is that of van Nostrand and colleagues (5). In their study, patients who could not tolerate climbing one flight of stairs without severe dyspnea had a postoperative mortality of 50% versus 10% for those with better tolerance. Other studies have since correlated positively the ability to climb two or three flights of stairs to reduced postoperative morbidity rates (4,6).

In an attempt to improve the preoperative assessment of patients with impaired pulmonary function, more formalized exercise tests have been shown to provide better insight into the outcome after resection. In 1987, Bechard and Wetstein (7) tried to correlate exercise $O_2$ consumption ($M\dot{V}O_2$) with postoperative morbidity and mortality. Stratification on the basis of exercise performance showed a 29% mortality and a 43% morbidity in patients with a $M\dot{V}O_2$ less than 10 ml/kg/min. Patients with an $M\dot{V}O_2$ less than 20 but greater than 10 ml/kg/min had a 10,7 % morbidity and there were no deaths. No patients with an $M\dot{V}O_2$ greater than 20 ml/kg/min sustained any morbidity or died (p < 0.001). In a similar study, Bolliger et al. (8) showed that maximal oxygen uptake ($\dot{V}O_2$ max)< 60% of predicted was highly predictive of complications in lung resection candidates whereas a $\dot{V}O_2$ max value > 75% of predicted was an excellent predictor of an uneventful postoperative course irrespective of the extent of resection.

In 1997, Ninan et al (9) reported on the use of an easily performed standardized exercise oxymetry outpatient test which they used to assess patients undergoing lung resection. Room air oxymetry was measured at rest and during exercise on a stair-stepper apparatus which provided uniform resistance to stepping. Oxygen saturation was noted at 10, 20, and 30 steps considered to be the equivalent of 3 flights of stairs. Resting saturation less than 90% or desaturation greater than or equal to 4% during exercise significantly predicted longer intensive care unit stay (p = 0.0002) and incidence of major morbidity. In a similar study from Toronto (10) Rao et al. compared the relative ability of standardized exercise oxymetry and FEV1 to predict morbidity and mortality after lung resection. Exercise oxymetry more reliably predicted home oxygen requirements (p < 0.001), need of admission to the intensive care unit (p < 0.05), prolonged hospital stay (p <0.01), and respiratory failure (p < 0.05).

## Rationale of Rehabilitation

There are many opinions on this subject but only one randomized trial has ever been conducted (11). In that trial, patients were first identified as high risk by their pulmonary function studies. Group I received aggressive pre- and postoperative pulmonary care and group II received the standard of care. The group that received aggressive pulmonary care intervention had less morbidity compared with the non-aggressive group.

The main goal of rehabilitation is to increase patient's endurance and exercise performance via exercise training. This increase is likely to result in more effective cough and increased respiratory muscle strength which in turn will lead to a lower incidence of major postoperative events. Other important components of preoperative rehabilitation in lung cancer patients include optimization of medication management, nutrition, and psychosocial support. If the patient is a current smoker, immediate cessation of smoking and delay of surgery for at least 3-4 weeks should be undertaken. It is to be noted that this delay in surgery is unlikely to significantly reduce chances for a long-term cure.

## Components of Rehabilitation

In most centers that have rehabilitation programs for patients undergoing lung cancer surgery, preoperative evaluation includes the six minute walk test where the patient walks as far as he can during the allotted time. A record is made of the distance covered, number of steps, oxygen saturation, heart rate, and oxygen requirements. The stair climbing test is done by having the patient climb two flights or as many steps as he can. Patients are monitored with continuous oxymetry and supplemental oxygen is administered if necessary to maintain saturation above 88% (12). If a patient desaturates despite a six liter canula, an oxygen reservoir device (oxymizer) is used to deliver increased oxygen delivery during inspiration (12). In St. Louis, the patient also rates the intensity of each exercise with perceived exaction scale which is a modified Borg scale with numbers from 6 to 20.

Most rehabilitation programs for patients awaiting lung cancer surgery are home based. The duration and intensity of exercise training depends on the severity of the COPD, patient conditioning and motivation, level of apprehension and anxiety and sensitivity to sensation of dyspnea. The form of exercise is directed toward activities that involve large muscles or that mimic activities that the patient does every day (13). For instance, patients are instructed to walk rather than cycle and activities involving upper extremities such as lifting are considered less

important. Patients are provided with a log book where they can record dates of exercise, distances walked, and heart rate.

Occasionally, patients will be referred to a supervised pulmonary rehabilitation program for a period of 3-8 weeks preoperatively. In such cases, exercise guidelines include having the patient exercise at least 5 days per week with the goal of thirty minutes of continuous walking on the treadmill.

# Rehabilitation Prior to Surgery for End-Stage Lung Disease

## Background

Historically, application of giant bullae was the first operation advocated for the relief of dyspnea in COPD patients. Patients were improved if the bulla occupied at least one third of the volume of the hemithorax and was compressive of adjacent lung. Better results were also obtained if the underlying emphysema was not too severe and if the compressed lung had potential for function as documented by adequate perfusion (14) and dynamic ventilation. Although a number of authors have reported improvements in lung volume flow rates, dyspnea, and exercise tolerance postoperatively, indications for bullectomy are infrequent mostly because the ideal candidate is seldom seen.

On the contrary, generalized non bullous emphysema is a progressive, disabling disease that affects almost two million people in the United States (15). Its prevalence is rising, especially among women whose tobacco usage has steadily increased since World War II. The prognosis of patients with COPD is related to a number of factors including decreasing FEV1 on serial testing. In patients with severe disease characterized by an FEV1 less than 30% of predicted, the 1-year and 5-year survival rates average 90% and 40% respectively (16-18). In addition to poor survival, the consequent need for repeated admissions to hospital and ongoing supervision have resulted in a major impact on the utilization of health care resources. Fortunately, these figures have led to new modes of therapy both medical and surgical. Controlled trials of graded exercise, for instance, have demonstrated significant improvements in exercise tolerance and capacity, and dyspnea (19-23). In one such trial, Goldstein et al (22) evaluated the effects of 2 months of intensive rehabilitation followed by a further 4 months of out-patient supervision in patients with COPD. When compared to a control group who received conventional community care, patients who underwent rehabilitation experienced significant improvements in their exercise tolerance as measured by the 6-minute walk test (p = 0.0067), subjective dyspnea (p=0.0061), fatigue (p = 0.0507), and emotional function (p = 0.0150). There is also some evidence that a patient's quality of life and sense of well-being are enhanced as a result of rehabilitation although important improvements may not occur in either spirometric values or gas exchange indices (21,23,24-26).

In 1957, Brantigan and Mueller (27) reported the procedure of LVRS as an innovative surgical approach for the management of emphysema. The operation was aimed at reducing lung volume by resecting functionless tissue. The objective was that the improved elastic recoil of the remaining smaller lung would enhance ventilation by placing the muscles of respiration such as the diaphragm and intercostals at an improved mechanical advantage. The procedure was soon abandoned because of high operative mortality but was resurrected in 1995 by Cooper (28) who did so after careful meticulous planning and thought (29). His initial report on 20 patients showed that after bilateral LVRS, the mean FEV1 improved by 82%, residual volume (RV) was significantly reduced, and patients noted a marked relief in dyspnea, improvement in QL, and exercise tolerance. Since then, the results of numerous studies have been reported and, at present, enough data is available to demonstrate that LVRS can be performed with acceptable morbidity and mortality, and that it improves the respiratory status and QL in end-stage emphysema patients, at least in the short term (30).

Lung transplantation has also become a viable option for some patients with COPD with two-year survival rates now exceeding 75%. Unfortunately, the shortage of donor organs and the age restriction renders transplantation inaccessible to most COPD patients.

## Rationale of Rehabilitation

Preoperative rehabilitation is the norm at most centers performing LVRS and indeed it is considered in some institutions as the most important component of the entire program of LVRS (31). Often surgery is refused to patients who are unable to complete preoperative rehabilitation or are unable to achieve the targeted goals. In 1996, Cooper also stated that a final decision to proceed with the operation (LVRS) is only made after satisfactory completion of the rehabilitation program (32).

In 1997, Kesten (2) nicely summarized the rationale for the use of rehabilitation before LVRS (Table 15.1).

In general, the primary goal of preoperative rehabilitation is to improve the strength and aerobic conditioning of patients, making surgery less traumatic and postoperative recovery faster. Some patients might improve with exercise to such a degree that they no longer need or desire surgery. Similarly, patients not motivated enough for rehabilitation or not compliant with the program are likely to struggle throughout the recovery period and therefore should not have surgery. It should be noted that at some institutions, patients are encouraged to enroll in a rehabilitation program although surgeons will proceed with surgical interventions even if the patient cannot meet the specific goals (33).

It is understood that patient conditioning as measured by the six-minute walk test does improve significantly with rehabilitation while the level of dyspnea and measured pulmonary function do not.

Table 15.1 Possible Rationale for Pulmonary Rehabilitation Prior to LVRS (Reprinted From Kesten S, Clinics in Chest Medicine 1997, Ref 2)

| Potential results of rehabilitation | Outcome |
| --- | --- |
| Satisfactory improvement in symptoms | May eliminate desire or need for surgery |
| Non compliance, poor motivation, inability to exercise | Eliminates poor candidates for LVRS |
| Improved nutrition, mental health, exercise tolerance | Decreased risk of postoperative morbidity and increased likelihood of positive outcome |

In their 1996 paper, Cooper et al (32) showed that with preoperative rehabilitation the distance walked during the 6-minute walk test improved from 856 feet to 1110 feet. A further improvement to 1280 feet was noted at 3 months postoperatively. In an interesting study, Crina et al (34) compared the benefits of rehabilitation alone to rehabilitation followed by LVRS. After 8 weeks of pulmonary rehabilitation, the authors noted that pulmonary function tests remained unchanged but that there was a trend toward a higher 6-minute walk distance. Bilateral LVRS further improved static lung function, gas exchange and QL compared with rehabilitation alone. Similar findings were observed by Pompeo and coll (35) who randomized 60 patients eligible to LVRS to receive either LVRS (N = 30) or comprehensive pulmonary rehabilitation. Dyspnea index, $PaO_2$, and exercise capacity improved more after LVRS than after rehabilitation whereas pulmonary function improved only after LVRS.

Another rationale for rehabilitation is the impact that these programs are likely to have on the nutritional deficits often observed in patients with severe COPD (36). In the published data of Wilson and coworkers (36) on 779 patients with stable COPD, the authors found that in 25% of patients the body weight was < 90% of ideal body weight. This depleted state was found to be associated with a higher incidence of infection and with abnormalities in both the tumoral and cell-mediated immune responses. In 1999, Mazolewski et al (37) looked at the impact of nutritional status on the outcome after LVRS. Fifty-one patients were included in the analysis and 50% of them had a deficient nutritional status identifiable by BMI, but not by standard nutritional indexes. This impaired nutritional status was associated with increased morbidity following LVRS. The authors concluded that repletion of nutritional deficiencies in patients with a low BMI prior to operation may decrease morbidity and length of stay in the hospital.

### Components of Rehabilitation

In most centers, the targeted goals of rehabilitation are of 30 consecutive minutes on a bicycle at 1.5 mph and of 30 consecutive minutes on a treadmill at 1.0 mph. These objectives are carried out within a supervised structured rehabilitation program for a minimum of 8-10 weeks prior to surgery. During exercise, the patient's pulse and oxygen saturation are monitored and supplemental oxygen is given as necessary to maintain saturation at more than 90%. An evaluation is sent regularly to the physician so that progress can be monitored. Patients may also be asked to do exercise arm ergometry in order to improve the strength of their upper extremities.

## Location of the Program

In 1994, Wijkstra and coworkers (21) developed a rehabilitation program at home. They studied 43 patients and found a highly significant improvement in the rehabilitation group compared to the control group for dimensions, dyspnea, emotion, and mastery. Although lung function showed no changes, the exercise tolerance improved significantly in the rehabilitation group thus demonstrating the feasibility and usefulness of home care rehabilitation.

Since LVRS is only done at a few centers, home care rehabilitation should be very useful in the cohort of patients requiring this type of intervention. Debigaré and colleagues evaluated the efficacy of a minimally supervised home-based exercise program in this context (38). Twenty-three patients were recruited and the authors were able to demonstrate significant increases in 6 MWD (p < 0.001), quality of life (p < 0.005), peak work rate (p < 0.05), peak $O_2$ consumption (p < 0.05), endurance time (p < 0.005) and muscle strength. The training frequency was 5 times/week for 10 to 12 weeks and supervision was done by a weekly phone call during which the progression of the training was verified. The authors concluded that in motivated patients, home training is effective and allows the training of patients in regions where supervised training programs are not available.

## Conclusion

In summary, it is clear that rehabilitation is effective to increase patient endurance and reduce postoperative morbidity. It is also clear that much has to be done with lung cancer patients who most of the time go on to surgery unprepared. By documenting the efficacy of exercise training in such individuals, it is possible that one will show a decrease in the incidence of pulmonary complications which are the leading causes of postoperative deaths. In this context, it is probably very timely to carry out a prospective randomized trial looking at rehabilitation followed by surgery versus surgery alone in lung cancer patients.

# References:

1. American Thoracic Society: Pulmonary rehabilitation. *Am Rev Resp Dis* 1981;124:663-666.
2. Kesten S: Pulmonary rehabilitation and surgery for end-stage lung disease. *Clinics in Chest Medicine* 1997;18:173-181.
3. Parker SL, Tong T, Bolden S et al: Cancer statistics, 1997. *CA Cancer J Clin* 1997;47:5-27.
4. Olsen GN: Pulmonary physiologic assessment of operative risk. In Shields TW (ed.): General Thoracic Surgery, Malvern PA, William and Wilkins 1994; pp279-287.
5. Van Nostrand D, Kjelsberg MO, Humphrey EW: Preresectional evaluation of risk from pneumonectomy. *Surg Gynec and Obst* 1968;127:306-310.
6. Pate P, Tenholder MF, Griffin JP et al: Preoperative assessment of the high-risk patient for lung resection. *Ann Thorac Surg* 1996;61:1494-1500.
7. Bechard D and Wetstein L: Assessment of exercise oxygen consumption as preoperative criterion for lung resection. *Ann Thorac Surg* 1987;44:344-349.
8. Bolliger CT, Jordan P, Soler M et al: Exercise capacity as a predictor of postoperative complications in lung resection candidates. *AMJ Respir Crit Care Med* 1995;151:1472-1480.
9. Ninan M, Sommers KE, Landreneau RJ et al: Standardized exercise oxymetry predicts postpneumonectomy outcome. *Ann Thorac Surg* 1997;64:328-333.
10. Rao V, Todd TRJ, Kruus A et al: Exercise oxymetry versus spirometry in the assessment of risk prior to lung resection. *Ann Thorac Surg* 1995;60:603-609.
11. Stein M and Cassara EL: Preoperative pulmonary evaluation and therapy for surgery patients. *JAMA* 1970;211:787-790.
12. Biggar D: Personal communication from the University of Washington rehabilitation program, St. Louis.
13. Wilson DJ: Pulmonary rehabilitation exercise program for high-risk thoracic surgical patients. *Chest Surg Clin of North Am* 1997;7:697-706.
14. Foreman S, Weil H, Duke R et al: Bullous disease of the lung; physiologic improvement after surgery. *Ann Int Med* 1968;69:757-767.
15. Lung disease data 1995, New York, NY: American Lung Association, 1996.
16. Traver GA, Cline MG, Burrows B: Predictors of mortality in chronic obstructive pulmonary disease. *Am Rev Resp Dis* 1979;119:895-902.
17. Burrows B, Bloom JN, Traver GA, Cline MG: The course and prognosis of different forms of chronic airways obstruction in a sample from the general population. *N Engl J Med* 1987;317:1309-1314.
18. Postma DS, Sleiter HJ: Prognosis of chronic obstructive pulmonary disease: the Dutch experience. *Am Rev Respir Dis* 1989;140:S100-105.
19. Cockroft AE, Saunders MJ, Berry G: Randomized controlled trial of rehabilitation in chronic respiratory disability. *Thorax* 1981;36:200-203.
20. O'Donnell DE, Webb KA, McGuire MA: Older patients with COPD: benefits of exercise training. *Geriatrics* 1993;48:59-62.
21. Wijkstra PJ, Van Altena R, Kraan J et al: Quality of life in patients with chronic obstructive pulmonary disease improves after rehabilitation at home. *Eur Respir J* 1994;7:269-273.
22. Goldstein RS, Gort EH, Stubbing D et al: Randomized controlled trial of respiratory rehabilitation. *Lancet* 1994;344:1394-1397.
23. Reardon J, Awad E, Normandin E et al: The effects of comprehensive out-patient pulmonary rehabilitation on dyspnea. *Chest* 1994;105:1046-1052.
24. Ries AL, Ellis B, Hawkins RW: Upper extremity exercise training in chronic obstructive pulmonary disease. *Chest* 1988;93:688-692.
25. Weiner P, Azgad Y, Ganam R: Inspiratory muscle training combined with general exercise reconditioning in patients with COPD. *Chest* 1992;102:1351-1356.
26. O'Donnell DE, McGuire M, Samis L, Webb KA: The impact of exercise reconditioning on breathlessness in severe chronic airflow limitation. *Am J Respir Crit Care Med* 1995;152:2005-2013.
27. Brantigan OC, Mueller E: Surgical treatment of pulmonary emphysema. *Am Surg* 1957;23:789-804.
28. Cooper JD, Trulock EP, Triantafillou AN et al: Bilateral pneumectomy (volume reduction) for chronic obstructive pulmonary disease. *J Thorac Cardiovasc Surg* 1995;109:106-119.
29. Kaiser L: Lung volume reduction surgery, *Cur Prob Surg*, April 2000, p 262-317.
30. Naunheim KS, Ferguson MK: The current status of lung volume reduction operations for emphysema. Current Review, *Ann Thorac Surg* 1996;62:601-612.
31. Miller JI, Lee RB, Mansour KA: Lung volume reduction surgery: lessons learned. *Ann Thorac Surg* 1996;61:1464-1469.
32. Cooper JC, Patteson GA, Sundaresan RS et al: Results of 150 consecutive bilateral lung

volume reduction procedures in patients with severe emphysema. *J Thorac Cardiovasc Surg* 1996;112:1319-1330.

33. McKenna RJ Jr., Brenner M, Gelb AF et al: A randomized prospective trial of stapled lung reduction versus laser bullectomy for diffuse emphysema. *J Thorac Cardiovasc Surg* 1996;111: 317-322.

34. Criner GJ, Cordova FC, Furukawa S et al: Prospective randomized trial comparing bilateral lung volume reduction surgery to pulmonary rehabilitation in severe chronic obstructive pulmonary disease. *Am J Respir Crit Care Med* 1999;160:2018-2027.

35. Pompeo E, Marino M, Nofroni I et al: Reduction pneumoplasty versus rehabilitation in severe emphysema: a randomized study. *Ann Thorac Surg* 2000;70:948-954.

36. Wilson DO, Rogers RM, Hoffman RM: Nutrition and chronic lung disease. *Am Rev Resp Dis* 1985;132:1347-1365.

37. Mazolewski P, Turner JF, Baker M et al: The impact of nutritional status on the outcome of lung volume reduction surgery. A prospective study. *Chest* 1999;116:693-696.

38. Debigaré R, Maltais F, Whittom F et al: Feasibility and efficacy of home exercise training before lung volume reduction. *J Cardiopulm Rehab* 1999;19:235-241.

# Chapter 16

# Update on Coronary Artery Bypass Surgery and Rehabilitation

Paul Dubach, MD, Jonathan Myers, PhD, Sebastian Sixt, MD, Claudia Mosimann, MD, Switzerland and USA

More than 200,000 coronary artery bypass graft (CABG) procedures are performed annually in the United States. Structured programs of cardiac rehabilitation have become an accepted adjunct to CABG for optimizing the surgical result (1,2). Improved survival has not been demonstrated by a controlled trial of exercise training after CABG, although benefits have been observed in functional capacity, graft patency and psychological characteristics after rehabilitation (2-6). Historically, rehabilitation programs after CABG have not differed from those for patients with CAD without prior cardiac surgery, even though there are physiologic and cognitive sequelae unique to the surgical act and the cardiopulmonary bypass (7-11). The approach to rehabilitation after CABG has changed recently in that the initial steps of the comprehensive approach to rehabilitation are performed early in the cardiac surgery wards before and after the operation; today, these steps should be an integral part of treatment in the CABG patient. This paper focuses on newer concepts related to exercise training after CABG, reviews pertinent studies, provides an overview of problems unique to CABG patients undergoing rehabilitation, and discusses the potential impact of new surgical techniques on cardiac rehabilitation.

## Issues Unique to the CABG Patient in Cardiac Rehabilitation

The most important issues that can influence outpatient rehabilitation after CABG are the amount of myocardial damage occurring during surgery, graft patency, cardiopulmonary bypass-related complications, and wound healing problems.

## Myocardial Damage During Cardiac Surgery

Resting regional perfusion defects are improved after CABG in at least 65% of patients (12), and coronary flow reserve returns to normal in many patients (13). Thus, myocardial perfusion and function are normally improved after CABG. Peri-operative myocardial infarction (MI) is usually related to inappropriate medical management rather than to coronary artery disease or to the CABG operation per se (14). The prevalence of MI therefore varies widely and is dependent upon the criteria used; it generally ranges between about 2% and 5% (15). Peri-operative infarctions are normally small, but when quantitatively more than trivial, they indicate a higher risk for mortality (16). Damage from a period of ischemia may result in a variable and sometimes prolonged period of both systolic and diastolic dysfunction without muscle necrosis. This is commonly termed myocardial stunning or hibernation (17).

In over 90% of patients, myocardial function is unchanged or even improved after CABG (18). For the vast majority of patients, myocardial performance thus allows mobilization and rehabilitation immediately after surgery. In 2% to 5% of patients however, the degree of myocardial damage after cardiac surgery can be significant (15). The infarct size, post-operative ejection fraction, and the presence or absence of congestion will ultimately determine the timing of rehabilitation in these patients. In most cases however, only a small increase in creatine kinase is noted (16). Several authors have demonstrated that the risk of early ambulation and progressive mobilization in patients with a small uncomplicated myocardial infarction without CABG is minimal (19,20). There do not appear to be compelling reasons to manage patients with a small myocardial infarction occurring during cardiac surgery differently. Clearly, most patients with myocardial damage that occurs during CABG can be discharged within days after surgery. If however, the myocardial damage has been considerable, or if there are symptoms or signs of congestion or serious rhythm disturbances, ambulation and discharge of these patients must be tailored individually (21).

## Graft Patency

Nikai and co-workers studied the influence of exercise training on graft patency in 155 patients (4). The patients were divided (not randomized) into a control (n=60) or an exercise group (n=55). Patients in the exercise group were informed about the importance of exercise training before the operation. The rehabilitation program started immediately after open heart surgery and lasted seven weeks. Patients in the control group were instructed not to perform activities beyond those of daily living. After the study period, cardiac catheterization was repeated. Three out of 180 grafts (2%) were occluded in the exercise group, but 36 out of 178 (20%) were occluded in the control group (p<0.05). Factors related to graft patency after CABG were examined by multivariate analysis. Post-operative double product, cardiac index, stroke index, left ventricular end-diastolic pressure, and training efficacy were found to be correlated with graft patency (p<0.01). The authors concluded that exercise training should begin as early as possible after CABG and may improve graft patency.

## Cardiopulmonary Bypass-Related Complications

Some adverse neural and behavioral outcomes are an inevitable result of the total circulatory arrest required during CABG (7-10). In addition, with advances in surgical techniques and anesthesia, CABG is now being performed in patients with more serious comorbid conditions, such as hypertension and diabetes, as well as in older patients who may be at higher risk for complications. Although patients in their 70's and 80's tolerate the procedure well and generally have excellent outcomes, the inclusion of patients at higher risk has led to an appreciation for the serious and potentially fatal neurological difficulties that can be associated with CABG. The neural and behavioral

outcomes range from the well-documented incidence of stroke to the less well-defined postoperative delirium, cognitive difficulties, and depression. Thus, the clinical focus post-operatively now includes both effects of CABG on the brain and thought processes as well as its effect on the myocardium. Specific cognitive and neurologic sequellae of CABG include the following (9):

### Stroke

Stroke is a well-recognized complication of CABG. The reported frequency ranges from 0.8 to 5.2% (22,23). Models to predict those most at risk of post-CABG stroke have focused on cardiovascular factors such as hypertension, diabetes, peripheral vascular disease, age and evidence of previous cerebrovascular disease (24). Identification of high risk patients, localization of arteriosclerotic plaques, and subsequent modification of the surgical procedure can decrease the rate of stroke (25).

### Postoperative Delirium

The reported frequency of delirium in the immediate post-operative period ranges between 10 and 28% (26). Whether patients with delirium develop later cognitive deficits related to CABG is unknown (9).

### Cognitive Changes

Advances in anaesthetic and surgical techniques have led to the assumption that post-operative cognitive decline is currently less common than in previous years. The benefits of such technological advances however, may be offset by the inclusion of older patients with greater comorbidity. The extent to which post-operative cognitive dysfunction occurs is dependent upon measurement techniques, timing of the assessment, statistical methods and pre-operative cognitive performance (9). Short-term changes are generally related to memory loss, which has been reported to have an incidence ranging between 33% and 83% (27). Long-term changes have included difficulties in tasks such as following directions, playing chess, or making calculations (28). No precise data exist regarding the incidence of long-term cognitive changes.

### Depression

Depression is commonly reported after cardiac surgery, with an incidence of up to 25% (29). Depression appears unrelated to change in cognitive performance (30), but newly acquired depression is associated with increased mortality and poorer cardiovascular outcomes after CABG (9).

### Mechanisms of Neurological Sequelae

Two major mechanisms have been proposed to explain post-operative brain injury: intraoperative hypotension and multiple emboli. Genetic susceptibility may also have a role (31,32).

### Biochemical Markers of Central-Nervous-System Injury

Two biochemical markers related to CABG have recently received attention: S-100 protein and neuron-specific enolase. These markers can be detected in cerebrospinal fluid or blood (33). Whether either of these markers correlates with long-term cognitive changes after CABG however, is unknown.

## Rehabilitation-Related Issues After CABG

Complete wound healing, including osseous consolidation after conventional trans-sternal thoracotomy usually takes about 6 weeks. Therefore, the following precautions are recommended during rehabilitation: 1) exercise with uncontrolled motion of the shoulders and arms should be avoided (especially in osteoporotic sternum or chronic lung disease); 2) an upper limit of 10 kg is generally apropriate for resistence training; and 3) swimming should be allowed only once the sternotomy and saphenous vein procurement wounds are completely dry (34).

In a series of 340 patients who underwent cardiac surgery and subsequently entered a supervised cardiac rehabilitation program, a total of 32 patients (9.6%) underwent surgical re-intervention during rehabilitation (34). The interventions included sternum repair (2 patients), evacuation of pleura (17 patients), pericardial effusion (4 patients), and revision of the saphenous vein procurement site (9 patients). A questionnaire sent to the patients revealed that a significant proportion suffered from minor problems caused by the procurement of the saphenous vein. Although major wound complications were rare, impaired or delayed healing as well as discomfort were reported to be as high as 20% and were sometimes responsible for delaying the start of cardiac rehabilitation. Overall, cardiac complications were responsible for interruption of phase II rehabilitation in 3.2%, whereas surgery-related complications were responsible for early discharge from rehabilitation in 5.2% of patients (34,35).

Minimal invasive harvest techniques have recently been developed. They offer many advantages over the traditional approach; aside from cosmetic issues, healing is accelerated and post-operative discomfort is markedly reduced (36). These minimally-invasive techniques have the potential to reduce surgery-related dropouts from rehabilitation, although studies are not yet available assessing this issue.

## Studies on Cardiac Rehabilitation After CABG

The body of data that has been reported assessing the effects of exercise rehabilitation on exercise capacity, return to work, or quality of life in patients who have undergone bypass surgery is now considerable. Some of the recent papers that have influenced recent changes in attitude toward rehabilitation after CABG are discussed in the following.

Engelmann and co-workers (37) published their experience with so-called "fast-track recovery after CABG" in 1994. The fast track recovery protocol involves the following principles: 1) pre-operative education; 2) early extubation; 3) methylprednisolone sodium succinate before the operation followed by dexamethasone for 24 h post-operatively; 4) prophylactic digitalization; 5) accelerated rehabilitation; 6) early discharge; and 7) follow-up at one week, four, twelve and twenty-four months postoperatively. Two hundred eighty patients following the fast track protocol were compared with 282 patients following routine management after CABG. At one week, four weeks, twelve months and twenty-four months follow-up, the rates of infection, mortality and readmission were similar in both groups. However, the duration of stay in the intensive care unit was significantly shorter and discharge significantly earlier in the fast-track group compared with patients with routine management. Forty-eight per cent of the patients in the fast group were discharged within 3 to 5 days after operations, compared with only 26% among the routine care group (P<0.001).

Krohn and co-workers (38) discharged almost 80% of their patients within 5 days after cardiac surgery. In 240 consecutive patients, the median length of hospital stay after cardiac surgery was 4 days. The operations included CABG, aortic valve replacement and mitral valve operations. Six patients (2.5%) were rehospitalized within 6 months after discharge and five patients (2.1%) were rehospitalized 6 to 24 months after discharge. They concluded that a longer initial hospitalization would not have improved the rates of rehospitalization.

Only a few studies have been published assessing the influence of the timing of rehabilitation on the course of recovery after CABG. Dubach and co-workers (39) assessed the influence of residential rehabilitation on exercise performance beginning one month compared with two months after cardiac surgery. Forty-two patients after CABG were randomly assigned to an exercise (n=22) or a control group (n=20). Cardiopulmonary exercise tests were performed three times in each group during the two-month study period: at baseline, after one month of training or usual care, and at the end of the two months. During the first month, patients in the control group were asked not to perform activities beyond those of daily living, whereas patients in the exercise group underwent active rehabilitation. After one month there was a cross-over: patients in the control group had active rehabilitation and patients in the exercise group were asked not to perform activities beyond those of daily living. A significant increase in peak $\dot{V}O_2$ was observed across testing periods within each group. However, there was no significant interaction between groups. In other words, two months after cardiac surgery the increase in peak $\dot{V}O_2$ was similar in both groups, regardless of the timing of rehabilitation. The authors concluded that rehabilitation is equally beneficial whether begun early (one month) or late (two months) after surgery.

Köhler and coworkers (40) studied the influence of length of stay in the hospital after cardiac surgery before beginning outpatient rehabilitation on the outcome of rehabilitation. Comparing age, end-diastolic volume index, left ventricular ejection fraction, number of stenosed coronary arteries, number of bypass grafts, level of initial physical activity, body mass index, and total cholesterol/HDL ratio, no significant differences were found in outcomes after rehabilitation among patients who entered the rehabilitation program in the early postoperative period (mean one week), after 15-28 days, or later than 28 days. They concluded that rehabilitation in most of patients could start as early as one week after cardiac surgery.

Artinian found no differences in the recovery patterns after CABG relative to age or gender (41,42). Carroll (43) reported on the importance of self-efficacy expectations in elderly patients recovering from CABG. Circuit weight training starting 19 months after cardiac surgery did not improve peak $\dot{V}O_2$ after 10 weeks of training in a controlled

study, but was well tolerated (44). Stevens and Hanson compared the influence of supervised and unsupervised exercise training programs on exercise capacity after CABG. They concluded that unsupervised exercise can be performed safely and results in similar functional improvements compared with supervised exercise after uncomplicated CABG (45). Waites and coworkers compared the functional and physiologic status of active and dropout CABG patients in a rehabilitation program. They found that CABG patients maintaining participation in rehabilitation had greater improvements in peak $\dot{V}O_2$ and treadmill time, smoked less, were less often rehospitalized, and were more fully employed than those who dropped out (46). However, this study was uncontrolled.

Engblom and coworkers investigated the influence of rehabilitation on quality of life and return to work 5 years after CABG in a controlled, randomized study (47). The rehabilitation program included four phases. The first phase lasted two days and took place two weeks before the open heart surgery. It focused on general information about the surgery, recovery, and the rehabilitation program ahead. The second period started 6 to 8 weeks after the operation and lasted three weeks. It was based on exercise training but also included instruction in risk factor modification and psychosocial intervention. Refresher courses took place 8 months (third phase) and 30 months (fourth phase) after surgery and lasted two days and one day, respectively. They found that symptoms, use of medications, exercise capacity, and depression scores did not differ between patients randomized to the trained and control groups. Five years after CABG, the patients in the rehabilitation group reported less restriction in physical mobility and more patients perceived their health and overall life situation more favorably compared to control patients. Return to work was lower in control patients after 3 years but not after 5 years. The authors concluded that a cardiac rehabilitation program after CABG may induce a perception of improved health. However, the influence of rehabilitation on return to work was limited.

Only a few studies have assessed the influence of rehabilitation on neurobehavioural sequelae after CABG, including depression and emotional stress. Perski and coworkers followed 142 patients (43 "distressed"; 99 "non-distressed") in a cross-sectional study using a comprehensive 4-week residential rehabilitation program consisting of daily exercise, lectures about CAD and risk factors, psychosocial support, and nutrition counseling (5). They found that the emotionally distressed patients were highly successful in improving their functional status and reducing risk factors but less successful in returning to work. Both groups had a significant improvement in psychological well being. The authors also reported that systematic evaluation and treatment of emotional distress before CABG may result in a reduction in serious cardiac events after surgery (6).

## Impact of New Surgical Techniques on Cardiac Rehabilitation

Newer and less invasive surgical techniques have been developed to lessen surgery-related complications such as chest wall instability and wound infections, and to avoid cardiopulmonary bypass by operating on the beating heart. These techniques could have an important impact on the management of these patients, including cardiac rehabilitation.

The most important factors affecting the degree of invasiveness in cardiac surgery are the surgical approach itself and the cardiopulmonary bypass. The surgical approach is characterized largely by the length of the incision and the associated degree of trauma to tissue, the amount of loss of blood, and degree of residual pain. More serious complications such as sternitis and mediastinitis can also differ with the surgical approach. The cardiopulmonary bypass is known to be related to important changes in neurocognitive and psychosocial function (7-10). The main goals of the less invasive techniques are therefore to: 1) reduce surgical trauma; 2) minimize manipulation of the ascending aorta; and 3) avoidance of the morbidity associated with the cardiopulmonary bypass process.

There are four categories of less invasive cardiac surgery that differ in terms of access to the myocardium, whether or not extracorporeal circulation is used, the type of instruments, and the method of visualization (48):

- Coronary artery bypass surgery via sternotomy without extracorporeal circulation (coronary artery surgery on the beating heart).
- Limited or modified surgical approaches (T or L sternotomy, anterolateral minithoracotomy) using conventional techniques and instruments with conventional or endovascular cardiopulmonary bypass.
- MIDCAB (minimallly invasive direct coronary artery bypass, where a thoracoscopally har-

vested arterial bypass is anastomosed to the left anterior descending artery on the beating heart).
- Port-Access surgery (surgery performed through ports or other small intercostal incisions that are no wider than 4 cm). Cardiopulmonary bypass is instituted via a femoral approach.

## Summary

The mayor changes that have occurred regarding rehabilitation after CABG in recent years include the timing of rehabilitation, changes in pre- and post-operative management (shifting the focus from the status of the heart itself to the effects of CABG on the brain and thought process), and the important interaction between the advances in surgical techniques, rate of healing, and reduction in hospital stay. For many years outpatient rehabilitation was recommended no earlier than 4-6 weeks following cardiac surgery. While data in the literature are rather sparse at present, they do suggest that outpatient rehabilitation can begin as early as one week after open heart surgery without influencing sternal infections, mortality, or readmissions. Recently, evidence has demonstrated that early rehabilitation can improve graft patency after CABG. However, age, operative complications, and co-morbidities must be considered individually for each patient when determining the beginning of outpatient rehabilitation. Studies have confirmed the efficacy of such programs for both genders and for all ages. It has also been observed that unsupervised training has a similar effect on increasing exercise capacity as supervised exercise.

Changes in the pre- and post-operative management of patients with CABG as well as new surgical techniques have dramatically reduced hospital stays and improved the understanding of non-cardiac problems after surgery. Improved pre-operative management includes the dissemination of information to both patients and relatives about the surgery and the postoperative period. Today, there is a greater appreciation for quality of life and the neurobehavioural problems after CABG. This has meant a greater emphasis on the evaluation and treatment of emotional stress before surgery, and a greater understanding of the importance of risk assessment for postoperative stroke with appropriate modification of the surgical procedure. Cardiac surgery is becoming less invasive, and new technology will increasingly enable the surgeon to operate on the heart without sternotomy or cardiopulmonary bypass. Patients are increasingly being discharged after 2 to 4 days and resuming their normal physical activities within 1 to 2 weeks. These new surgical techniques have facilitated a more rapid transition from the hospital to beginning ambulation, and rehabilitation will likely become an integral part of treatment for patients undergoing these less invasive procedures.

# References

1. American heart association. 1989 Heart facts. Dallas: American Heart Association 1989.
2. Smith HC, La Von NH, Gupta S, et al.: Employment status after coronary artery bypass surgery. *Circulation* 1982; 65(Suppl II).
3. Keon WJ, Sherrard H: Early release after cardiac surgery. In: Yacoub MH, Carpentier A, eds. Annual of cardiac surgery. London: Rapid Science Publishers; 1997:71-7.
4. Nakai Y, Katoaka Y, Bando M, et al.: Effects of physical exercise training on cardiac function and graft patency after coronary artery bypass grafting. *J Thorac Cardiovasc Surg* 1987; 93:65-72.
5. Perski A, Osuchowski K, Andersson L, et al.: Intensive rehabilitation of emotionally distressed patients after coronary by-pass grafting. *J Intern Med* 1999; 246:253-263.
6. Persik A, Feleke E, Andersson G, et al.: Emotional distress before coronary bypass grafting limits the benefits of surgery. *Am Heart J* 1998; 136:510-7.
7. Ayanian J, Guadagnoli E, Cleary P: Physical and psychosocial functioning of women and men after coronary artery bypass surgery. *JAMA* 1995; 274(22):1767-70.
8. Roach GW, Kanchuger M, Mangano CM, et al.: Adverse cerebral outcomes after coronary bypass surgery. *N Engl J Med* 1996; 335:1857-63.
9. Selnes OA, Goldsborough MA, Borowicz LM, et al.: Neurobehavioural sequelae of cardiopulmonary bypass. *Lancet* 1999; 353:1601-6.
10. Newman MF, Kirchner JL, Phillip–Bute B, et al.: Longitudinal assessment of neurocognitive function after coronary-artery bypass surgery. *N Engl J Med* 2001; 344:395-402.
11. Froehlicher V, Myers J, Follensbee W, et al.: Exercise and the heart, 3rd edn. Chicago: Mosby, 1993.
12. Rubenson DS, Tucker CR, London E, et al.: Two-dimensional echocardiographic analysis of segmental left ventricular wall motion before and after coronary artery bypass surgery. *Circulation* 1982; 66:1025.
13. Wilson RJ, Macus ML, White CW: Effects fo coronary bypass surgery and angioplasty on coronary blood flow and flow reserve. *Prog Cardiovasc Dis* 1988; 31:95.
14. Bulkley BH, Hutchins GM: Myocardial consequences of coronary artery bypass surgery: the paradox of necrosis in areas fo revascularization. *Circulation* 1977; 56:906.
15. Obermann A, Kouchoukos NT, Makar YN, et al.: Perioperative myocardial infarction after coronary bypass surgery. *Cleve Clin Q* 1978; 45:172.
16. Brindis RG, Brundage BH, Ullyot DJ, et al.: Graft patency in patients with coronary artery bypass operation complicated by preoperative myocardial infarction, *J Am Coll Cardiol* 1984; 3:55.
17. Braunwald E, Kloner RA: The stunned myocardium: prolonged postischemic ventricular dysfunction. *Circulation* 1982; 66:1146.
18. Pantely G, Morton M, Rahimtoola SH: Effects of successful uncomplicated valve replacement on ventricular hypertrophy, volume, and performance in aortic stenosis and in aortic incompetence. *J Thorac Cardiovasc Surg* 1978; 75:383.
19. Sivarajan ES, Bruce RA, Aimes MJ, et al: In-hospital exercise after myocardial infarction does not improve treadmill performance. *N Engl J Med* 1981; 305:357-62.
20. Bloch A, Maeder J, Haissly J, et al.: Early mobilization after myocardial infarction: a controlled study. *Am J Cardiol* 1974; 34:152-7.
21. Dubach P, Myers J, Wagner D: Optimal timing of phase II rehabilitation after cardiac surgery. *Eur Heart J* 1998; 19;O35-7.
22. Martin WRW, Hashimoto SA: Stroke in coronary bypass surgery. *Can J Neurol Sei* 1982; 8:21-26.
23. Breuer AC, Furlan AJ, Hanson MR, et al.: Central nervous system complications of coronary artery bypass graft surgery: prospective analysis of 421 patients. *Stroke* 1983; 14:682-87.
24. Newmann MF, Wolfmann R, Kanchuger M, et al.: Multicenter preoperative stroke risk index for patients undergouing coronary artery pypass graft surgery. *Circulation* 1996; 94:II74-80.
25. Wareing TH, Davila-Roman VG, Daily BB, et al.: Strategy for the reduction of stroke incidence in cardiac surgical patients. *Ann Thorac Surg* 1993; 55:1400-8.

26. Van Der Mast RC, Roest FHJ: Delirium after cardiac surgery: a critical review. *J Psychosom Res* 1996; 41:13-30.

27. Savageau JA, Stanton BA, Jenkins CD, et al.: Neuropsychological dysfunction following elective cardiac operation, II: a six-month reassessment. *J Thorac Cardiovasc Surg* 1982; 84:595-600.

28. Klonoff H, Clark C, Kavanagh-Gray D, et al.: Two-year follow-up study of coronary bypass surgery: psychologic status, employment status, and quality of life. *J Thorac Cardiovasc Surg* 1989; 97:78-85.

29. Langeluddecke PM, Fulcher G, Baird D, et al.: A prospective evaluation of the psychosocial effects of coronary artery bypass surgery. *J Psychosom Res* 1989; 33:37-45.

30. McKhann GM, Borowicz LM, Goldsborough, et al.: Depression and congnitive decline after coronary artery bypass. *Lancet* 1997; 349:1282-84.

31. Newmann MF, Croughwell ND, Blumenthal JA, et al.: Predictors of cognitive decline after cardiac operation. *Ann Thorac Surg* 1995; 59:1326-30.

32. Moody DM, Bell MA, Johnston WE, et al.: Brain micoemboli during cardiac surgery or aortography. *Ann Neurol* 1990; 28:477-86.

33. Missler U, Wiesmann M, Friedrich C, et al.: S-100 protein and neuron-specific enolase conentrations in blood as indicators of infarction volume and prognosis in acute ischemic stroke. *Stroke* 1998; 28:1956-60.

34. Carrel T, Mohacsi P: Optimal timing of rehabilitation after cardiac surgery: the surgeon's view. *Eur Heart J* 1998; 19:O38-41.

35. Van Camp SP, Peterson RA: Cardiovascular complications of outpatients cardiac rehabilitation programs. *J Am Med Assoc* 1986; 256:1160-3.

36. Tevaearai HL, Müller XM, von Segesser LK: Minimal invasive harvest of the saphenous vein for coronary artery bypass grafting. *Ann Thorac Surg* 1997; 65:119-21.

37. Engelman RM, Rousou JA, Flack E, et al.: Fast-track revovery of the coronary bypass patient. *Ann Thorac Surg* 1994; 58:1742-6.

38. Krohn BG, Kay JH, Meney MA, et al.: Rapid sustained recovery after cardiac operations. *J Thorac Cardiovasc Surg* 1990; 100:194-7.

39. Dubach P, Myers J, Dziekan G, et al.: Effect of residential cardiac rehabilitation following bypass surgery. *Chest* 1995; 108:1434-9.

40. Köhler E, Karoff M, Körfer R, et al.: Stationäre Behandlungszeiten und körperliches Leistungsvermögen nach aorto-koronarer Bypassoperation, nach Herzklappenersatz sowie nach Myokardinfarkt. *Kardiol* 1995, 84:911-20.

41. Artinian NT, Duggan CH: Sex difference in patient recovery patterns after coronary artery bypass surgery. *Heart Lung* 1995;24:483-94.

42. Artinian NT, Duggan C, Miller P, et al.: Age differences in patient recovery patterns following coronary artery bypass surgery. *Am J Crit Care* 1993; 2:453-61.

43. Carroll DL: The importance of self-efficacy expectations in elderly patients recovering from coronary artery bypass surgery. *Heart Lung* 1995; 24:50-9.

44. Maiorana AJ, Briffa TG, Goodman C, et al.: A controlled trial of circuit weight training on aerobic capacity and myocardial oxygen demand in men after coronary artery bypass surgery. *J Cardiopulmonary Rehabil* 1997; 17:239-47.

45. Stevens R, Hanson P: Comparision of supervised and unsupervised exercise training after coronary bypass surgery. *Am J Cardiol* 1984; 53:1524-28.

46. Waites TF, Watt EW, Fletcher GF. Comparative functional and physiologic status of active and dropout coronary bypass patients of a rehabilitation program. *Am J Cardiol* 1983; 51:1087-90.

47. Engblom E, Korpilahti K, Hämäläinen H, et al.: Quality of life and return to work 5 years after coronary artery bypass surgery. *J Cardiopulmonary Rehabil* 1997; 17:29-36.

48. Vanermen H: What is minimally invasive cardiac surgery. *J Card Surg* 1998; 13:268-74.

49. Minale C, Reifschneider HJ, Schmits E, et al.: Single access for minimally invasive aortic valve replacment. *Ann Thorac Surg* 1997; 64:120-3.

# PART VII

# Selecting and Screening Patients for Rehabilitation

# Chapter 17

# Exercise Testing in the New Millennium

Katerina Shetler, Victor Froelicher MD, USA

As we go into the third Millennium, health care continues to experience unusual pressures to change. These pressures are largely financial responding to a progressive increase in the proportion of the gross national product expended in health care services. After several years of flattening of the costs due to managed care, 1998 saw an increase again. While managed care held costs down at least temporarily, more Americans than ever are without health insurance and yet we are again facing unsustainable cost increases. Reimbursements for procedures are being further decreased by HCFA, leading to the American College of Cardiology suing this governmental agency. The standard exercise test reimbursement when performed in the doctor's office has dropped to $126. Because of this, cardiologists favor adding echocardiography to the test or just deciding on whether to perform cardiac catheterization from the medical history.

Quite frankly, it is often difficult to teach our cardiology fellows how to do the exercise test as they would rather have it done by nurses or physician's assistants. While it appears that 50% of internists and family practitioners are performing exercise tests, it is difficult to assure that they are properly trained. Clinicians must learn so much these days that it is a problem for them to spend enough time to become comfortable doing the test. In fact, they are most comfortable in doing the test in low risk patients who probably need the test the least.

However, many physicians have learned from experience that the exercise test complements the medical history and physical examination and it remains the second most commonly performed cardiological procedure next to the ECG. The renewed efforts to control costs will undoubtedly win more over to this group of enlightened physicians. Convincing evidence that treadmill scores enhance the diagnostic and prognostic power of the exercise test

will add to this movement. In addition, there is increasing evidence that measurement of expired gases improves the prognostic power of the test in certain groups of patients.

The practitioners performing the exercise test appear to be changing. Cardiologists in general are less interested in anything related to the ECG and are moving to other modalities. This is at least partly explained by financial pressures. As George Bernard Shaw said 80 years ago: "the Doctor does the test he is paid (the most) for". Attempts to decrease medical expenditures by targeting commonly done procedures, has devalued the ECG and standard exercise test. Unfortunately, these attempts have driven practice toward the more expensive modalities that will just increase in volume and cause even greater increases in health care costs. It would have been better to apply the guidelines for reimbursement according to appropriately ordered tests rather than use financial forces that can be misdirected.

With internists and family practitioners becoming the main performers of the standard exercise test efficient training is critical since they have so much to learn within a period of limited time. Also, the approach of the non-cardiologist to testing is usually more practical than the specialist and our guidelines and books do not meet their needs. For specialty concepts to be adopted by generalists they must be taught from their unique perspective.

Recent changes in medical knowledge have impacted the exercise test. First, all of diagnostic testing is being evaluated by standardized rules. Biostatiticians have nicely presented a set of rules that allow diagnostic technologies to be properly evaluated before they are adopted for practice (1,2,3). Perhaps the practitioner does not need to understand limited challenge, work up bias and appropriate patient selection for studies, but he/she should at least appreciate that these concepts are now being applied in evidence-based guidelines that tell us what tests we should perform and when. When critically assessed often new technologies such as electron beam computer tomography (EBCT) are not found to have better diagnostic characteristics than the standard exercise test (4). The AHA/ACA Statement on EBCT do not recommend this new test for diagnosing obstructive coronary artery disease (CAD) because of its low specificity (5). It appears that EBCT provides no incremental value to the prognostic Framingham Score* or the National Cholesterol Education Program. The meta-analysis presented in the EBCT statement demonstrated a high sensitivity of EBCT for CAD, a much lower specificity, and an overall predictive accuracy of 70%. The statement concluded that EBCT has a predictive accuracy approximately equivalent but not superior to alternative methods for diagnosing CAD.

The guidelines should have a great impact on test utility and medical practice in general. In addition, they provide the best source of educational material about their subjects. While most books or articles are based on the opinion of one person, the guidelines require the consensus of many experts. It is the best source of knowledge for the practitioner regarding how to perform and interpret the exercise test.

The ACC/AHA guidelines have had significant changes since their initial release (6). The last rendition acknowledged that the ST segments have the same diagnostic power when right bundle branch block is present as when the ECG is normal. In addition, they stated that the exercise test has the same diagnostic characteristics in women when age and symptoms place them in the intermediate probability of disease. Also, they stated that imaging studies are not necessarily indicated when less than one millimeter of ST depression is present on the resting ECG. Finally, the re-analysis of the meta-analysis data considering the newer studies that removed

work up bias and did not use target heart rates indicates that the sensitivity of the exercise ECG is lower than previously thought (about 50%) while the specificity is higher (over 90%) (7).

## Scores

An important advance in exercise testing is the use of scores. First, clinical scores or classification tables should be used to identify patients with an intermediate probability of CAD who should be tested. Secondly, exercise test scores can incorporate clinical and non-ECG data with exercise test data to improve the diagnostic and prognostic characteristics of the standard exercise test. The limited sensitivity of the standard exercise ECG test (about 50%) for detection of coronary artery disease has stimulated increased use of noninvasive stress imaging technologies. An alternative to the use of more expensive tests is the more efficient use of available data. Statistical techniques that combine the patient's medical history, symptoms of chest pain, hemodynamic data, and exercise ECG response have been demonstrated to better predict CAD than a single ECG criterion like ST segment depression (8). Diagnostic and prognostic predictive accuracy increase when multiple pieces of information from the patient's clinical history and the treadmill test are integrated. Studies have shown that the diagnostic value of exercise testing can be improved by considering several factors in the test interpretation (9,10,11,12,13) but issues remain about their portability (14).

Scores can also provide a management strategy for patients with possible CAD. This is done by placing patients into three categories of risk rather than just dichotomizing them as positive or negative (Table 17.1). Low-risk patients have an excellent

*Framingham risk model is based on levels of blood pressure, cholesterol, high-density lipoprotein (HDL)

**Table 17.1   Paradigm for the Clinical Reaction to the Estimated Probability of CAD**

| | Risk for clinically significant CAD (50% or greater occulusion) |
|---|---|
| Low risk | Patient reassured symptoms most likely not due to CAD |
| Intermediate risk | Require other tests, such as stress echo, nuclear, or angiography to clarify diagnosis; antianginal medications tried. |
| High risk | Antianginal treatment indicated; intervention clinically appropriate; angiography may be required |

prognosis and may be risk-stratified by the treadmill test. This patient cohort can be managed safely with watchful waiting as well as symptomatic medical therapy without further testing. High-risk patients should be considered candidates for more aggressive management that may include cardiac catheterization. In patients with an intermediate-risk treadmill score, myocardial perfusion imaging and other tests appears to be of value for further risk stratification (15).

## Pretest Scores

The exercise ECG test is the recommended test for diagnosing coronary artery disease in patients at intermediate risk (6). In the Guidelines, the classification is enabled through a table considering age, gender and chest pain characteristics (6). (Table 17.2) Morise et al (16) proposed a clinical score for categorizing patients with suspected coronary disease and normal resting electrocardiograms into similar probability groups. The Morise score is calculated as follows:

Age code + Angina pectoris code · 5
+ diabetes · 2 + hypertension
+ smoking now + hypercholesterolemia
+ family history of CAD + obesity

Where age less than 40 equals 3, age between 40 to 55 equals 6 and age more than 55 equals 9. For es-

trogen status, 3 points were subtracted for positive and 3 points were added for estrogen negative status. Typical chest pain equals 5, atypical chest pain equals 3, non-anginal chest pain equals 1 and no chest pain equals zero. For diabetes mellitus, 2 points were added and 1 point was added for each of the other 5 risk factors (Hypertension, present smoking, hypercholestrolemia, family history CAD and obesity). Whether this score is more discriminating than the table has not been demonstrated.

## Diagnostic Scores

In order to derive diagnostic scores, statisticians recommend multivariable analysis, a statistical technique that separates subjects into two groups. Clinical investigators have commonly used two types of analysis: discriminate function and logistic regression analysis. Logistic regression has been preferred since it models the relationship to a sigmoid curve (which often is the mathematical relationship between a risk variable and an outcome) and its output is between zero and one representing the probability of disease being present (i.e., from zero to 100% probability of the predicted outcome). In addition, in the logistic regression analysis dichotomous and continuous variables can be considered together. Thus, the output of a discriminate function is a unitless numerical score while a logistic regression provides an actual probability. The general linear

**Table 17.2 Pre Test Probability of Coronary Disease By Symptoms, Gender and Age**

| Age | Gender | Typical/definite angina pectoris | Atypical/probable angina pectoris | Non-anginal chest pain | Asymptomatic |
|---|---|---|---|---|---|
| 30-39 | Males | Intermediate | Intermediate | Low (10%) | Very low (<5%) |
| | Females | Intermediate | Very low (<5%) | Very low | Very low |
| 40-49 | Males | High | Intermediate | Intermediate | Low |
| | Females | Intermediate | Low | Very low | Very low |
| 50-59 | Males | High (>90%) | Intermediate | Intermediate | Low |
| | Females | Intermediate | Intermediate | Low | Very low |
| 60-69 | Males | High | Intermediate | Intermediate | Low |
| | Females | High | Intermediate | Intermediate | Low |

High = 90%   Intermediate = 10-90   Low = <10%   Very Low = <5%

*There is no data for patients younger than 30 or older than 69 but it can be assumed that coronary artery disease prevalence increases with age.

logistic regression model used takes the following form:

$$\text{Probability (0 to 1)} = 1/(1 + e^{-(a+bx+cy....)})$$

Where a is the intercept, b and c are coefficients, and x and y are variable values. Forward selection is used with entry at a significance level >.05. The model separates patients with and without a given outcome (CAD) which is assessed by means of the area under a receiver-operating-characteristic (ROC) curve, which ranges from 0 to 1, with 0.5 corresponding to no discrimination (i.e., random performance), 1.0 to perfect discrimination, and values less than 0.5 to worse-than-random performance.

## Comparison of Clinical and Exercise Test Variables

In an extensive review, Yamada and colleagues (8) listed the variables (Table 17.3) chosen as predictors of disease in 24 studies that considered exercise test and clinical variables to predict presence of any angiographic disease.

All of the studies found gender to be significant and 94% of the studies found presenting chest pain symptoms to be significant for predicting the presence of angiographic disease. Other clinical and exercise test variables were less consistently predictive of disease.

Detrano et al presented one of the first well validated scores; they included 3549 patients from eight institutions who underwent exercise testing and angiography between 1978 and 1989 (17). Disease was defined as greater than 50% diameter narrowing in at least one major coronary arterial branch and the prevalence of disease according to this criterion was 64%. They considered a total of 15 clinical and exercise variables, which contributed significant and independent information to disease probability and had been judged clinically relevant by a panel of cardiologists as candidates for logistic regression. The Detrano equation is listed below:

$$1.9 + (0.025 \cdot \text{Age}) - (0.6 \cdot \text{Gender})$$
$$- (0.11 \cdot \text{Symptoms}) - (0.05 \cdot \text{METs})$$
$$- (0.02 \cdot \text{Maximal heart rate})$$
$$+ (0.36 \cdot \text{Exercise induced angina})$$
$$+ (0.59 \cdot \text{mm ST depression})$$

Gender was coded as 1 for female and -1 for male. Symptoms were classified into four categories: typical, atypical, nonanginal pain and no pain and coded

**Table 17.3  Predictors of Disease Presence in 24 Studies That Considered Exercise Test and Clinical Variables to Predict Presence of Any Angiographic Disease***

| Variables | Significant predictor | |
|---|---|---|
| Gender | 20/20 | 100% |
| Chest pain symptoms | 17/18 | 94% |
| Age | 19/27 | 70% |
| Elevated cholesterol | 8/13 | 62% |
| Diabetes mellitus | 6/14 | 43% |
| Smoking history | 4/12 | 33% |
| Abnormal resting ECG | 4/17 | 24% |
| Hypertension | 1/8 | 13% |
| Family history of CAD | 0/7 | 0% |
| ST segment slope | 14/22 | 64% |
| ST segment depression | 17/28 | 61% |
| Maximal HR | 16/28 | 57% |
| Exercise capacity | 11/24 | 46% |
| Exercise induced angina | 11/26 | 42% |
| Double product | 2/13 | 15% |
| Maximal systolic BP | 1/12 | 8% |

with values of 1, 2, 3 and 4, respectively. Exercise angina was coded as 1 for presence and -1 for absence.

Morise et al studied a total of 915 consecutive patients without a history of prior myocardial infarction or coronary artery bypass surgery who were referred to the exercise lab at West Virginia University Medical Center between June 1981 and December 1994 for evaluation of coronary disease (18). All patients had coronary angiography within 3 months of the exercise test. The same angiographic criterion was used and the prevalence of disease was 41%. The following is their logistic regression equation:

$$-.12 + (4.5 \cdot [-3.61 + (0.076 \cdot \text{Age})$$
$$- (1.33 \cdot \text{Gender}) + (0.64 \cdot \text{Symptoms})$$
$$+ (.65 \cdot \text{Diabetes}) + (0.28 \cdot \text{Smoking})$$
$$- (1.46 \cdot \text{Body Surface Area}) + (.50 \cdot \text{Estrogen})$$
$$+ (0.33 \cdot \text{Number of Risk Factors})$$
$$- (.40 \cdot \text{Rest ECG})]) + (0.37 \cdot \text{mm ST depression})$$
$$+ (1.02 \cdot \text{ST slope}) - (0.37 \cdot \text{Negative ST})$$
$$- (0.02 \cdot \text{Maximal heart rate})$$

Gender was coded as 1 for female and 0 for male. Symptoms were classified into four categories: typical, atypical, nonanginal pain and no pain and coded with values of 4, 3, 2 and 1, respectively. Diabetes was coded as 1 if present and 0 if absent. Smoking was coded as 2 for current smoking, 1 for any prior smoking and 0 for never smoked. Estrogen was coded as 0 for males, 1 for estrogen negative (postmenopausal and no estrogen) and -1 for estrogen positive (premenopausal or taking estrogen). Risk factors included history of hypertension, hypercholesterolemia and obesity (BMI $\geq$ 27 kg/m$^2$). Rest ECG was coded as 0 if normal and 1 if there were QRS or ST-T wave abnormalities. mm ST depression was coded as 0 for women. ST Slope was coded as 1 for downsloping and 0 for upsloping or horizontal. Negative ST was coded as 1 if ST depression was less than 1 mm depression horizontal or downsloping, or ST depression was less than 1.5 mm upsloping.

In an attempt to make the scores more portable, we used a consensus approach. Data from 718 male patients at two university-affiliated Veterans Affairs medical centers who underwent exercise testing and coronary angiography within 3 months of an exercise test was analyzed (19). After development of a model for predicting pre-exercise test probability for CAD, the exercise test variables were considered along with the pre-exercise score as candidates for a second stepwise logistic regression. Pre-exercise Test Equation:

$$-2.1 + (0.03 \cdot age) - (0.4 \cdot symptoms) \\ + (0.8 \cdot diabetes) + (0.4 \cdot hypercholesterolemia) \\ + (0.01 \cdot pack\text{-}years) \\ + (0.7 \cdot resting\ ST\ depression\ in\ mm)$$

Postexercise Test Equation.

$$-1.2 + (3.3 \cdot pretest) \\ + (0.5 \cdot exercise\ ST\ depression\ in\ mm) \\ + (0.6 \cdot ST\ slope) + (0.16 \cdot METs) \\ - (0.5 \cdot exercise\ angina)$$

Only four exercise variables were independent predictors: exercise ST depression, ST slope, exercise capacity in METs, and the presence of angina during exercise. Pretest was a number between 0 and 1 generated by the pretest equation.

A probability score was calculated for each patient using the LB-PA equation and the two other equations developed in different populations [Morise et al (18) and Detrano et al (17)]. Since the patients in the intermediate group would be sent for further testing and would eventually be correctly classified, the sensitivity of the consensus approach was 94% and specificity was 92%. The percent of correct diagnosis increased from the 67% for standard exercise ECG analysis and from the 77% for multivariable predictive equations alone to >90% correct diagnoses for the consensus approach. The consensus approach avoids the need to calibrate the equations for disease prevalence, and it avoids some of the problems associated with missing data, differences in the definition of collected variables, and even angiographic interpretation and criteria. In addition, the consensus approach is best applied utilizing a computer program such as EXTRA to simplify the process of calculating the probability of coronary artery disease (20).

Simplified scores derived from multivariable equations have been developed for pre-test estimates of disease and for prognosis; they require physicians to only add points. To develop such a score but from treadmill testing, data from 2 VA Medical Centers was analyzed. The score derived was then validated in 476 males from another institution. METs were eliminated in the model by maximal heart rate since they were highly correlated.

Our simplified score is calculated as follows:

$$6 \cdot Maximal\ Heart\ Rate + 5 \cdot ST\ depression\ code \\ + 4 \cdot age\ code + Angina\ Pectoris\ code \\ + Hypercholesterolemia\ code + Diabetes\ code \\ + Treadmill\ angina\ index\ code$$

Patients were assigned into three groups. The group with low probability of CAD was defined as having a score of less than 40, intermediate a score between 40 and 60 and high probability as a score above 60. The prevalence of any CAD in the low probability group was 27%, 62% in the intermediate and 92% in the high probability group which was comparable to the validation group with 22%, 58% and 92% in low, intermediate and high probability groups respectively. The score showed good portability and requires use of simple coding that can be carried on index cards. (Table 17.4)

## Prognostic Scores

Several studies have incorporated multiple exercise variables into a simple prognostic score to extract the maximum information available and to allow the clinician to summarize the most important information from the test without using complex regression formulas. The most accepted of these is the Duke Treadmill score since it can be used both for

**Table 17.4   Coding of the Variables for the Score for Men**

| Variables | Enter variable | Code | Add points |
|---|---|---|---|
| Maximal heart rate | | Less than 200 bpm = 5; 100-130 = 4; 130-160 = 3; 160 to 190 bpm = 2; 190-220 = 1; more than 220 = 0 | × 6 = |
| St depression | | 0–1 mm = 0; 1-2 mm = 3; more than 2 mm = 5 | × 5 = |
| Age for men | | 0 to 40 = 0; 40-55 = 3; more than 55 = 5 | × 4 = |
| Angina pectoris | | Definite AP = 5; probable = 3; non-cardiac = 1; None = 0 | |
| Hypercholestrolem ia | | Yes = 5; No = 0 | |
| Diabetes | | Yes = 5; No = 0 | |
| Treadmill angina index | | None = 0; angina occurred = 3; reason for stopping = 5 | |

Total points:

prognosis (21) and diagnosis (22). Mark and colleagues developed the Duke treadmill score using data collected from the 2842 hospitalized patients with known or suspected CAD, all of whom had a catheterization (23). The score was subsequently validated in 613 outpatients evaluated before the decision for cardiac catheterization as well as in several other centers. The Duke score is based on three variables: the amount of ST depression, exercise capacity and whether or not angina occurred during the test or was the reason for stopping. This score should be calculated as part of the final report of every exercise test where it is appropriate. This can be done using a nomogram or by a computer. Some of the commercial treadmill systems automatically calculate it. The Duke treadmill score was calculated as follows:

$$\text{Exercise time} - (5 \cdot \text{ST depression}) - (4 \cdot \text{treadmill angina index})$$

Exercise time is measured in minutes, ST depression is measured in millimeters, and the treadmill angina index is coded from 0 to 2. A value of 0 was assigned if angina was absent, 1 if typical angina occurred during exercise, and 2 if angina was a reason the patient stopped exercising. The final score ranges from +15 or greater (corresponding to a patient who exercise through stage 5 without angina or ST changes to –25 or less (corresponding to a patient who stops exercising at 3 minutes or less because of angina and who has 4 mm of ST depression. The high-risk group are defined by a score less or equal to –11, moderate-risk group with score

ranging from –10 to +4 and low-risk with score more or equal to +5. Patients with a predicted average annual cardiac mortality rate less or equal 1% per year can be managed medically without the need for cardiac catheterization. Patients with predicted average annual cardiac mortality rate more or equal to 3% per year should be referred for cardiac catheterization. Patients with predicted average annual cardiac mortality rate of 1% to 3% per year, including those with suspected LV dysfunction, should have either cardiac catheterization or exercise imaging study (24). (Table 17.5)

In addition to providing accurate prognostic estimates, the Duke Treadmill Score also provides valuable information about the presence and severity of coronary disease. According to Shaw at al, the Duke Treadmill Score was effectively diagnostic for significant and severe CAD. For low-risk patients 60% had no coronary stenosis > 75% and 16% had single-vessel > 75% stenosis. More than 80% of high-risk patients had 2-vessel coronary dis-

**Table 17.5   Survival According to Risk Groups Based in Duke Treadmill Score**

| Risk group, score | % of total | 4-year survival | Annual mortality, % |
|---|---|---|---|
| Low (≥5) | 62 | 0.99 | 0.25 |
| Moderate (–10 to 4) | 34 | 0.95 | 1.25 |
| High (<–10) | 4 | 0.79 | 5.0 |

ease with left anterior descending involvement or more severe disease (22). Iskandrian and colleagues reported that almost 50% of low-risk treadmill score patients had no or single-vessel coronary disease, whereas 75% of high-risk patients had multivessel disease in a series of 834 patients undergoing myocardial perfusion imaging (25).

Clinical presentation, performance in diagnostic tests and prevalence of coronary artery disease is different between men and women presenting with chest pain. Treadmill testing has been reported to have a lower accuracy for diagnosis of chest pain in women due to an increase rate of false-positives. Researchers at Duke University Medical Center (26) collected data from 3225 patients referred for evaluation of chest pain and underwent exercise treadmill test and cardiac catheterization. Of these, 30% (976) were women. Analysis showed that predictions for women should be interpreted within the context of lower pretest risk for both diagnostic and prognostic stratification. Women and men differed significantly in mean Duke Treadmill Score (DTC), disease prevalence (32% in men vs. 72% in women), and 2-year mortality (1.9% in women, 4.9% for the men). Two-year mortality for women was 1.0%, 2.2% and 3.6% respectively for low, moderate, high risk DTS groups. Two year mortality for men was 1.7%, 5.8% and 16.6%, respectively for low, moderate and high risk DTS groups. Although many low risk men can be managed without additional invasive testing, this is true for both low and moderate risk women. Although overall women had better survival, the DTS performed actually better in women than in men for excluding disease.

Froelicher and colleagues have created a prognostic VA score using 2546 patients from Long Beach Veterans Administration Hospital (27). In contrast to the Duke score which is strictly exercise-based, clinical data were included also. Using multivariable Cox regression analysis, four variables with the best predictive power were chosen: history of congestive heart failure or digoxin use, a score for the change in systolic blood pressure during exercise, exercise capacity (METs), and exercise-induced ST depression. The score that was derived from the survival analysis was:

$$5 \cdot (\text{congestive heart failure or digoxin use [yes = 1, no = 0]})$$
$$+ \text{ exercise induced ST depression in millimeters}$$
$$+ \text{ change in systolic blood pressure score} - \text{METs}$$

Where systolic blood pressure score was equal to 0 for increase of systolic blood pressure greater than 40 mmHg during exercise test, 1 for increase of 31 to 40 mm Hg, 2 for increase of 21 to 30 mm Hg, 3 for increase of 11 to 20, 4 for increase of 0 to 11 mmHg and 5 for a reduction below standing systolic pre-exercise blood pressure. ST depression is measured in millimeters. Three groups were formed in which –2 indicated low risk, –2 to 2 indicated moderate risk, and greater than 2 indicated high risk. The annual cardiovascular mortality was less than 2% for low-risk (77% of population), 7% for moderate risk (18% of cohort) and 15% for high-risk groups (6% of patients).

## Resting ST Depression and Exercise Testing

Exercise testing of patients with ST-T abnormalities on the resting electrocardiogram was traditionally thought to be problematic. Recent studies have shown that resting ST segment depression does not affect the overall diagnostic accuracy of the exercise test. In a large study from our lab, sensitivity of the treadmill test increased in patients with resting ST segment depression (71 + 7% vs. 42 + 4%) and specificity decreased (52 + 9% vs. 87 + 3%) (28). Kwok et al demonstrated that the Duke treadmill score can effectively risk-stratify patients with ST-T abnormalities on the resting ECG. When patients with ST-T abnormalities were classified into risk groups according to Duke Score, there were significant overall differences among the risk groups for all outcome endpoints. The 7-year event-free survival was 94%, 88%, and 69% for the low-, intermediate-, and high- risk groups, respectively. More patients with ST-T changes were classified as high risk (5% vs. 2%) and their 7-year survival was lower than that of the control population high-risk patients (76% versus 93%) (29).

## Exercise Testing and Prognosis in the Elderly

The decline in function that accompanies aging is a consequence of age-related decrements in cardiovascular, pulmonary, and musculoskeletal structure. Ultimately, these result in impaired physical function in the elderly (30). While the Duke treadmill score was validated in patients in the age range when CAD first appears, data is limited in the elderly. To determine the prognostic value of the treadmill test in the elderly, researchers from the Mayo

Clinic and the Olmsted Medical Group compared the prognostic value of the test in patients less than 65 and older than 65 years of age. Elderly (n = 2593) and younger (n = 514) patients who underwent treadmill exercise testing between 1987 and 1989 were identified retrospectively and followed up for 6 years. Compared to younger patients, elderly patients had more comorbid conditions, a higher prevalence of abnormal ST depression (28% vs. 9%) and achieved lower workloads (6.0 METs vs. 10.7 METs). A poor exercise capacity and angina during the exercise test were associated with future cardiac events. Exercise-induced ST depression did not carry significant value in the elderly and was associated with future cardiac events only in younger patients. An increase of 1 MET in the workload was associated with a 14% decrease in risk for a cardiac event in younger patients and with a 18% risk reduction among the elderly. After adjustment for clinical factors, there was a strong inverse association between exercise capacity and outcome. Workload achieved was the only treadmill exercise testing variable that provided prognostic information for mortality and cardiac events. In the elderly, exercise capacity was also inversely associated with the likelihood of nursing home placement (31).

Studies of exercise capacity and exercise conditioning in selected groups of elderly subjects have demonstrated a diminished exercise capacity compared with that of younger subjects but a similar relative ability to improve aerobic capacity with a conditioning program (32). Exercise training is widely recommended as a valuable tool in prolonging longevity as well as the quality of life of elderly patients.

## Patients With Congestive Heart Failure

Prognostic studies have shown the usefulness of cardiopulmonary exercise testing in heart failure assessment, particularly in selecting those who may benefit from cardiac transplantation (33). Exercise capacity determined by peak ventilatory oxygen uptake ($\dot{V}O_2$), has been shown to complement other clinical and invasive markers of disease severity, including ejection fraction, pulmonary capillary wedge pressure, type of heart failure, and cardiac index. Peak $\dot{V}O_2$ less than 10 mL/kg per minute identifies a group of patients with a particularly poor 1-year prognosis (1-year mortality rate, 24% to 77%). Patients in whom the peak $\dot{V}O_2$ is greater than 14 mL/kg per minute have a 1-year survival

rate similar to that of patients receiving transplantation (>90%). This suggests that transplantation can be deferred in these patients. A recent study by Myers et al (34) determined that measured $\dot{V}O_2$ is more powerful than estimated $\dot{V}O_2$ in predicting prognosis. Cardiopulmonary exercise test was more important in assessing risk in patients with chronic heart failure than right heart catheterization.

Elderly patients with CHF have a high mortality with the majority dead within two years. As in younger patients, VE/$\dot{V}CO_2$ slope and peak $\dot{V}O_2$ carry significant prognostic information (35). Despite the fact that older subjects with CHF have lower exercise capacities, the discriminatory power of cardiopulmonary exercise test remains the same in risk stratification as it is in the younger patients (36).

## Localization

The data available supports the concept that the major ST shift with ischemia is down the long axis of the left ventricle and is due to global subendocardial ischemia. Another words, ST depression does not localize the blocked coronary artery. ST elevation is another matter but it is relatively rare. The local effect of right ventricular ischemia could cause elevation over the right-sided leads but even perfusion scanning could not validate this. The norms for the right-sided ST response need to be determined by appropriate study and the Athens study must be validated before right-sided leads are utilized clinically to diagnose ischemia (37).

## Heart Rate

The heart rate in recovery is largely controlled by vagal tone that returns very quickly after exercise during which the sympathetic system predominates after exercise (38). The level of exercise training is the major controller of the rate of heart rate drop and this may be indirectly linked to disease. The autonomic dysfunction of chronotropic incompetence is related to left ventricular dysfunction and not ischemia and thus may predict prognosis in groups of patients where CHF or LV dysfunction are not excluded. It should not be helpful in predicting angiographic findings. The main concern is that so many things affect the vagal and sympathetic tone balance that it cannot be a good marker. Interestingly, in follow up studies, the Cox hazard function picks METs over maximal heart rate while angiographic correlate studies using logistic regression pick maximal heart rate over METs (8). They are so interrelated that both are never chosen but substitute nicely for each other.

The ST Heart rate index is attractive theoretically but statistically flawed (39). A ratio requires that both numerator and denominator have equal weights for prediction. This clearly is not the case for ST depression and heart rate. First, the ranges and units are totally different and secondly, when heart rate and ST depression are entered into logistic regression (or any multivariable model) they have totally different weights. The only way to deal with the potential variables for prediction of angiographic disease is to put them into a mathematical model and allow them to be selected or not and to be weighted as to their predictive power if they are chosen.

## Exercise Testing Post–Myocardial Infarction

Meta-analyses of the prognostic value of exercise testing post-MI, one pre (40) and one post (41) the advent of the thrombolysis era, confirm the value of testing. However, there are other benefits of performing the test (42). Submitting patients to exercise testing post MI can expedite and optimize their discharge from the hospital. The patient's response to exercise, their work capacity, and limiting factors at the time of discharge can be assessed by the exercise test. An exercise test prior to discharge is important for giving patient guidelines for exercise at home, reassuring them of their physical status, and determining the risk of complications. It provides a safe basis for advising the patient to resume or increase his or her activity level and return to work. The test can demonstrate to the patient, relatives, or employer the effect of the MI on the capacity for physical performance. Psychologically, it can cause an improvement in the patient's self-confidence by making the patient less anxious about daily physical activities (43). The test has been helpful in reassuring spouses of post MI patients of their physical capabilities. The psychological impact of performing well on the exercise test is impressive. Many patients increase their activity and actually rehabilitate themselves after being encouraged and reassured by their response to this test.

Exercise testing is useful in activity counseling after hospital discharge. It is also an important tool in exercise training as part of comprehensive cardiac rehabilitation, where it can be used to develop and modify the exercise prescription, assist in providing activity counseling, and assess the patient's response into, and progress in, the exercise training program. For all these reasons, the ACC/AHA guidelines call for exercise testing post-MI (44).

One consistent finding in the post MI exercise test studies that included a follow up for cardiac end points is that patients who met whatever criteria set forth for exercise testing were at lower risk than patients not tested. This finding supports the clinical judgment of the skilled clinician. In the first meta-analysis, only an abnormal SBP response or low exercise capacities were significantly associated with a poor outcome (40). These responses are so powerful because they can be associated with either ischemic events or CHF events.

The DUKE meta-analysis compared the available noninvasive tests results to outcomes in patients recovering from acute-myocardial infarction (41). Studies published from 1980 to 1995 had to fulfill these criteria: only MI patients, most patients enrolled after 1980, tested within 6 weeks of MI, follow-up rates greater than 80%, and having outcome prevalence rates for test results, and only the latest results were considered if there were multiple reports from the same institution. Sensitivity, specificity, and predictive values were calculated for test results for 1-year outcomes (cardiac death, cardiac death or reinfarction). Univariable and summary odds ratios (OR) were calculated for test results. The qualifying reports (n=54) included 19,874 patients and three-quarters were retrospective (76%) and a third were small samples with less than 5 deaths. One-year mortality in the studies ranged from 2.5% for pharmacologic stress echocardiography to 9.3% for exercise radionuclide angiography studies consistent with population differences. Positive predictive values (the percentage of those with an abnormal test that have the outcome during follow up) for most noninvasive risk markers were less than 10% for cardiac death and less than 20% for death or reinfarction. Electrocardiographic, symptomatic, and scintigraphic markers of ischemia (ST-segment depression, angina, a reversible defect) were less sensitive (average about 44%) for identifying morbid and fatal outcomes than markers of both left ventricular dysfunction and ischemia (exercise duration, exertional hypotension, peak left ventricular ejection fraction). The positive predictive value of predischarge noninvasive testing is low. Markers of left ventricular dysfunction or both dysfunction and ischemia were better predictors than markers of myocardial ischemia alone.

The GISSI-2 database has enabled reevaluation of the prognostic role of exercise testing in patients who have received thrombolysis (45). Exercise tests were performed on 6296 patients at an average of 28 days after randomization for thrombolysis post MI. The test was not performed on 3923 patients (40%) because of contraindications. The test was positive for ischemia in 26% of the patients, negative in 38%, and non-diagnostic in 36%. Among the patients with an ischemic test result, 33% had symptoms, whereas 67% had silent myocardial ischemia. The mortality rate was 7.1% among patients who did not have an exercise test and 1.7% for those with an ischemic test, 0.9% for those who had a normal test, and 1.3% for those with non-diagnostic tests. In an adjusted analysis, symptomatic induced ischemia, ischemia at a sub maximal workload, low work capacity, and abnormal systolic blood pressure were independent predictors of 6-month mortality (relative risks 2.5, 2.3, 2, and 1.9, respectively). However, when these variables were considered simultaneously, only symptomatic induced ischemia and low work capacity were confirmed as independent predictors of mortality (Cox hazard ratio of 2 and 1.8, respectively) (46).

The two meta-analyses summarized above of 30 studies including over 20,000 patients found that poor exercise capacity and abnormal SBP response were more predictive of adverse cardiac events after myocardial infarction than measures of exercise-induced ischemia. While the majority of the studies included were performed prior to the reperfusion era, similar results were found in the GISSI report that considered 6000 patients who received thrombolysis.

## Conclusions

It is important to consider these precepts regarding exercise testing methodology:

- The treadmill protocol should be adjusted to the patient and one protocol is not appropriate for all patients.
- Report exercise capacity in METs not minutes of exercise.
- Hyperventilation prior to testing is not indicated but can be utilized at another time if a false positive is suspected.
- ST measurements should be made at ST0 (J-junction) and ST depression should only be considered abnormal if horizontal or downsloping.

- Patients should be placed supine as soon as possible post-exercise with a cool down walk avoided in order for the test to have its greatest diagnostic value.
- The three-minute recovery period is critical to include in analysis of the ST response.
- Measurement of systolic blood pressure during exercise is extremely important and exertional hypotension is ominous; at this point, only manual BP measurement techniques are valid.
- Age-predicted heart rate targets are largely useless because of the wide scatter for any age; a relatively low heart rate can be maximal for a given patient and submaximal for another. Thus, a test should not be considered non-diagnostic if a percentage of age-predicted maximal heart rate (i.e., 85%) is not reached.
- The Duke Treadmill score should be calculated automatically on every test.
- Other predictive equations should be considered as part of the treadmill report.

To insure the safety of exercise testing and reassure the non-cardiologist performing the test, the following list of the most dangerous circumstances in the exercise testing lab should be considered:

- Testing patients with aortic valvular disease or obstructive hypertrophic cardiomyopathy (ASH or IHSS) should be done with great care. Aortic stenosis can cause cardiovascular collapse and it may be extremely difficult to resuscitate them because of the outflow obstruction; IHSS can become unstable due to arrhythmia. Because of these conditions, a physical exam including assessment of systolic murmurs should be done before all exercise tests. If a significant murmur is heard, an echocardiogram should be considered before performing the test.
- The most important indicator of a possible adverse event is a drop in systolic blood pressure.
- When patients exhibit ST segment elevation without diagnostic Q-waves this can be associated with dangerous arrhythmias and infarction; it occurs in about one out of 1000 clinical tests.
- A cool down walk is advisable when a patient with an ischemic cardiomyopathy exhibits severe chest pain due to ischemia (angina pectoris) since the ischemia can worsen in recovery.

- A cool down walk is advisable when a patient develops exertional hypotension accompanied by ischemia (angina or ST depression) or when it occurs in a patient with a history of CHF, cardiomyopathy or recent MI.
- A cool down walk is advisable when a patient with a history of sudden death or collapse during exercise develops PVCs, which become frequent.
- Appreciation of these circumstances can help avoid any complications in your exercise lab.

In the next millennium medical instrument manufacturers, should become more involved in helping physicians use proper methodologies and correct interpretation. Since the guidelines have standardized these areas the manufacturers will not be medico-legally liable. Calculation of scores and computerized reports should become the standard for equipment performance (47). Recently we have shown that the scores do as well as expert cardiologists in estimating disease (48). Over reading services for all ECG functions should become readily available utilizing the Internet. Both of these advances will assist the practitioner in performing the exercise test optimally. In regard to equipment, the next decade should bring inexpensive web-enabled devices that will bring sophisticated exercise testing to the Doctor's office with little initial expense. Neither the patient nor the physician will be paying for expensive equipment but just the service. This largely depends upon broadband Internet access in the doctors' office and acceptance of a new financial paradigm for the medical instrument industry.

# References

1. Philbrick JT, Horowitz, Feinstein AR. Methodological problems of exercise testing for coronary artery disease: groups, analysis and bias. *Am J Cardiol* 1989;64:1117-1122.
2. Reid M, Lachs M, Feinstein A. Use of Methodological Standards in Diagnostic Test Research. *JAMA* 1995;274:645-651.
3. Guyatt GH. Readers' guide for articles evaluating diagnostic tests: What ACP Journal Club does for you and what you must do yourself. *ACP Journal Club* 1991;115:A-16.
4. Froelicher VF, Fearon W, Ferguson C, West J, Hedenreich P. Lessons learned from studies of the standard exercise test? *CHEST* 1999; 116:1442-1451.
5. O'Rourke R, Brundage B, Froelicher V, Greenland P, Grundy S, Hachamovitch R, Pohost G, Shaw L, et al. American College of Cardiology/American Heart Association Expert Consensus Document on Electron-Beam Computed Tomography for the Diagnosis and Prognosis of Coronary Artery Disease. (ACC/AHA Expert Consensus Document). *Circulation* 2000;102(1):126-140.
6. Gibbons RJ, Balady GJ, Beasley JW, et al. ACC/AHA guidelines for exercise testing: executive summary. A report of the American College of Cardiology/American Heart Association Task Force on Practice Guidelines (Committee on Exercise Testing). *J Am Col Card* 1997(30);260-311.
7. Froelicher VF; Lehmann KG; Thomas R; Goldman S; Morrison D; Myers J; Dennis C; Shabetai R; Do D; Froning J. The electrocardiographic exercise test in a population with reduced workup bias: diagnostic performance, computerized interpretation, and multivariable prediction. Veterans Affairs Cooperative Study in Health Services #016 (QUEXTA) Study Group. Quantitative Exercise Testing and Angiography. *Ann Intern Med* 1998 Jun 15;128(12 Pt 1):965-74
8. Yamada H, Do D, Morise A, Froelicher V. Review of Studies Utilizing Multi-variable Analysis of Clinical and Exercise Test Data to Predict Angiographic Coronary Artery Disease. *Progress in CV Disease*, 1997; 39:457-481.
9. Kansal S; Roitman D; Bradley EL Jr; Sheffield LT. Enhanced evaluation of treadmill tests by means of scoring based on multivariate analysis and its clinical application: a study of 608 patients. *Am J Cardiol* 1983 Dec 1;52(10):1155-60.
10. Fisher LD; Kennedy JW; Chaitman BR; Ryan TJ; McCabe C; Weiner D; Tristani F; Schloss M; Warner HR Jr. Diagnostic quantification of CASS (coronary artery surgery study) clinical and exercise test results in determining presence and extent of coronary artery disease. A multivariate approach.
11. Hollenberg M; Budge WR; Wisneski JA; Gertz EW Treadmill score quantifies electrocardiographic response to exercise and improves test accuracy and reproducibility. *Circulation* 1980 Feb;61(2):276-85.
12. Cohn K; Kamm B; Feteih N; Brand R; Goldschlager N. Use of treadmill score to quantify ischemic response and predict extent of coronary disease. *Circulation* 1979 Feb;59(2):286-96.

13. Berman JL; Wynne J; Cohn PF. A multivariate approach for interpreting treadmill exercise tests in coronary artery disease. *Circulation* 1978 Sep;58(3):505-12.

14. Laupacis, Andreas MD; Sekar, Nandita MD; Stiell, Ian G. MD. Clinical Prediction Rules: A Review and Suggested Modifications of Methodological Standards. [Review] *JAMA* 1997; 277(6):488-494.

15. Hachamovitch R, Berman D, Kiat H, Cohen I, Cabico A et al. Exercise Myocardial Perfusion SPECT in Patients Without Known Coronary Artery Disease. Incremental Prognostic Value and Use in Risk Stratification. *Circulation* 1996;93(5):905-914.

16. Morise A, Haddad J, Beckner D. Development and Validation of a Clinical Score to estimate the Probability of Coronary Artery Disease in Men and Women Presenting with Suspected Coronary Disease. *Am J Med*. 1997;102:350-356.

17. Detrano R, Bobbio M, Olson H, et al. Computer probability estimates of angiographic coronary artery disease: Transportability and comparison with cardiologists's estimates. *Comp & Bio Res* 1992; 25:468-485.

18. Morise AP, Detrano R, Bobbio M and Diamond GA. Development and Validation of a Logistic Regression - Derived Algorithm for Estimating the Incremental Probability of Coronary Artery Disease Before and After Exercise Testing. *JACC* 1992; 20:1187-96.

19. Do D, West J, Morise A, Atwood E, Froelicher V. A Consensus Approach to Diagnosing Coronary Artery Disease Based on Clinical and Exercise Test Data. *Chest* 1997;11(6):1742-1749.

20. Shiu P, Froelicher V. EXTRA: An Expert System for Exercise Testing Utilizing Consensus to Predict Coronary Disease. *J Inv Card* 1998; 2(6):21-26.

21. Mark DB, Shaw L, Harrell FE, Jr., et al. Prognostic value of a treadmill exercise score in outpatients with suspected coronary artery disease. *N Engl J Med* 1991;325(12):849-53.

22. Shaw LJ; Peterson ED; Shaw LK; Kesler KL; DeLong ER; Harrell FE Jr; Muhlbaier LH; Mark DB. Use of a prognostic treadmill score in identifying diagnostic coronary disease subgroups. Circulation 1998 Oct 20;98(16):1622-30

23. Mark D, Hlatky M, Harrell F, Kerry L et al. Exercise Treadmill Score for Predicting Prognosis in Coronary Artery Disease. *Ann Intern Med* 1987;106:793-800.

24. Gibbons R, Chatterjee K, Daley J, Douglas J et al. ACC/AHA/ACP-ASIM Guidelines for the Management of Patients with Chronic Stable Angina: Executive Summary and Recommendations (Committee on Management of patients With Chronic Stable Angina). *Circulation* 1999;99:2829-2848.

25. Iscandrian AS, Ghods M, Helfeld H, Iscandrian B et al. The Treadmill exercise score revised: coronary arteriographic and thallium perfusion correlates. *Am Heart J*. 1992;124:1581-1586.

26. Alexander K, Shaw L, Delong E et al. Value of Exercise Treadmill Testing in Women. *J Am Coll Cardiol* 1998;32(6):1657-64.

27. Morrow K, Morris C, Froelicher V, Hideg A et al. Prediction of Cardiovascular Death in Men Undergoing Noninvasive Evaluation for Coronary Artery Disease. *Ann Intern Med* 1993;118:689-695.

28. Fearon W, Lee D, Froelicher V. The Effect of Resting ST Segment Depression on the Diagnostic Characteristics of the Exercise Treadmill Test. *J Am Coll Cardiol* 2000;35:1206-11.

29. Kwok JM, Miller TD, Christian TF, Hodge DO, Gibbons RJ. Prognostic Value of a Treadmill Exercise Score in Symptomatic Patients with Nonspecific ST-T Abnormalities on Resting ECG. *JAMA*;1999:282(11):1047-53.

30. Brechue W, Pollock M. Exercise training for coronary artery disease in the elderly. *Clinics in Geriatric Medicine* 1996;12(1):207-229.

31. Goraya T, Jacobsen S, Pellikka P, Miller T, Khan A, Weston S, et al. Prognostic Value of Treadmill Exercise Testing in Elderly Persons. *Ann Intern Med* 2000;132:862-870.

32. Ades P, Grunvald M. Cardiopulmonary Exercise testing before and after conditioning in older coronary patients. *Am Heart J* 1990; 120:585-589.

33. A Symposium: Consensus Recommendations for the Management of Chronic Heart Failure. *Am J Cardiol* 1999;83(2):2A-38A.

34. Myers J, Gullestad L, Vagelos R, Do D et al. Clinical, Hemodynamic, and Cardiopulmonary Exercise Test Determinants of Survival in Patients Referred for Evaluation of Heart Failure. *Ann Intern Med* 1998;129(4):286-293

35. Davies LC, Francis DP, Piepoli M, Scott AC et al. Chronic Heart Failure in the Elderly: Value of Cardiopulmonary Exercise Testing in Risk Stratification. *Heart* 2000;83(2):147-151.

36. Ades P, Grunvald M. Cardiopulmonary Exercise Testing Before and After Conditioning in Older Coronary Patients. *Am Heart J* 1990; 120:585-589.

37. Michaelides A, Psomadaki Z, Dilaveris P, et al. Improving detection of coronary artery disease by exercise electrocardiography with the use of right precordial leads. *New England Journal of Medicine* 1999;340:340-345.

38. Lauer MS, Francis GS, Okin PM, Pashkow FJ, Snader CE, Marwick TH. Impaired chronotropic response to exercise stress testing as a predictor of mortality. *JAMA* 1999;281(6):524-9.

39. Lachterman B, Lehmann KG, Neutel J, Froelicher VF. Comparison of the ST/heart rate index to standard ST criteria for analysis of the exercise electrocardiogram. *Circulation* 1990; 82:44-50.

40. Froelicher VF, Perdue S, Pewen W, Risch M. Application of meta-analysis using an electronic spreadsheet to exercise testing in patients with myocardial infarction. *Am J Med* 1987; 83:1045-1054.

41. Shaw LJ; Peterson ED; Kesler K; Hasselblad V; Califf RM. A metaanalysis of predischarge risk stratification after acute myocardial infarction with stress electrocardiographic, myocardial perfusion, and ventricular function imaging. *Am J Cardiol* 1996 Dec 15;78(12):1327-37

42. Madsen EHJ 2000;

43. Ewart CK, Taylor CB, Reese LB, DeBusk RF. Effects of early postmyocardial infarction exercise testing on self-perception and subsequent physical activity. *Am J Cardiol* 1983;51:1076-1080.

44. Ryan TJ; Anderson JL; Antman EM; Braniff BA; Brooks NH; Califf RM; Hillis LD; Hiratzka LF; Rapaport E; Riegel BJ; Russell RO; Smith EE; Weaver WD. ACC/AHA guidelines for the management of patients with acute myocardial infarction: executive summary. A report of the American College of Cardiology/American Heart Association Task Force on Practice Guidelines (Committee on Management of Acute Myocardial Infarction). *Circulation* 1996 Nov 1;94(9):2341-50

45. Villella A; Maggioni AP; Villella M; Giordano A; Turazza FM; Santoro E; Franzosi MG. Prognostic significance of maximal exercise testing after myocardial infarction treated with thrombolytic agents: the GISSI-2 data-base. *Lancet* 1995 Aug 26;346(8974):523-9

46. Piccalo G, Pirelli S, Massa D, Cipriani M, Sarullo FM, DeVita C. Value of negative predischarge exercise testing in identifying patients at low risk after acute myocardial infarction treated by systemic thrombolysis. *Am J Cardiol* 1992;70:31-33.

47. Atwood JE; Do D; Froelicher V; Chilton R; Dennis C; Froning J; Janosi A; Mortara D; Myers J. Can computerization of the exercise test replace the cardiologist? *Am Heart J* 1998 Sep;136 (3):543-52

48. Can Physicians Diagnose Coronary Disease as well as Scores? Michael Lipinski, Eddie Atwood, Lars Osterberg, , Barry Franklin, Jeff West, Victor Froelicher, AHA Scientific Sessions, 1999

# Chapter 18

# Doppler Echocardiography for Stratification of Patients Wtih Heart Failure

Pier Luigi Temporelli, MD, Italy

## Introduction

Despite recent advances in medical and surgical therapy of chronic heart failure (CHF), this disease process still has high annual mortality rates, and consequently, its management represents a major challenge in day to day medical practice. Although many clinical indices have been used to estimate the severity of CHF, all have limitations on the account of heterogeneity and complexity of the syndrome.

## Left Ventricular Dysfunction

Although early investigators were interested by the abnormalities of systolic function to explain the signs and symptoms of heart failure, it has become increasingly clear that abnormalities of diastolic function also play a major role (1).

Left ventricular (LV) diastolic performance, characterized by two distinct parameters—relaxation and compliance—was initially evaluated by direct measurements of intracardiac pressures, cardiac catheterization being the standard technique for measurement of filling pressures and rate of LV relaxation. It is not practical, however, to use cardiac catheterization for diagnosis or for serial longitudinal follow-ups, mainly because the technique is invasive and sometimes associated with such complications as pneumothorax, infection, arrhythmia and bleeding.

Doppler echocardiography has now become a reliable, reproducible and practical noninvasive method for the diagnosis and longitudinal follow-up of patients with LV dysfunction and CHF. During the past decade, numerous studies have related Doppler mitral flow velocity patterns to left ventricular and pulmonary capillary wedge pressure (PWP) recordings, and a number of transmitral filling abnormalities referable to hemodynamic phenomena have been identified (2-8). Despite the complexity of diastolic function and the multiplicity of factors influencing LV filling, experimental and clinical studies have clearly demonstrated that the major determinant of mitral flow velocity is the transmitral pressure gradient.

In the clinical setting, two diastolic properties (the rate of LV relaxation and compliance) appear to be particularly important determinants of transmitral pressure gradient. In fact, two distinct abnormal flow velocity profiles correlate with specific types of LV diastolic dysfunctions and different filling pressures. The pattern of reduced early rapid filling wave, increased or normal atrial wave (E/A ratio usually <1), prolonged isovolumic relaxation time and deceleration time (DT) of early filling is due to impaired or delayed LV relaxation, reflecting a slower rate of decline in the LV pressure. This pattern is usually associated with normal or near normal left atrial pressure and is frequently observed in patients with LV hypertrophy, systemic hypertension, coronary artery disease and in elderly patients with dilated cardiomyopathy and CHF who do not have severely elevated PWP. The second filling pattern, which is termed *restrictive*, is characterized by a short or normal isovolumic relaxation time, an increased rapid filling wave, a reduced DT of early filling and a decreased velocity at atrial contraction (increased E/A ratio, usually ≥2). This pattern is believed to be related to markedly increased LV stiffness resulting from myocardial or pericardial factors and it is usually seen in patients with more advanced heart disease and increased left atrial pressure.

Besides these two well defined patterns of LV filling, a third abnormal mitral flow velocity profile has been described and this pattern is termed *pseudonormal* indicating that although the ratio of mitral E and A velocities appears normal, abnormalities of LV diastolic properties are present. In this situation, abnormal relaxation and increased chamber stiffness have opposing effects on LV filling, and when both of these abnormalities are present simultaneously, an elevated left atrial pressure, from increased chamber stiffness, normalizes the early diastolic transmitral pressure gradient and velocity despite the impaired LV relaxation. As a consequence, the transmitral pattern appears to be normal (E/A >1) although it is actually pseudonormal. In this setting, the ability of the Doppler flow velocity profile to predict diastolic abnormalities and LV filling pressure may be significantly reduced. This limitation is particularly relevant in more symptomatic patients with systolic dysfunction where noninvasive methods of estimating LV filling pressure would be of great clinical importance. In these patients, it has been recently demonstrated that the DT of early filling is the most powerful predictor of PWP (9).

Although several mitral Doppler variables are independent predictors of PWP, peak flow velocities (both E and A wave) and their ratio are only modestly correlated with PWP. By contrast, a very close negative correlation (r = −0.90) has been found between DT and PWP. Because this relation appears linear for values of 8 to 35 or 40 mm Hg, DT may be used to estimate the absolute PWP between these values. Values <8 mm Hg appear to be less accurate, but this is not clinically relevant. Although the correlation between E/A ratio and PWP is weaker (r 0.65), the mitral flow velocity pattern (as defined by the E/A ratio) is able to identify patients with different degrees of LV dysfunction. However, Doppler-derived mitral DT of early filling, irrespective of the filling pattern, provides a simple and accurate noninvasive method of estimating and monitoring PWP in patients with severe LV systolic dysfunction and CHF, whether the patient is in sinus rhythm (9) or in atrial fibrillation (10). In addition, the prognostic value of mitral DT of early filling has clearly been demonstrated. More specifically, a short (≤125 ms) mitral DT has been found to be a powerful independent predictor of poor prognosis in both symptomatic and asymptomatic patients with LV dysfunction (11). In a study carried out on a large number of patients with severe LV systolic dysfunction (with or without clinical heart failure) Doppler-derived mitral DT of early filling emerged as the most powerful independent predictor of future events (all-cause mortality and hospitalization for congestive heart failure) among demographic, his-

toric, clinical, echocardiographic and mitral Doppler variables. Over a 4-year follow-up period, mortality occurred in 45% of patients with ≤125 ms DT as compared with 13% of patients with >125 ms DT.

In view of the dynamic nature of LV filling, deceleration time and restrictive pattern may vary over time due to changes in LV filling pressures; in other words, an optimal therapeutic regimen may reverse a restrictive pattern and normalize a short DT. Interestingly, a recent study has shown that in clinically stable patients with CHF, a significant prolongation of an initially short (<125 ms) DT may be obtained after 6 months of optimized oral therapy and this improvement clearly identified patients with more favorable outcomes (12). In that study it was also noted that higher risks for fatal outcomes could be predicted through noninvasive variables such as persistently short DT, moderate to severe tricuspid regurgitation, lack of change in ejection fraction over time and LV end-systolic volume at entry. All of these parameters were independent prognostic indicators, while persistent short DT was the single best predictor of cardiac mortality. Over a 4-year follow-up period, cardiac death occurred in 48% of patients with DT persistently <125 ms after 6 months of optimized medical therapy while it occurred in only 14% of patients showing a significant prolongation of a short DT after such therapy. Furthermore, persistently short DT was shown to be the most important predictor of both hospital admissions for worsening heart failure and cumulative cardiac events (death, urgent transplant and hospital admission for heart failure). It was also noted that although at univariate analysis E/A ratio >2 and its variation over time were significantly associated with a worse outcome, at multivariate analysis they did not prove to be independent prognostic indicators. On the contrary, a persistently short (<125) early DT (associated with an E/A ratio <2 in 26% of patients) was found to be the single most powerful indicator of poor prognosis, whereas a prolongation of an initially short DT, which was usually accompanied by a significant reduction in E/A ratio, was associated with a 66% risk reduction of cardiac mortality.

## Right Atrial Pressure

The estimation of right atrial pressures (RAP) is also required for the diagnosis, management, and monitoring of various pathologic hemodynamic conditions. Right heart catheterization allows an accurate measurement of RAP, but it is expensive and not without risks, particularly if prolonged monitoring of this value is needed. Therefore, an alternative and less invasive method for estimation of RAP is highly desirable in the context of clinical practice. In the past decade, several attempts have been made to noninvasively estimate RAP, and echocardiography has always been considered the most reliable tool. Morphologic parameters such as respiratory motion of the inferior vena cava, its respiratory diameters and percent collapse (caval index), left hepatic vein diameter or right atrial dimension (areas, volumes) were initially studied. More recently, functional measurements such as left hepatic or tricuspid flow variables have also been considered. Some of these indexes, however, offer only semiquantitative measurements of RAP, and have failed to demonstrate any prognostic value. Although highly sensitive and specific, other methods are only useful in selected groups of patients because of technical or clinical limitations pertaining to the mode of measurement.

On the basis of the well known and close correlation between Doppler transmitral flow and left ventricular filling pressure, i.e. mean left atrial pressure, it has been hypothesized that the same correlation might exist in the cavities of the right heart. Through the analysis of Doppler tricuspid velocity profile and mean RAP (Swan-Ganz catheter) recorded simultaneously in patients with severe LV systolic dysfunction and CHF, it has been shown that acceleration rate of early tricuspid flow is the most powerful and accurate predictor of mean RAP, both in patients in sinus rhythm and in those with atrial fibrillation (13), irrespective of whether the recordings are at baseline or after acute loading manipulations. As this parameter provides a quantitative estimate of RAP, it gives an accurate noninvasive prediction of systolic pulmonary artery pressure, by adding the RAP value to the right atrium-ventricular gradient derived through the widely accepted modified Bernoulli equation. Ideed, in a recent preliminary analysis (14) of patients with CHF and LV systolic dysfunction, RAP by pulsed Doppler yielded an accurate quantitative estimation of a wide range (from 15 to 79 mm Hg) of systolic pulmonary pressure values (r = .98).

## Pulmonary Vascular Resistance

Assessment of pulmonary vascular resistance (PVR) is an essential component of orthotopic heart transplantation recipient evaluation, and threshold values have been identified that predict poor outcomes both early and late after heart transplantation. The presence of elevated PVR (≥3 Wood units) is an indication for serial right heart catheterization and assessment of pulmonary vascular reactivity before heart transplantation. However, serial right heart catheterization is logistically difficult in outpatients receiving anticoagulant therapy, and data obtained from this procedure are susceptible to interpretive errors, especially in patients with pericardial disease. The accurate noninvasive estimation of PVR represents the ongoing challenge of Doppler echocardiography.

## Summary

Doppler echocardiography has emerged as a noninvasive modality which can be used to assess diastolic filling. There is little doubt that in patients with LV dysfunction and CHF, it is now possible to estimate filling pressures, guide therapy and predict prognosis by analyzing mitral flow velocity curves. Transmitral Doppler derived DT of early filling seems to be the key to the noninvasive assessment of LV filling pressures and diastolic dysfunction in heart failure. In addition, Doppler echocardiographic estimates of several hemodynamic variables in patients with advanced heart failure are now accurate and reproducible. Not too far in the future, the time will come when Doppler echocardiography will replace heart catheterization in the bedside approach to patients with CHF.

## References

1. Grossman W. Diastolic dysfunction in congestive heart failure. *N Engl J Med* 1991;325:1557-64.
2. Appleton CP, Hatle LK, Popp RL. Relation of transmitral velocity patterns to left ventricular diastolic function: new insights from a combined hemodynamic and Doppler echocardiographic study. *J Am Coll Cardiol* 1988; 12:426-40.
3. Stoddard MF, Pearson AC, Kern MJ, Ratcliff J, Mrosek DG, Labovitz AJ. Left ventricular diastolic function: comparison of pulsed Doppler echocardiographic and hemodynamic indexes in subjects with and without coronary artery disease. *J Am Coll Cardiol* 1989; 13:327-36.

4. Vanoverschelde JJ, Raphael DA, Robert AR, Cosyns JR. Left ventricular filling in dilated cardiomyopathy: relation to functional class and hemodynamics. *J Am Coll Cardiol* 1990; 15:1288-95.

5. Giannuzzi P, Shabetai R, Imparato A et al. Effects of mental exercise in patients with dilated cardiomyopathy and congestive heart failure. An echocardiographic Doppler study. *Circulation* 1991;83 (suppl II):II 155-165.

6. Nishimura RA, Appleton CP, Redfield MM, Ilstrup DM, Holmes DR Jr, Tajik AJ. Noninvasive Doppler echocardiographic evaluation of left ventricular filling pressures in patients with cardiomyopathies: a simultaneous Doppler echocardiographic and cardiac catheterization study. *J Am Coll Cardiol* 1996;28:1226-33.

7. Nishimura RA, Tajik AJ. Evaluation of diastolic filling of left ventricle in health and disease: Doppler echocardiography is the clinician's Rosetta stone. *J Am Coll Cardiol* 1997;30:8-18.

8. Pinamonti B, Di Lenarda A, Sinagra G, Camerini F, and the Heart Muscle Disease Study Group. Restrictive left ventricular filling pattern in dilated cardiomyopathy assessed by Doppler echocardiography: clinical, echocardiographic and hemodynamic correlations and prognostic implications. *J Am Coll Cardiol* 1993;22:808-15.

9. Giannuzzi P, Imparato A, Temporelli PL et al. Doppler-derived mitral deceleration time of early filling as a strong predictor of pulmonary capillary wedge pressure in postinfarction patients with left ventricular systolic dysfunction. *J Am Coll Cardiol* 1994;23:1630-7.

10. Temporelli PL, Scapellato F, Corrà U, Eleuteri E, Imparato A, Giannuzzi P. Estimation of pulmonary capillary wedge pressure by transmitral Doppler in patients with chronic heart failure and atrial fibrillation. *Am J Cardiol* 1999;83:724-7.

11. Giannuzzi P, Temporelli PL, Bosimini E et al. Independent and incremental prognostic value of Doppler-derived mitral deceleration time of early filling in both symptomatic and asymptomatic patients with left ventricular dysfunction. *J Am Coll Cardiol* 1996;28:383-90.

12. Temporelli PL, Corrà U, Imparato A, Bosimini E, Scapellato F, Giannuzzi P. Reversible restrictive left ventricular diastolic filling with optimized oral therapy predicts a more favorable prognosis in patients with chronic heart failure. *J Am Coll Cardiol* 1999;31:1591-7.

13. Scapellato F, Eleuteri E, Temporelli PL, Imparato A, Corrà U, Giannuzzi P. Doppler-derived acceleration rate of right ventricular early filling as a measurement of RAP in chronic heart failure secondary to ischemic or idiopathic dilated cardiomyopathy. *Am J Cardiol* 1998; 81:513-5.

14. Temporelli PL, Scapellato F, Corrà U, Eleuteri E, P. Giannuzzi. Accurate non-invasive estimation of systolic pulmonary artery pressure by Doppler echocardiography in chronic heart failure. *Eur Heart J* 1999;20 (Supplement):200.

Chapter 19

# Usefulness of the Timed Walking Test: An Alternative to the GXT In Cardiac Rehabilitation

William G. Herbert, PhD, Lee M. Pierson, MS, USA

## Introduction and Purpose

Symptom-limited graded exercise testing with electrocardiographic monitoring (GXT) on the treadmill or cycle ergometer provide an excellent means for understanding the cardiopulmonary and metabolic pathophysiology that may contribute to deficits in functional capacity. Results of GXTs aid medical decision-making relative to cardiac diagnoses, return to physical work, risk stratification for subsequent cardiac mortality, and counseling for activity levels (1,2). In cardiac rehabilitation, the GXT has long been considered an essential tool for establishing levels of exercise supervision, prescribing intensities for training, and evaluating the outcomes of care (1-4). Contemporary practice guidelines in the United States continue to reflect nearly a universal consensus that the GXT or some very similar objective measure of exercise capabilities be performed for each patient in conjunction with their participation in cardiac rehabilitation. Furthermore, the guidelines stipulate that these assessments be performed for each patient at entry and repeated at appropriate time points along the course of rehabilitation. The year 2000 recommendations on core components of cardiac rehabilitation from the AHA/AACVPR (5) even advocate that these exercise evaluations include "assessment of heart rate and rhythm, signs, symptoms, ST-segment changes, and exercise capacity." Several of the guidelines indicate that the GXT is instrumental in determining which patients may safely exercise, which need intensive monitoring, what should be the intensity of their aerobic exercise, or even if and when resistance training should be initiated (3,4,6,7).

In 1994, the AACVPR conducted a survey to determine practice patterns in a 20% sample of it's member facilities from 39 locations across the US, Canada,

& Mexico (8). Fifty-two percent of the 199 respondent centers reported that they tracked functional capacity outcomes; 85% of these centers did so using the GXT. Another small survey conducted in the early 1990s in the Mid-Atlantic US region showed that ~80 percent of all cardiac and pulmonary rehabilitation centers used GXTs to conduct their exercise evaluations (9). However, 43 percent of the pulmonary rehabilitation centers in that survey used either 6- or 12-min walk tests instead of the GXT (9).

Since the advent of healthcare reform in the 1990's and even earlier, cardiac rehabilitation programs have been accepting more and more patients without having the results from standardized GXTs to use in programming for incoming patients. When exercise test data has been available from other sources, these typically have been inadequate for meeting the needs for rehabilitation, e.g. nonstandard submaximal exercise data collected in conjunction with cardiac imaging studies or results of GXTs in which a few stages were performed, with missing information or poorly defined endpoints. Such test results or inability of rehabilitation professionals to perform and recover costs for these tests themselves has increasingly compromised the ability of programs to accurately establish the individual patient's exercise capacity, goals, risk status, or set specific intensities for aerobic training. Recently, this dilemma has generated vigorous dialogue among professionals, particularly about perceived necessity, safety, accountability for outcomes, and medico-legal risks surrounding the issue of conducting GXTs in day-to-day cardiac rehabilitation practice (10-12).

Given these circumstances, the purpose of this paper is three-fold: 1) to briefly review the current cardiac rehabilitation guidelines to clarify expectations of the profession for providing exercise evaluation; 2) provide a viewpoint on the values and limitations of the GXT for meeting these assessment needs and; 3) discuss in some detail the evidence on walking tests as a means for satisfying the specific exercise evaluation needs unique to this field. The paper concludes with recommendations relative to optimizing the application of walking tests in cardiac rehabilitation.

## Review of Related Literature

### Current Practice Guidelines

Several national organizations in the US have recently updated their cardiac rehabilitation practice guidelines. To a certain extent, these publications help influence attitudes and approaches in other nations as well (3-5,7,13). The American College of Sports Medicine (3) is specific about the need for exercise evaluation prior to cardiac patients beginning moderate-vigorous exercise. However, their most recent guideline includes some flexibility relative to how this may be accomplished: 1) often, it is not be feasible to conduct GXTs on patients who enter cardiac rehabilitation programs; 2) for some, the GXT may not even be medically appropriate, e.g. recent hospital discharge or evaluations delayed for economic reasons; 3) submaximal exercise tests increasingly are being utilized instead. The ACSM position on this matter, however, includes the proviso that whenever exercise programs for patients are implemented without preliminary (formal) exercise testing, medical supervision, i.e. continuous exercise ECG and BP monitoring should be provided (3).

Last year, the American Heart Association jointly with the AACVPR published a position statement on core components of cardiac rehabilitation (5). This document calls for obtaining exercise test (results) or some other standard measure of exercise capacity before patients begin exercise, repeated testing if changes in condition warrant, and assessment of rate, rhythm, signs, symptoms, ST-changes, and exercise capacity as part of the procedure (5,7). In a recent AHA scientific advisory on assessment of functional capacity in clinical and research applications, the AHA offered further support for use of exercise testing in cardiac rehabilitation (14). Needs cited include quantifying functional capacity for use in developing exercise prescriptions, evaluating exercise-training outcomes; specifically for revascularization patients, this guideline also recommends exercise testing for confirming completeness of post-surgical outcomes and periodically updating exercise prescriptions (14).

Finally, the most recent AACVPR practice guideline supports exercise testing of patients entering cardiac rehabilitation, with a distinct preference for the GXT (7). Reasons cited include stratification both for risk of exercise-induced complications and disease progression; in this case, METpk from the exercise test is indicated as a pivotal component to separate patients into high vs. low risk strata (high vs. low risk is < 5 vs. >7 METs). Other reasons cited include guiding the exercise prescription and selecting those patients who need medical supervision for exercise (5,7). Taken collectively, these guidelines confirm the consensus that formal and objective exercise evaluation should be performed in cardiac rehabilitation. Individualized monitoring during such exercise evaluations is clearly an expectation, as are applications of the results for safety-related decisions, exercise prescription, and accountability for outcomes central to rehabilitation treatment.

### Usefulness of the GXT in Cardiac Rehabilitation.

In cardiac rehabilitation, certainly part of the motivation for conducting GXTs is rooted in accumulating evidence suggesting that prognosis is better, even in those with CAD, when one's functional (aerobic) capacity is higher (15,16). Thus, the ability of programs to document the benefits of their exercise training protocols in terms of raising and preserving a patient's functional capacity is widely regarded as important. It is helpful to question the evidence on how effectively the GXT measures not only functional capacity in cardiac patients, but also the extent to which it serves cardiac rehabilitation as a effective tool for exercise prescription, forecasting risk of exercise-induced complications, and measuring exercise training outcomes?

On the question of assessing functional capacity, the GXT has a number of problems and limitations. First, it is unusual in practice even when testing healthy individuals in a rigorous research protocol to discern a true $\dot{V}O_2$max from data collected in the GXT, i.e. most test results do not show evidence of a plateau in $\dot{V}O_2$ at peak effort wherein the external load is continually increasing (17). Reasons for this failure to find an upper limit to oxygen transport capabilities continue to be debated and it raises legitimate questions about what really are the limiting factors (18-20). Few cardiac rehabilitation programs are able to perform GXTs with gas exchange measurements, yet it is common practice to translate a peak speed, grade, or time into an index of metabolic capacity through use of prediction equations for $\dot{V}O_2$pk or METpk (3). These prediction equations have limited precision and their use adds to any error in estimating the aerobic capacity of a patient. These errors are attributable to variations in exercise biomechanics, body size, or sluggish $O_2$ kinetics as patients with more severe cardiopulmonary disease transition to reach higher stages of the GXT, e.g. depressed ventricular function (21). Finally, test validity may be compromised by prior practice, patient motivation or anxiety, choice of protocol, and handrail holding which may reduce the actual external demand and result in gross overestimations of the patient's exercise capacity (21). Even if precision of assessing or predicting $\dot{V}O_2$pk with the GXT is optimized, it should be questioned whether this measure has sufficient generalizability to allow meaningful judgments about a patient's physical capabilities in activities important to their daily lives. To illustrate, Guyatt and coworkers (22) evaluated exercise capacity by cycle ergometry in the laboratory, by walking performance over ground, and by patient perceptions on a functional status questionnaire. This study showed that the laboratory measure (GXT) had virtually no association with the scores on the other two indicators of functional capacity among these low-fit patients with chronic cardiopulmonary disease. So, if one major objective of a cardiac rehabilitation fitness measure is to assess physical capacity for and confidence in performing challenging physical activities of daily living, the usefulness of the GXT may be quite limited.

Due to many of the issues identified in the foregoing paragraph and to task specificity considerations, the GXT also has limited usefulness for prescribing exercise with patients. To illustrate some of these limitations, consider the study of Milani et al (23) who evaluated $\dot{V}O_2$ at maximal and submaximal levels for treadmill in 15 cardiac patients. These investigators found that widely used prediction formulas for estimating oxygen uptake in treadmill testing either under- or over-estimate the measured $\dot{V}O_2$, typically by 0.4 - 0.8 METs at submaximal loads and 1-2 METs at maximal loads (23). In another study with clear implications exercise prescription, Brubaker et al (24) conducted maximal GXTs with two groups of Phase III cardiac patients (N = 15 and 25; METpk = 6-8). They compared heart rates and perceived exertion scores from the treadmill tests against the same measures collected during ambulation exercise in a gymnasium. In the ambulation exercise the patients completed a brief warm-up and then self-paced their exercise to hold perceived exertion constant; their heart rates unobtrusively were recorded at the same time by Polar® devices at 2-minute intervals. At matched heart rates, the patients reported significantly higher perceived exertion scores during the over ground exercise (gym), thus showing a limited ability to directly translate a prescribed heart rate-perceived exertion guideline from a GXT to the patients' exercise training environment.

With regard to use of the GXT in risk stratification, METpk appears in several of the most important published models for risk appraisal in cardiac rehabilitation. Is this measure effective in discriminating among those who will have exercise-induced complications? Indirectly at least, Paul-Labrador et al. (25) evaluated this issue in a series of 239 cardiac rehabilitation patients over 2.5 years. All patients had GXTs and assessments of cardiac ejection fraction and these data were used to stratify them for risk of exercise-induced events according to four different sets of clinical guidelines. Twelve cardiovascular events occurred, all of which required use of a crash cart; these included episodes of chest pain and hypotension. Five of the event patients required hospitalization, but none had cardiac arrests, myocardial infarctions, or deaths. The low event rate (2.3/1,000 patient-hours of exercise) restricted statistical power relative to the findings, but despite this limitation the only trend for any variable to be different in the event patients was *smoking*. Thus, the four major risk stratification models in which METpk from the GXT is a prominent predictor variable were of minimal value in predicting which patients would have exercise-induced complications

How effective is the GXT in providing a measure of exercise training outcomes for patients in cardiac rehabilitation? Lavie and Milani (26), in part, investigated this question in a series of 500 consecutive CAD patients who participated in an outpatient exercise program. They assessed maximal GXT responses and quality of life measures before and 12 weeks after aerobic exercise training. METpk improvements derived from prediction formulas grossly overestimated functional capacity improvement in both younger and older patients alike. Measured improvements in $\dot{V}O_2$pk, ventilatory threshold, and quality of life physical functioning scores were comparable (15-20 percent improvement after training), but generally were only half as great as the METpk scores obtained by prediction from peak speed/grade on the GXT (26).

In a retrospective study in our laboratory, we used pre- and post-training GXT data to estimate changes in aerobic fitness after 5-8 months of thrice-weekly exercise training at 60-90 percent of apparent maximal heart rate in 60 cardiac outpatients (27). One GXT measure was METpk predicted from metabolic equations applied to speed and grade from the highest stages of the pre- and post-training GXTs. RatePressure Product at 5 METs (RPP5METs), from the same pre- and post-training GXTs, also was evaluated as a submaximal measure of fitness. The RPP5METs scores were obtained by linear regression and only subjects with records showing at least three GXT stages and a strong linear relation between heart rate, blood pressure, and MET level at each stage were included in the analysis. Both measures indicated significantly higher aerobic fitness as a result of training when the data were evaluated in a group analysis. Average improvements based on the METpk scores were nearly twice as high as those estimated from RPP5METs (25 vs. 13.6 percent). When data for individual change scores were evaluated, however,

the disparity in these two markers became more apparent. In this analysis, we correlated change scores for each patient to assess concordance of these two measures; there was essentially no relationship between these two sets of scores ($r^2 = 0.08$). Lastly, we transformed and rescaled these individual change scores into what one of three possible clinical outcomes of training: improvement, decline, or no change. For the measure of METpk, a meaningful change was accepted as an increase or decrease after training of >1 MET; the threshold for a meaningful change after training in RPP5METs was set at >10 percent. Figure 19.1 shows the substantial disparity in outcomes when the data are evaluated in the third way and these findings leave open to question just what is the most meaningful and objective way to represent the effects of rehabilitation exercise for these patients. None of these patients had GXT endpoints limited by signs/symptoms or medical decisions leading to early termination of the tests; no patients

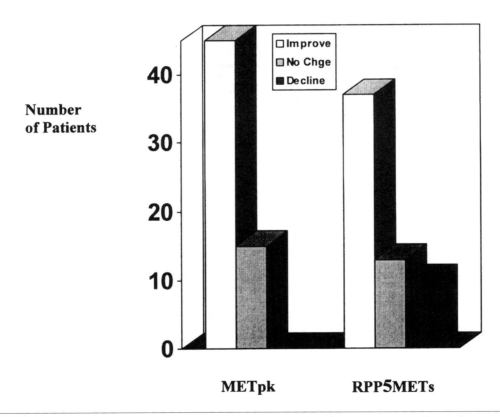

**Figure 19.1**   Comparison of changes in aerobic fitness in cardiac rehabilitation patients after endurance exercise training. METpk is a measure of change in fitness after training, as calculated from the highest speed/grade from the GXT tolerated by the patient. RPP5METs, is established by regression analysis from physiological data (heart rate and blood pressures) in the same GXTs. It is a submaximal exercise marker of aerobic fitness, minimally affected by patient motivation.

were included who had any changes in medications or clinical status over the training period. Thus, when a submaximal exercise marker of aerobic fitness is used to judge training outcome in this series of patients, 62 percent of the group showed meaningful improvement. In contrast, when change in METpk is used as the outcome, a measure affected by subjective endpoints, 85 percent of the patients made meaningful improvement and none showed any decline in fitness.

## Usefulness of Timed Walk Tests in the Cardiac Rehabilitation Setting

Thus, it can be argued that there is a clear need for alternatives to the GXT for exercise assessment needs in cardiac rehabilitation. These must be meaningful to professionals and patients alike, inexpensive, psychometrically sound, and commensurate with widely accepted practice guidelines. Timed walking tests for specified periods of 6 to 12 minutes (6MWT to 12MWT) performed over ground or on a treadmill increasingly are being accepted for this purpose. Very recently, the North Carolina Cardiac Rehabilitation Association adopted the 6MWT for its statewide outcomes project in 2001 (personal communication). Their test procedure requires that patients walk through a quiet indoor hallway or walking track of > 30 m (>100 ft). A chair is placed at mid-point in the straightaway of the course to allow temporary rest for any fatigued patients. A staff person observes the patient and calls out encouragement at 30-sec intervals and at time marks at 2, 4, and 6 minutes. Pre- and post-test perceived exertion scores, blood pressures, and heart rates are taken. For patients not able to walk or for programs without the necessary facilities, an

equivalent 6-minute test is performed on the Schwinn Air Dyne® ergometer; the odometer on Air Dyne® is used to quantify the work completed. NCCRA requires those programs that elect to participate in this outcomes project to do the walking test within the first week of each patient's start in rehabilitation and again at program discharge.

How effective are these tests in assessing exercise capabilities of patients with chronic diseases and conditions typical of those in cardiac rehabilitation programs, e.g. CAD, CHF, and COPD? How do these tests measure up to expectations of current practice guidelines, what are the costs and facility requirements, what about patient acceptance, accessibility, and safety? Recently, Steele (28) reviewed the published evidence on timed walking tests, as applied to exercise assessment of cardiopulmonary patients. The review addresses technical development of the tests, design modifications to increase relevance to limitations of chronic disease patients, and recommends a set of standard procedures consistent with published evidence on factors affecting measurement with patients (28). The idea of predicting aerobic capacity from distance covered in a finite time during over ground ambulation had its origins in Kenneth Cooper's work of the late 1960's (29). Cooper designed and validated the 12-minute walk-run test for distance that could be self-administered on any measured course, such as an outdoor track; it provided the apparently healthy and relatively fit adult with the means to estimate aerobic capacity and consider modifying their physical activity levels on the basis of population-based normative comparisons. The application of this approach for assessing exercise tolerance of chronic disease patients soon followed and then has accelerated over the past 15 years. Table 19.1 provides a brief but

**Table 19.1   Studies on Applications of Walking Tests in Chronic Disease Patients**

| Investigators | Year | Focus of study |
|---|---|---|
| McGavin et al. (30) | 1976 | Chronic bronchitis and practice effects |
| Guyatt et al. (31, 32) | 1984 1985 | Effects of encouragement and practice (habituation) on performance |
| Guyatt et al. (32) | 1985 | Validation with congestive heart failure (CHF) patients |
| Bittner et al. (33) | 1993 | Prognosis in patients with left ventricular dysfunction |
| Cahalin et al. (34) | 1995 | Validation in pre-lung transplant patients |
| Cahalin et al. (35) | 1996 | Validation and prognosis in advanced CHF patients |
| O'Keefe et al. (36) | 1998 | Reproducibility and responsiveness in elderly CHF patients |

representative list of published studies that have addressed psychometric issues and applications to specific diagnostic groups of chronic disease patients.

It is helpful at this point to summarize the key advantages and disadvantages of these walking tests. We offer the following impressions, partly based on our own interpretations of this literature, as well as the publications by Steele (28) and the recent AHA advisory on assessment of functional capacity (14). *Advantages:* virtually no costs involved; relevant to many daily activities and functional abilities; reproducible; well accepted by patients; responsive to surgical and medical interventions; requires minimal staff and training. *Weaknesses:* incapable of evaluating cardiopulmonary limitations and status changes over time, e.g. signs/symptoms, ECG changes; special facilities needed; only indirect monitoring (visual surveillance) possible during exercise; performance only modestly correlated to $\dot{V}O_2$pk from GXT; the results are influenced by practice and motivation; $\dot{V}O_2$pk can't be accurately estimated for patients with exercise capacities above ~5 METs; patients with lower limb impairment and obesity may not be able to perform the test; the test is incapable of demand high enough to evoke abnormalities in patients with latent cardiopulmonary signs and symptoms; a walk way with clear distance of at least 20-30 m (67-100 ft) is needed; a staff person must be assigned to watch and verbally encourage patient at time points defined by standardized procedures.

Two very recent publications, especially relevant to the application of the 6MWT in cardiac rehabilitation, deserve special attention in this discussion (37,38). This first of these by Roul et al. (37) reports the comparative values of the $\dot{V}O_2$pk vs. 6MWT for predicting CHF-related deaths or hospitalizations for CHF in a group of 121 patients (NYHA classes II/III). In this study, patients were evaluated in a cycle ergometer ramping test (GXT) for $\dot{V}O_2$pk and on a different occasion in a pedometer monitored best-effort 6MWT for distance. This cohort was followed for 1.5 + 1 yr, after which subjects were classified according to outcome: no event = 74 and CHF event = 47.

Main Findings: the two outcome groups were significantly different for $\dot{V}O_2$pk, but not 6MWT performance; $\dot{V}O_2$pk independently predicted survival, but 6MWT did not. ROC curve analysis for the subgroup with 6MWT scores of < 300 m (equivalent pace: <50 m/min or 2.0 mph) showed that distance walked effectively predicted the clinical outcome; the 6MWT scores were unrelated to $\dot{V}O_2$pk ($r^2 = 0.06$), unless the analysis was restricted only to those patients with 6MWT performances of <300 m ($r^2 = 0.42$) (37).

The study by Hamilton and Haennel (38) investigated the validity and reliability of the 6MWT in a group of 94 outpatients (mean age = 63 yr) participating in either rehabilitation or cardiac maintenance exercise programs. Data were available for 76 of these patients from their treadmill GXTs, apparently from the time at or near entry into these programs; functional capacities (METpk) were estimated from equations based on peak speed/grade rather than from gas exchange measurements. Soon thereafter, each patient performed three 6MWT, one/exercise session, on a 100 m rectangular path. Prior to the test a 10-min warm-up was performed and heart rate and blood pressure were measured immediately before and after the test. In general, the procedures were as recommended by Steele (28). Each patient also completed two different health-related quality of life questionnaires. Main Findings: The male patients walked ~10% further than the females and walking performances were shorter (worse) among the older subsets. Learning across the three 6MWTs resulted in an average improvement in performance by Test 3 of ~6%. Test-retest reliability was high as determined by an intra-class correlation coefficient of R = 0.97. The 6MWT was validated against $\dot{V}O_2$pk, as predicted from the end stage speed/grade of the GXT: r = 0.69. Scores for the 6MWT showed a moderate association with self-appraised scoring of abilities for physical functioning (r = 0.50-0.62). This high validity coefficient for prediction of $\dot{V}O_2$pk is surprising given that only 5 of 60 study patients had performance levels low enough (<300 m) to be in the range found valid by Raul et al. (37) Validity estimates are less certain when the criterion measure of aerobic capacity is an indirect one, in this study (38) being a prediction based on speed/grade. The results of this study do suggest that many of the patients in cardiac rehabilitation have functional capacities above the level at which Raul et al. (37) showed the 6MWT to perform reasonably well for prediction of aerobic capacity or prognostic purposes. In the Hamilton and Haennel (38) study, 72 percent of the patients had METpk values >6.

## Discussion

Thus, a quandary exists concerning a best solution to providing meaningful and economical approach to exercise evaluation in cardiac rehabilitation in the years ahead. Yet, the approaches employed must fully satisfy the multiple requirements for this process as described in the most up to date practice guidelines. These guidelines continue to express that objective exercise evaluation with medical monitoring is a minimal expectation for patients participating in exercise rehabilitation—both at the point of entry and again whenever prudent clinical judgment indicates that an exercise prescription needs updating or there is a change in clinical status. These guidelines are pivotal in determining the standard of care, at least in the United States, and failure to adhere arguably raises risks of harm to patients and to professionals and programs in the event of litigation arising from related personal injuries. While the standard GXT is the most-widely accepted method of satisfying these needs, the opportunities to do this testing in cardiac rehabilitation are disappearing and declining resources likely will further reduce its use in the future. We have discussed evidence in this article suggesting some of the technical concerns inherent in the GXT that limit its usefulness for exercise evaluation needs specific to cardiac rehabilitation. The timed walking test offers an appealing alternative and published data on its usefulness as an indicator of aerobic capacity in chronic disease patients is impressive, so long as the individuals do not have an exercise capacity >5 METs. The explanation for loss of validity in higher fit patients may be explained simply by the fact that ambulation on a level surface at velocities much higher than 100 m/min are biomechanically inconsistent with maintaining a consistent walking gait for the adult of average body size. Prediction of $\dot{V}O_2$ for ambulating at speeds of 100-134 m/min is made difficult by awkward mechanics and inter-patient variations in walking vs. running modes to complete a given distance. The illustration in Figure 19.2 assumes that in ambulating at a near constant effort for >6 minutes an individual's highest self-selected walking speed will be limited by their Ventilatory Threshold (assume 75 percent of individual $\dot{V}O_2$pk). So, if the average aerobic cost of the highest walking speed of 100 m/min is calculated to be just under 4 METs, then only for those patients with exercise capacities of <5 METs would the 6MWT be an aerobic challenge that would closely approximate the metabolic demand at peak effort in the GXT.

Some investigators (39-43) have developed 9-and 12-minute walking tests on self-powered treadmills, for patients which are similar in design to the 6MWT. Yamani et al. (41)(41), for instance, utilized this type of test to evaluate exercise capacity with CHF patients and control subjects, setting the grade at 7 degrees for all tests so that subjects at the up-

per end of the range for $\dot{V}O_2$pk could be challenged near their peak aerobic capacity while still ambulating within reasonable walking speeds. As a consequence, Yamani et al (41) were able to demonstrate that treadmill $\dot{V}O_2$pk was highly correlated to distance completed in the self-powered treadmill test, both among the control subjects and the CHF patients (r = 0.63 and 0.79, respectively). Beaumont et al (43) evaluated 10 low-fit male COPD patients in a self-paced 12-minute walking test and on a treadmill equivalent test in which the grade was kept at zero and the patients were encouraged to manipulate speed only to cover the greatest possible distance. This study showed that, for these patients, the over ground walking test and treadmill test performances were highly correlated (r = 0.90). Unlike procedures required to assure reliable performance with the over ground walking tests, only a single practice trial was needed on the treadmill test to assure test-retest reliability. Treadmill tests of these types (41,43)have an advantage over the 6MWT in that heart rate and blood pressure can be frequently assessed during exercise and the patient monitored for signs/symptoms and ST segment changes on the electrocardiogram. These measures continue to be regarded as essential in cardiac rehabilitation for detecting changes in patient status that might require medical follow up, safety of exercise, or developing an objective exercise prescription.

The following set of procedures might provide a valid and practical means of exercise assessment suitable for cardiac rehabilitation patients with a wide range of fitness levels. It is based on principles of the 6MWT, but employs predicted cumulative energy expenditure over a 6-minute walk at grade on the treadmill as a performance criterion, rather than distance covered. Acceptance in practice, however, would benefit by formal evaluation in clinical studies to examine validity, reliability, usefulness for risk stratification, etc.

1. Continue to risk stratify patients with current criteria (AACVPR, ACP, ACC, AHA, etc); include exercise capacity data in this process, whenever results of recent GXT are available and the clinical status of the patient has not changed;

2. Ask patients to estimate their exercise capabilities using one of the quickly administered questionnaires that have been validated for this purpose, e.g. the Duke Activity Status Index (DASI) (44) or the Veterans Specific Activity Questionnaire (VSAQ) (45,46), the latter being easily understood by patients and possible to

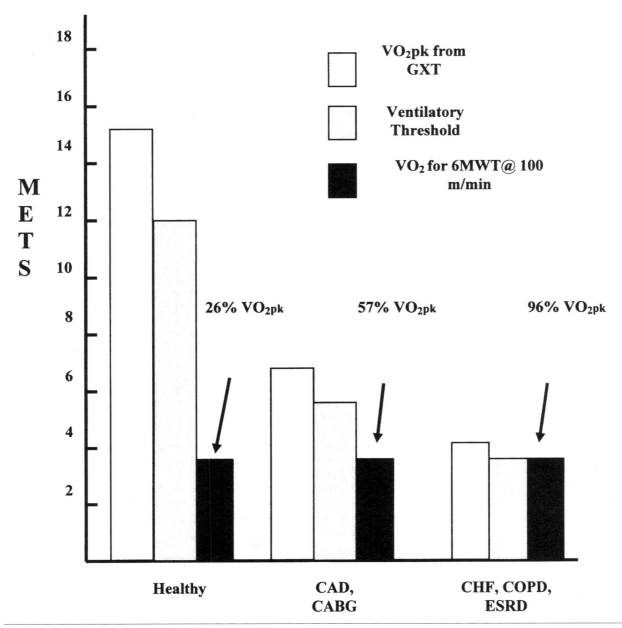

**Figure 19.2**   Possible reasons for limited value of the 6MWT in predicting aerobic capacity for many cardiac rehabilitation patients who have exercise capacities in excess of 5 METs. CAD = coronary artery disease; CABG = coronary artery bypass graft surgery; CHF = congestive heart failure; COPD = chronic obstructive pulmonary diseases; ESRD = end-stage renal disease.

complete and interpret in just a few moments;

3. Orient patient to the rehabilitation exercise program in the usual way, with sessions 1-3 allowing for orientation and titration of aerobic intensity on each training mode (exercise prescription);

4. During session two, using the treadmill exercise station, have the patient select a walking speed that is most comfortable for them—the

estimate of functional capacity from the DASI or VSAQ should be used as an aid in selecting a speed at zero grade which represents a predicted MET requirement (3) no higher than ~50% of the patient's apparent functional capacity;

5. After taking baseline measurements for heart rate and blood pressure in standing posture, the patient should perform a warm-up of 2

min at zero grade and the speed selected for the walking test;

6. Instruct, coach, and verbally queue the patient at time points, as recommended by Steele (28), conducting the test in a manner similar to the over ground 6MWT;

7. Unlike the standard 6MWT, the objective would be for the patient to reach the highest possible energy expenditure in 6 minutes by manipulating grade throughout the test, within limits of their signs, symptoms, and perceived capabilities. The treadmill used for this test would require a continuous readout of estimated cumulative kilocalories – several commercial-grade treadmills have programming and display capabilities to permit this information to be displayed;

8. Before and during exercise, monitor for ECG changes and signs/symptoms. Measure heart rate and blood pressure in exercise at 2 and 5 minutes. Use a slow walking pace for ~6 min recovery and continue assessing heart rate and blood pressure at appropriate points.

## Summary

The standard of care in cardiac rehabilitation mandates exercise assessment of individual patients before and over the course of exercise training. Practice guidelines advocate such testing to establish safe/effective limits for exercise intensity, stratify patients to make decisions on supervision and allocate resources, assess changes in status, and determine outcomes of care. Use of the maximal treadmill test with electrocardiography and other data suitable to meet these needs generally is no longer available to cardiac rehabilitation programs. Healthcare costs and the lack of resources in rehabilitation programs will continue to reduce the availability of GXTs. The timed walking test is an inexpensive and relevant means by which to meet several of the key needs for this setting; it is supported by reasonable evidence of validity and reliability, relevance to activities of daily living, and prognostic usefulness for patients who have very low fitness levels. However, the timed walk test has limited usefulness for a high percentage of cardiac rehabilitation patients with moderate or higher levels of fitness. The over ground walking test precludes monitoring of cardiopulmonary responses that are important for safety and establishing exercise prescriptions. The walking test fails to suf-

ficiently challenge the great majority of these patients to an aerobic intensity that might reveal latent myocardial or hemodynamic dysfunction, as is needed for setting activity limits or for prognosis. Future research is needed to develop and evaluate clinical useful and inexpensive alternatives to the over ground walk tests. Timed walk tests on self-propelled or motor driven treadmills have the potential to more fully satisfy the special needs for exercise evaluation in the rehabilitation setting and such tests merit investigation.

## References

1. Gibbons RJ, Balady GJ, Beasley JW, Bricker JT, Duvernov WF, Froelicher VF, et al. ACC/AHA Guidelines for Exercise Testing. A report of the American College of Cardiology/American Heart Association Task Force on Practice Guidelines (Committee on Exercise Testing). *J Am Coll Cardiol* 1997;30:260-311.

2. Mahler DA, Franco MJ. Clinical applications of cardiopulmonary exercise testing. *J Cardiopulm Rehabil* 1996;16:357-65.

3. ACSM. ACSM's Guidelines for Exercise Testing and Prescription. sixth ed. Philadelphia: Lippincott Williams & Wilkins, 2000.

4. AHCPR. Clinical Practice Guideline Number 17: Cardiac Rehabilitation. Washington, D.C.: U.S. Department of Health and Human Services, 1995:202.

5. Balady GJ, Ades PA, Comoss P, Limacher M, Pina IL, Southard D, et al. Core components of cardiac rehabilitation/secondary prevention programs: A statement for healthcare professionals from the American Heart Association and the American Association of Cardiovascular and Pulmonary Rehabilitation Writing Group. *Circulation* 2000;102:1069-73.

6. Balady GJ, Fletcher BJ, Froelicher ES, Hartley LH, Krauss RM, Oberman A, et al. AHA Medical/Scientific Statement. Cardiac rehabilitation programs. A statement for healthcare professionals. *Circulation* 1994;90:1602-1610.

7. AACVPR. Guidelines for Cardiac Rehabilitation and Secondary Prevention Programs. third ed. Champaign, IL: Human Kinetics, 1999.

8. Pashkow P, Ades PA, Emery CF, Frid DJ, Houston-Miller N, Peske G, et al. Outcome measurement in cardiac and pulmonary rehabilitation. AACVPR Outcomes Committee. American Association of Cardiovascular and Pulmonary

Rehabilitation. *J Cardiopulm Rehabil* 1995;15:394-405.

9. Weiser PC, Ryan KP. Tri-state region pulmonary rehabilitation survey. Delivery of exercise conditioning services. The Pulmonary Rehabilitation Committee, Tri- State Society for Cardiovascular and Pulmonary Rehabilitation. *J Cardiopulm Rehabil* 1996;16:175-82.

10. McConnell TR. Exercise prescription when the guidelines do not work. *J Cardiopulm Rehabil* 1996;16:34-7.

11. McConnell TR, Klinger TA, Gardner JK, Laubach CA, Jr., Herman CE, Hauck CA. Cardiac rehabilitation without exercise tests for post-myocardial infarction and post-bypass surgery patients. *J Cardiopulm Rehabil* 1998; 18:458-63.

12. Balady GJ. Exercise testing in cardiac rehabilitation. Is the engine running hot? *J Cardiopulm Rehabil* 1998;18:464-6.

13. Balady GJ, Chaitman B, Driscoll D, Foster C, Froelicher E, Gordon N, et al. Recommendations for cardiovascular screening, staffing, and emergency policies at health/fitness facilities. *Circulation* 1998;97:2283-93.

14. Fleg JL, Pina IL, Balady GJ, Chaitman BR, Fletcher B, Lavie C, et al. Assessment of functional capacity in clinical and research applications: An advisory from the Committee on Exercise, Rehabilitation, and Prevention, Council on Clinical Cardiology, American Heart Association. *Circulation* 2000;102:1591-7.

15. Blair SN, Connelly JC. How much physical activity should we do? The case for moderate amounts and intensities of physical activity. *Res Q Exerc Sport* 1996;67:193-205.

16. Blair SN, Kampert JB, Kohl HW, 3rd, Barlow CE, Macera CA, Paffenbarger RS, Jr, et al. Influences of cardiorespiratory fitness and other precursors on cardiovascular disease and all-cause mortality in men and women. *JAMA* 1996;276:205-10.

17. Myers J, Walsh D, Buchanan N, Froelicher VF. Can maximal cardiopulmonary capacity be recognized by a plateau in oxygen uptake? *Chest* 1989;96:1312-6.

18. Bassett DR, Jr., Howley ET. Maximal oxygen uptake: "classical" versus "contemporary" viewpoints. *Med Sci Sports Exerc* 1997;29:591-603.

19. Bassett DR, Jr., Howley ET. Limiting factors for maximum oxygen uptake and determinants of endurance performance. *Med Sci Sports Exerc* 2000;32:70-84.

20. Noakes TD. Maximal oxygen uptake: "classical" versus "contemporary" viewpoints: a rebuttal. *Med Sci Sports Exerc* 1998;30:1381-98.

21. Haskell WL, Savin W, Oldridge N, DeBusk R. Factors influencing estimated oxygen uptake during exercise testing soon after myocardial infarction. *Am J Cardiol* 1982;50:299-304.

22. Guyatt GH, Thompson PJ, Berman LB, Sullivan MJ, Townsend M, Jones NL, et al. How should we measure function in patients with chronic heart and lung disease? *J Chronic Dis* 1985;38:517-24.

23. Milani J, Fernhall B, Manfredi T. Estimating oxygen consumption during treadmill and arm ergometry activity in males with coronary artery disease. *J Cardiopulm Rehabil* 1996;16:394-401.

24. Brubaker PH, Rejeski JH, Law HC, Pollock WE, Wurst ME, Miller JH,.Jr. Cardiac patients' perception of intensity during graded exercise testing: Do they generalize to field settings? *J Cardiopulmonary Rehabil* 1994;14:127-133.

25. Paul-Labrador M, Vongvanich P, Merz CN. Risk stratification for exercise training in cardiac patients: do the proposed guidelines work? *J Cardiopulm Rehabil* 1999;19:118-25.

26. Lavie CJ, Milani RV. Disparate effects of improving aerobic exercise capacity and quality of life after cardiac rehabilitation in young and elderly coronary patients. *J Cardiopulm Rehabil* 2000;20:235-40.

27. Pierson LM, Ocel, J.V., Davis, S.E., Herbert, W.G. Alternatives for defining physical training outcomes using GXT data in cardiac rehabilitation. *Journal of Cardiopulmonary Rehabilitation* 1996;16:307.

28. Steele B. Timed walking tests of exercise capacity in chronic cardiopulmonary illness. *J Cardiopulm Rehabil* 1996;16:25-33.

29. Cooper KH. A means of assessing maximal oxygen intake. Correlation between field and treadmill testing. *JAMA* 1968;203:201-4.

30. McGavin CR, Gupta SP, McHardy GJ. Twelve-minute walking test for assessing disability in chronic bronchitis. *Br Med J* 1976;1:822-3.

31. Guyatt GH, Pugsley SO, Sullivan MJ, Thompson PJ, Berman L, Jones NL, et al. Effect of encouragement on walking test performance. *Thorax* 1984;39:818-22.

32. Guyatt GH, Sullivan MJ, Thompson PJ, Fallen EL, Pugsley SO, Taylor DW, et al. The 6-minute walk: a new measure of exercise capacity in patients with chronic heart failure. *Can Med Assoc J* 1985;132:919-23.

33. Bittner V, Weiner DH, Yusuf S, Rogers WJ, McIntyre KM, Bangdiwala SI, et al. Prediction of mortality and morbidity with a 6-minute walk test in patients with left ventricular dysfunction. SOLVD Investigators [see comments]. *JAMA* 1993;270:1702-7.
34. Cahalin L, Pappagianopoulos P, Prevost S, Wain J, Ginns L. The relationship of the 6-min walk test to maximal oxygen consumption in transplant candidates with end-stage lung disease. *Chest* 1995;108:452-9.
35. Cahalin LP, Mathier MA, Semigran MJ, Dec GW, DiSalvo TG. The six-minute walk test predicts peak oxygen uptake and survival in patients with advanced heart failure. *Chest* 1996;110:325-32.
36. O'Keeffe ST, Lye M, Donnellan C, Carmichael DN. Reproducibility and responsiveness of quality of life assessment and six minute walk test in elderly heart failure patients. *Heart* 1998;80:377-82.
37. Roul G, Germain P, Bareiss P. Does the 6-minute walk test predict the prognosis in patients with NYHA class II or III chronic heart failure? [see comments]. *Am Heart J* 1998;136:449-57.
38. Hamilton DM, Haennel RG. Validity and reliability of the 6-minute walk test in a cardiac rehabilitation population. *J Cardiopulm Rehabil* 2000;20:156-64.
39. Bristow MR, Gilbert EM, Abraham WT, Adams KF, Fowler MB, Hershberger RE, et al. Carvedilol produces dose-related improvements in left ventricular function and survival in subjects with chronic heart failure. MOCHA Investigators. *Circulation* 1996;94:2807-16.
40. Sparrow J, Parameshwar J, Poole-Wilson PA. Assessment of functional capacity in chronic heart failure: time- limited exercise on a self-powered treadmill. *Br Heart J* 1994;71:391-4.
41. Yamani MH, Wells L, Massie BM, Ammon S, Der E, Prouty K. Relation of the nine-minute self-powered treadmill test to maximal exercise capacity and skeletal muscle function in patients with congestive heart failure. *Am J Cardiol* 1995;76:788-92.
42. Yamani MH, Sahgal P, Wells L, Massie BM. Exercise intolerance in chronic heart failure is not associated with impaired recovery of muscle function or submaximal exercise performance. *J Am Coll Cardiol* 1995;25:1232-8.
43. Beaumont A, Cockroft A, Guz A. A self-paced treadmill walking test for breathless patients. *Thorax* 1985;40:459-464.
44. Hlatky MA, Boineau RE, Higginbotham MB, Lee KL, Mark DB, Califf RM, et al. A brief self-administered questionnaire to determine functional capacity (the Duke Activity Status Index). *Am J Cardiol* 1989;64:651-4.
45. Myers J, Do D, Herbert W, Ribisl P, Froelicher VF. A nomogram to predict exercise capacity from a specific activity questionnaire and clinical data. *Am J Cardiol* 1994;73:591-6.
46. Cook JW, Pierson, L.M., Herbert, W.G., Norton, H.J., Fedor, J.M., Kiebzak, G.M., Ramp, W.K., Robicsek, F. The influence of patient strength, aerobic capacity and body composition upon outcomes after coronary bypass grafting. *Thorac Cardiov Surg* 2001;49:89-93.

# Chapter 20

# Selecting COPD Patients for Rehabilitation

Claudio F. Donner, MD, Italy

In theory, candidates for rehabilitation programs can include all non smoking symptomatic COPD patients willing to participate. Prime candidates are however those with more severe deconditioning, muscle weakness and exercise intolerance. Current smokers resolved to quit must be helped in their smoking cessation efforts. Patients with a concomitant disease severely affecting their life expectation and current smokers unable to quit should be excluded from formal rehabilitation programs.

## Patient Evaluation and Selection for Rehabilitation Program

A global evaluation of the patient must be done within the conceptual frame of health status and functional assessment, including physical functioning, emotional functioning, sense of well-being, social functioning and social role (1).

Pulmonary function tests must be first carried out for a precise determination of the level of impairment. Impairment is severe when forced expiratory volume in one second ($FEV_1$) equals or is less than 40 percent of predicted, forced vital capacity (FVC) equals or is less than 50 percent of predicted and $FEV_1/FVC$ equals 40 % of predicted. The transfer factor for carbon monoxide (TL,CO) must also be determined and TL,CO values equal to or lower than 40 percent of predicted indicate severe impairment. A further step is the estimation of work capacity through exercise testing or by the analysis of maximal oxygen uptake (2). Arterial blood gases need to be looked at in severe cases. On occasion, nocturnal pulsoximetry may also be helpful to identify patients in need of formal polysomnography.

Other pathophysiological analyses such as those of pulmonary haemodynamics, measurements of respiratory muscle strength [maximal inspiratory and expiratory pressures, (MIP and MEP)], peripheral muscle force (isometric muscle tests) and pulmonary mechanics are generally limited to specialist settings, and carried out mainly for research purposes.

Quantification of dyspnea either directly (Modified Borg Scale, Visual Analogue Scale) or indirectly (dyspnea targeted activities) is important to evaluate individual programs in the clinical setting as well as for research purposes. Measurements of disability are mainly obtained through exercise tests (multistage incremental cardiopulmonary exercise test, single-stage endurance test, timed walk test, shuttle test), and performance tests in the occupational laboratory.

Handicap is influenced by subjective and environmental factors. An objective evaluation can, at least partly, be obtained through quality of life questionnaires, including evaluation of activities pertinent to daily living (3) (see chapter on outcome measurements).

## Selection and Tailoring of Rehabilitation Programs for Individual Patients

Rehabilitation programs must be adjusted to the individual patient, taking into account the disease and its severity as well as non-medical factors. Therefore, general guidelines rather than strict rules must be followed. Because rehabilitation deals in most cases with incurable diseases, good results cannot be achieved indefinitely. There is therefore a need for intensive rehabilitation over a period of time followed by periodical reinforcing sessions.

Planning and performance of rehabilitation programs must rely on team cooperation and effort. Chest physicians usually act as team coordinators and are responsible for patient evaluation (eligibility, formal consent, motivation, individual resources and needs, familial and social environment), individual prescriptions, supervision of staff and quality control of service providers (e.g. private companies supplying oxygen or equipment for mechanical ventilation). In order to facilitate the allocation of resources in difficult situations, the coordinator must on occasion also take care of the contact with third party payers such as local health authorities, and insurance companies.

Nurses are responsible for clinical monitoring, patient and relatives' education, administration of questionnaires, and assisting the coordinator in implementing the cooperative network of individuals participating regularly or occasionally in the program. Physiotherapists play an important role in conducting all the different forms of training such as general exercise, selective muscle group training, breathing retraining, and chest physiotherapy. In some countries, such as in the USA, the staff also includes specialized personnel such as respiratory therapists which are highly qualified for the assessment, intervention and outcome evaluation/follow up of respiratory rehabilitation.

Other specialized personnel can be added for specific purposes as determined by the coordinator. These include occupational therapists, psychologists, dieticians, social workers, and speech therapists.

## Rehabilitation Programs

### In-Patient Programs

In-patient rehabilitation is indicated for patients with unstable disease, patients requiring complex functional evaluation (e.g. full polysomnography, right heart catheterism), or patients with major mobility problems. These programs allow for comprehensive and individual diurnal assessment as well as stabilization or reversing of health-related physio- or psychopathological disabilities. They not only focus on obvious impairments and handicaps but also on the more hidden aspects of the disease which might influence the patient's health-related quality of life. In order to optimize the ability to perform daily living activities and coping skills, the patient's close relatives should be considered active participants in this process of rehabilitation.

### Selection for Inpatient Programs

Participation in in-patient programs is indicated for the following reasons:

1. Patients who need an integrated 24 hour supervised monitoring management plan including training, teaching of coping skills and other aspects of daily life functioning.
2. Patients in need of behavioral intervention to correct psycho-social disturbances.
3. Patients requiring specific interventional strategies such as nutritional therapy.
4. Patients who are scheduled for thoracic surgical procedures including lung transplantation (pre- and postoperative).
5. Patients leaving intensive care units with disabling respiratory problems or patients unable to be weaned off the respirator.
6. Patients who need to be assisted for long-term oxygen therapy or long-term home mechanical ventilation.
7. Patients for whom out-patient rehabilitation is not available or travel distances do not allow him to participate in intensive out-patient rehabilitation.

## Out-Patient Programs

In general, out-patient programs are reserved for patients with mild to moderate disability who can still lead an active life (social and often occupational), patients without transportation problems, and particularly patients where only periodic follow-ups are required. On occasion, patients with severe but relatively stable disease and patients on a waiting list for lung transplantation and lung volume reduction surgery can participate in outpatient programs. The specific objectives of out-patient rehabilitation are to alleviate dyspnea, increase exercise tolerance, educate patients, improve quality of life, and ensure a long-term commitment to regular physical activity. Each of these components requires regular evaluation.

### Selection for Out-Patient Programs

Patients with symptomatic COPD should be considered for out-patient rehabilitation under the following circumstances:

1. Patients with moderate or severe but stable disease already under optimal medical therapy.
2. Patients able to maintain an independent lifestyle.

3. Patients without major psychological problems
4. Patients without significant co-morbidities such as congestive heart failure, or metastatic cancer, etc. (2,4).

These criteria must be rigidly followed since outpatient rehabilitation programs are often based on exercise training.

## Phases of Rehabilitation Program

### Clinical Phase

The first objective of this phase is to properly assess the patient through history of his disease, tobacco exposure, clinical status, etc. It also includes determining the patient's level of motivation and availability, taking into account professional obligations, living arrangements, travel distances, etc.

The second objective of this phase is to determine the best choice of activity for individual patients in order to ensure long-term commitment to regular physical activity (5). This choice is based on pathophysiology [activities at a work rate inducing substantial lactic acidosis are preferable (6)], patient preference (physical activity must be enjoyable), and quality of exercise environment.

### Assessment Phase

This phase provides information which will be used as a reference for the final evaluation of the training program. It also allows for an individualized approach to training since it is during this phase that training intensity will be determined on the basis of the patient's physical potential.

Training intensity is usually defined on the basis of relative-percent heart rate. Unfortunately, this measurement, while valid for normal people and patients with coronary artery disease, is probably not so relevant for respiratory patients since these individuals are limited by their ventilatory, not by their cardiovascular function (7). For this reason, a reasonable strategy for COPD patients might be to adopt training protocols which have the same duration and frequency characteristics as those used for normal subjects and to select the maximal intensity which can be tolerated by the patient without cardiovascular side effects (8).

Exercise tests used to measure the anaerobic threshold require sophisticated equipment, gener-ally available only in specialized rehabilitation centers. A reasonable alternative is to use the dyspnea threshold (DT) to individualize exercise intensity because it has been shown that there is a close relationship between heart rate and DT (9). When DT determination is not possible, the 60% of the heart rate reserve ($HR_{max} - HR_{rest}$) can be used if $HR_{max}$ is measured during exercise. In most cases, the anaerobic threshold is equivalent to this percentage.

### Rehabilitation Phase

According to a recent meta-analysis, the minimum duration of most rehabilitation programs is three months (10). During that time, patients undergo 3 sessions of two and a half hours duration per week. These are approximately divided into 30 min of health education, 45 min of exercise training inside the center, 30 min of physical therapy and relaxation, and 45 min of gymnastics and/or outdoor exercise training. Four components play a major role during this rehabilitation phase:

1. Health education: the main objective of health education is to optimize patient's compliance with treatment, and to ensure long-term commitment to regular physical activity. At present, clearcut and definite evidence of the positive influence of education in COPD rehabilitation is still lacking (10).
2. Psychosocial support: although little is known about its mechanism of action, psychosocial support appears to be helpful in restoring coping skills and in learning stress management. Short term results show that dyspnea and anxiety are reduced but long-term results are still unknown. As an adjunct to exercise training, psychosocial support is effective in improving compliance, exercise tolerance and health-related quality of life (10).
3. Exercise training: an important priority is to ensure that exercise intensities as determined in the laboratory are used during actual training. Exercise intensities are monitored through cardio-frequency-meters and programmed alarm systems in order to make sure that predetermined targets of heart rate (+5 beats/min) are being reached.

Practically, indoor training, on a bicycle or treadmill, is usually advised. It is however important that the patient understands that he/she should carry out other activities such as outdoor walking. Indeed, outdoor activities are usually enjoyable and in general the more enjoyable the activity, the better the compliance will be. At least during indoor training, repeated periods of exercise are preferable to a single longer period of the same duration (5). The "best" modalities for training sessions (e.g. repeated periods of exercise versus single long period, high intensity/short duration versus low intensity/long duration training) have not yet been determined (8).

4. Specific muscle training: At present, there is no data that has shown significant clinical benefit for ventilatory muscle training over general exercise alone (10, 11). However, peripheral muscle training improves exercise capacity and quality of life, and for that reason, it should be included in all rehabilitation programs intended for COPD patients (12).

### Follow-Up

Regular laboratory evaluation is of major importance not only to ensure readjustments of training intensity but also to discuss these improvements with the patient so that his motivation is reinforced.

Perhaps the most important goal of rehabilitation programs is to introduce the respiratory patient to a new lifestyle which includes regular physical activity. Indeed, one must try to develop and implement exercise maintenance programs that can be followed at home and maintained for the patient's remaining life.

## "Home Care" Rehabilitation

The objective of home care rehabilitation is to provide the best possible lifestyle at the lowest possible cost. Indeed a well-structured home care program can provide the patient with most of the therapeutic modalities available in the hospital setting, continued education and follow-up. The home care team is best supervised by a pulmonologist with or without the help of a general practitioner. It also includes trained personnel able to perform the role of nurses, physiotherapists and social workers. The extent of therapeutic modalities being used depends on the structure of each individual program (13-15).

### Primary Objectives of "Home Care" Rehabilitation

There are seven primary objectives of home care rehabilitation:

1. Support of the patient to incorporate recommended therapeutic measures to his/her housing and social situation.
2. Support of the patient and immediate family in servicing technical devices in case of dysfunction.
3. Involvement and training of caregivers in supportive measures in order to promote independence of the patient from third-party services and strengthen his/her social contacts.
4. Reinforcement of patient adherence to therapeutic regimens and intervention if compliance deteriorates.
5. Intervention during acute exacerbations of the underlying pulmonary disease.
6. Maintaining and further development of the skills and functional improvements that have been gained during the rehabilitation process.
7. Assessment of the success of therepeutic interventions as well as of the functional capabilities of the patient after an adequate time interval (3-6 months) with feedback being provided to institutions involved during the preceding or ongoing rehabilitation process.

In general, patients eligible for respiratory "home care" (3, 16, 17) include newly diagnosed and first-time hospitalized patients not eligible for outpatient rehabilitation programs after their discharge from acute care centers. It also includes patients discharged with new respiratory equipment, patients with recurrent exacerbations and repeated hospitalizations, patients with ongoing exacerbations treated at home, anxious, confused, and forgetful patients, patients formally included in inpatient or outpatient rehabilitation programs, and end-stage patients who would rather stay home.

### Justification of Home Care Rehabilitation

Rehabilitation of a mobile patient in his home due to lack of adequate inpatient or outpatient programs may be justified in developing countries or in remote areas lacking adequate transport facilities.

Additional comorbidities such as mental disorders, or dependence on technical and social measures only available in home care programs may also make a patient unsuitable for institutionalized rehabilitation.

In general, therapeutic interventions in "home care" programs are similar to those available in institutionalized rehabilitation programs. They include technical and personal support such as home visits by physicians, respiratory, occupational, and speech therapists, physiotherapy, nutritional, social and psychiatric counseling.

### Advantages and Disadvantages of "Home Care" Rehabilitation

The main advantage of "home care" rehabilitation is the fact that the patient is treated in his own environment (18,19). Therefore, any adjustments can be made promptly on the basis of personal observations by health care professionals. It is important to define the duration of home care support (short, mid-, long-term) as well as the frequency of home visits based on individual needs and characteristics of home treatment.

Compared to inpatient rehabilitation, home mechanical ventilation after successful training is cost-effective (20,21). Unfortunately, controlled studies comparing costs or outcome between "home care" and formalized rehabilitation programs in patients with respiratory diseases are not yet available. A recent Cochrane review on "hospital-at-home" concluded that health outcomes are not improved in comparison with inpatient hospital care. Patient satisfaction is increased but the caregiver's satisfaction is not (22).

There are several disadvantages to home care rehabilitation and these include:

1. Individual treatments done at home may require increased manpower and therefore may cost more.
2. The accepted standard procedures of treatment by a whole rehabilitation team may not be possible in the home setting.
3. The exchange of opinions and experiences with other patients, the social contacts, and the availability of a wider range of means for education, training and treatment are more limited.

In pulmonary patients, home care rehabilitation is considered more of an adjunct to outpatient programs or after inpatient programs than an appropriate substitute to formalized rehabilitation programs (23).

## Practical Aspects of Selection of Components in COPD Rehabilitation Programs

The last part of this review will focus on practical aspects of the selection of program components in COPD rehabilitation, based on the Author's experience at the Rehabilitation Centers of the S. Maugeri Foundation (24, 25). It should be reemphasized that in COPD, scientific evidence of efficacy is currently limited to a few program components (10).

In mild to moderate COPD, education and psychological support are most important to maintain proper life-style and cope with disability, in particular with regard to smoking habits (26), nutritional status and interpersonal relationships. General exercise training or training of selected muscle groups is recommended (10,27,28), and chest physiotherapy can be considered in the hypersecretive patients. Occupational therapy can be valuable in those still leading an active life. The obese chronic bronchitic patient and the underweight emphysematous individual with loss of muscle mass should be referred to the dietician.

Good results have been obtained in terms of improved exercise endurance, reduced dyspnea, better quality of life, and reduced health care utilization after rehabilitation (24,25). In severe COPD, chronic respiratory failure is a frequent complication requiring long-term oxygen therapy (LTOT) and/or mechanical ventilation. The components already outlined for less severe patients can be applied to more severe cases but the exercise protocols must be adjusted (e.g. self paced walking instead of bicycle ergometer). Supplemental oxygen during training should be considered to relieve dyspnea when substantial desaturation occurs.

For the treatment of acute exacerbations, several options are available depending on the level of impairment of gas exchange. These include oxygen-therapy and non-invasive ventilation, either in the negative or positive mode. Intensive care expertise and facilities may be required when intubation is needed. Rehabilitation may also be of some importance in helping to wean a patient off the respirator. This is done through airway humidification and clearance, breathing exercises, mobilization and prevention of incorrect postures, and nutritional supplementation.

Participation of caregivers in educational sessions during home management is essential for the most disabled patients (e.g. tracheostomized patients, ventilator-dependent patients), in order to improve their skills in managing the equipment or in emergency situations.

Finally, I would like to underscore the use of specific outcome measurements in planning and evaluating programs of pulmonary rehabilitation. In fact, the concept of evidence-based pulmonary rehabilitation is now well established and specific knowledge about the effectiveness of separate components with respect to outcome is available.

On the basis of the foregoing, rehabilitation programs currently represent an essential part of the clinical management of patients with chronic obstructive pulmonary disease.

# References

1. Fishman AP. Pulmonary rehabilitation research. *Am J Respir Crit Care Med* 1994; 149:825-833.
2. American Thoracic Society. Standards for the diagnosis and care of patients with chronic obstructive pulmonary disease (COPD) and asthma. *Am Rev Respir Dis* 1987; 136:225-244.
3. Donner CF, Muir JF, and the Rehabilitation and Chronic Care Scientific Group of the European Respiratory Society. Selection criteria and programs for pulmonary rehabilitation in COPD patients. *Eur Respir J* 1997; 10:744-757.
4. Hodgkin JE. Pulmonary rehabilitation: definition and enertial components. In Pulmonary rehabilitation. JE Hodgkin, GL Connors, CW Bell eds. JB Lippincott Company, 2nd edition 1993; p. 1-14.
5. Varray A, Préfaut CH. Exercise training in patients with respiratory disease: procedures and results. *Eur Respir Rev* 1994; 5 (25): 51-58.
6. Patessio A, Ioli F, Donner CF. Exercise prescription. In: Principles and Practice of Pulmonary Rehabilitation. R Casaburi, TL Petty eds. WB Saunders Company, Philadelphia 1993; pp 322-335.
7. Olopade CO, Beck KC, Viggiano RW, Staats BA. Exercise limitation and pulmonary rehabilitation in chronic obstructive pulmonary disease. *Mayo Clin Proc* 1992; 67: 144-157.
8. Patessio A, Casaburi R, Préfaut C, Folgering H, Donner CF. Exercise training in chronic lung disease: exercise prescription. *Eur Respir Mon* 1997; 6:129-146.
9. Lachman A, Sanna A, De Coster J, Sergysels R. Evaluation of dyspnea during exercise in COPD patients. *Am Rev Respir Dis* 1990; 141: A830.
10. Lacasse Y, Guyatt GH, Goldstein RS. The components of a respiratory rehabilitation program. A systematic overview. *Chest* 1997; 111:1077-1088.
11. Smith K, Cook D, Guyatt GH, Madhavan J, Oxman AD. Respiratory muscle training in chronic airflow limitation: a meta-analysis. *Am Rev Respir Dis* 1992; 145:533-539.
12. Decramer M, Donner CF, Schols AMWJ. Rehabilitation. *Eur Respir Mon* 1998; 7:215-234.
13. Donner CF, Pesce L, Zaccaria S, Erbetta M, Mazzetti D. Organization of respiratory home care in Italy. *Monaldi Arch Chest Dis* 1993; 48: 468-472.
14. Muir JF, Voisin C, Ludot A. Organization of home respiratory care: the experience in France with ANTADIR. *Monaldi Arch Chest Dis* 1993; 48: 462-467.
15. Haggerty MC, Stockdale Woolley R, Nair S. Respi-Care. An innovative home care program for the patient with chronic obstructive pulmonary disease. *Chest*. 1991; 100: 607-612.
16. Sahn SA, Petty TL. Results of a comprehensive rehabilitation program for severe COPD. In: Lung Biology in Health and Disease: Chronic Obstructive Pulmonary Disease. TL Petty ed. Marcel Dekker Inc, New York, 1978; pp 203-220.
17. Donner CF, Howard P, Robert D. Patient selection and techniques for home mechanical ventilation. European Respiratory Society Rehabilitation and Chronic Care Scientific Group. *Monaldi Arch Chest Dis* 1993; 48: 40-47.
18. Wijkstra PJ, Van Altena R, Kraan J, Otten V, Postma DS, Koeter GH. Quality of life in patients with chronic obstructive pulmonary disease improves after rehabilitation at home. *Eur Respir J* 1994; 7: 269-273.
19. Crockett AJ, Moss JR, Cranston JM, Alpers JH. The effects of home oxygen therapy on hospital admission rates in chronic obstructive airways disease. *Monaldi Arch Chest Dis* 1993; 48: 445-446.
20. Bach JR. Comprehensive rehabilitation of the severely disabled ventilator-assisted individual. *Monaldi Arch Chest Dis* 1993; 48: 331-345.
21. Bach JR, Intintola P, Alba AS, Holland IE. The ventilator-assisted individual. Cost analysis of institutionalization vs rehabilitation and in-home management. *Chest* 1992; 101: 26-30.

22. Shepperd S, Iliffe S. Effectiveness of hospital at home compared to inpatient hospital care. Cochrane Review, 18 Nov 1997. In: The Cochrane Library. Oxford: Update Software. Reported by Masters PA. Review: Hospital-at-home care does not improve patient health outcomes. Evidence-based Medicine, November/December 1998, p. 181.

23. Walters MI, Edwards PR, Waterhouse JC, Howard P. Long term domiciliary oxygen therapy in chronic obstructive pulmonary disease. *Thorax* 1993; 48: 1170-1177.

24. Ambrosino N, Vitacca M, Rampulla C. Standards for rehabilitative strategies in respiratory diseases. *Monaldi Arch Chest Dis* 1995; 50:293-318.

25. Donner CF, Lusuardi M. Pulmonary rehabilitation. In: Brambilla C, Costabel U, Naeije R, Rodriguez-Roisin R, eds. Pulmonary Diseases. McGraw-Hill Publishing Company UK, London, 1999, ch. 59, pp. 577-584.

25. Anthonisen NR, Connett JE, Kiley JP, Altose MD, Bailey WC, Buist AS, Conway WAJ, Enright PL, Kanner RE, O'Hara P, Owens GR, Scanlon PD, Tashkin DP, Wise RA. Effects of smoking intervention and the use of an inhaled anticholinergic bronchodilator on the rate of decline of FEV1. The lung health study. *JAMA* 1994; 272:1497-1505.

26. Lake FR, Henderson K, Briffa T, Openshaw J, Musk W. Upper limb and lower limb exercise training in patients with chronic airflow limitation. *Chest* 1990; 97:1077-1082.

27. Martinez FJ, Vogel PD, Dupont DN, Stanopoulos I, Gray A, Beamis JF: Supported arm exercise vs. unsupported arm exercise in the rehabilitation of patients with severe chronic airflow obstruction. *Chest* 1993; 103:1397-1402.

# Chapter 21

# Who Responds to Exercise Training? Are We Asking the Proper Questions?

Marc Decramer, MD, PhD, Belgium

Chronic obstructive pulmonary disease (COPD) is a slowly progressive disorder characterised by irreversible airflow obstruction and enhanced annual decline in lung function (1). At present, only smoking cessation has been shown to affect the decline in lung function (2). Inhaled corticosteroids cause a small increment in lung function and quality of life, without, however, affecting the annual decline in lung function (3,4). One of the most important findings in the ISOLDE study was the demonstration of an accelerated decline in health status in COPD patients with moderate to severe airflow obstruction.

Although they have been available for several decades, pulmonary rehabilitation programs have become increasingly popular in the treatment of COPD during the last few years. Indeed, the "State of the Art" review written by Lertzman and Cherniack and published in 1976 identified 184 references, clearly demonstrating significant interest in this field more than 20 years ago (5). This method of treatment is therefore not new although what can be expected from pulmonary rehabilitation programs has now become much clearer. This information comes from several randomised well-designed clinical trials conducted over the last 10 years which have showed that pulmonary rehabilitation does improve health status and functional exercise capacity in COPD patients. This new information is also based on a multitude of observations indicating that exercise capacity correlates poorly with airflow obstruction in COPD patients, and that associated phenomena such as deconditioning and muscle weakness are important in generating symptoms. In light of these observations, more clarity may also emerge on how candidates for a pulmonary rehabilitation program should be selected and this will be addressed in this review.

This manuscript will essentially focus on two important questions: 1) What can be expected from a rehabilitation program? 2) How should candidates for pulmonary rehabilitation be selected?

## What Can Be Expected From a Pulmonary Rehabilitation Program?

Several studies published over the past ten years have answered a number of important questions related to what can be expected from pulmonary rehabilitation programs. It is now abundantly clear that pulmonary rehabilitation reduces symptoms (6), improves exercise tolerance (7, 8, 9) and improves the quality of life of COPD patients (8, 9). This latter benefit was recently reviewed in a meta-analysis written by Lacasse et al. (10). In their analysis, quality of life had been measured in 12 out of 14 trials although only two validated instruments (transitional dyspnea index and chronic respiratory disease questionnaire (CRDQ)) were used. The CRDQ was used in four trials (8, 11, 12, 13). As a whole, quality of life improved in all four of its dimensions (dyspnea, fatigue, emotional function and mastery) and the average increase exceeded the minimal clinical important difference for all dimensions. For dyspnea and mastery the minimal effect also exceeded the minimal clinically important difference (MCID) set at 0.5 points on a Likert type score comprising 7 points. Examples of effects of rehabilitation on 6-MWD and health status (14) are shown in Figures 21.1 and 21.2.

Four important trials were too recently published to be included in the meta-analysis (7, 9, 15, 16, 17). The first of these trials did not show an improvement in quality of life, but it demonstrated an improvement in dyspnea and fatigue (15). The absence of a positive effect on quality of life is likely due to

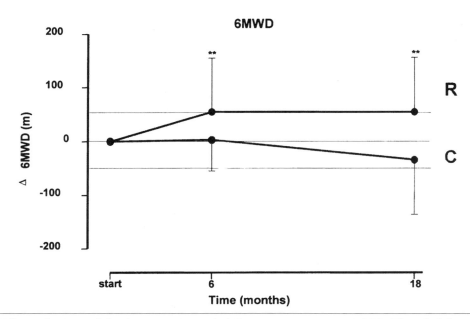

**Figure 21.1**    Effects of a 6 month lasting outpatient rehabilitation program on 6-MWD. The rehabilitation group is represented in red (R) and the control group (C) in blue. The effect clearly exceeds the minimal clinically important difference of about 55 meters, shown by the pink line. From Troosters et al. (14). ** p < 0.01.

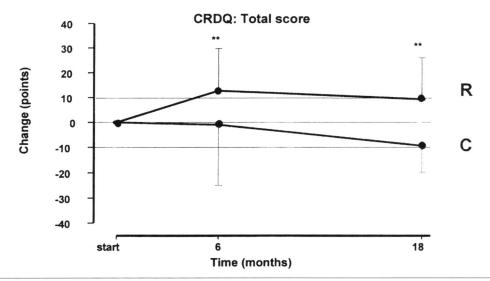

**Figure 21.2**    Effects of a 6 month lasting outpatient rehabilitation program on health status measured with the CRDQ. The rehabilitation group (R) is represented in red and the control group (C) in blue. The effect clearly exceeds the minimal clinical important difference shown by the pink line. The effects on the total score are shown, similar effects were obtained in the four subdomains. From Troosters et al. (14). ** p < 0.01.

the fact that a generic quality of life instrument (quality of well-being scale) likely to be less sensitive than disease-specific instruments was used. Two of the 4 other trials used the St.George's Respiratory Questionnaire (SGRQ) in combination with the CRDQ and both found a positive effect of rehabilitation although in one study the effect may have been less pronounced in patients with severe dyspnea (16). The last trial used the Sickness Impact Profile (SIP) and documented that both 8 weeks of rehabilitation and lung volume reduction surgery (17) improved quality of life. Three months of additional rehabilitation did not improve quality of life further in non surgical patients while LVRS did.

It is noteworthy that the SIP is a generic instrument that may lack sensitivity. In addition, it should be noted that in that trial, the effect of rehabilitation on functional exercise capacity was exceedingly small and averaged only 16 meters. This value is considerably less than the predicted effect of rehabilitation on functional exercise capacity which on the average is 54 meters (10). This may indicate that either patients had already done some rehabilitation before the 8 week program, thus resulting in better conditioning before the program even started or that the program was too short lasted and not intense enough. This observation is of considerable importance because similar findings were described in the NETT-trial (18).

It is now well established that improvements in exercise capacity and quality of life, obtained after rehabilitation are poorly related (14, 19). In a recent study, we were able to show a reasonably close relationship between improvement in quality of life as measured with the CRDQ and improvement in muscle force following rehabilitation (14). This might indicate that muscle force is one of the key variables in pulmonary rehabilitation. As a rule, it is not necessary to improve exercise capacity in order to improve quality of life. Indeed, in 1992, Simpson et al. (11) showed that weight lifting exercises training of peripheral muscles without affecting exercise capacity improved all four dimensions of the CRDQ. Similarly, we recently showed that aerobic exercise training and peripheral muscle strength training both improved health status (measured by the CRDQ) to a similar extent in COPD patients (20).

Up until now, pulmonary rehabilitation has not been shown to significantly improve survival of COPD patients, although at least two studies have shown trends for improved survival (15, 21). In addition, two other studies (9,14) have demonstrated reductions in the number of hospital admissions and reductions in the number of hospital days. The study by Griffiths et al. (9) demonstrated a concomitant increase in the number of visits to the general practitioner indicating increased use of primary care facilities. These findings are all the more relevant since COPD patients are known to be high consumers of health care resources (22, 23).

## How Should We Select Candidates for Pulmonary Rehabilitation?

If pulmonary rehabilitation beneficially affects outcome variables in COPD patients, should we then admit all COPD patients into these programs or should we select patients? If so, how should patients be selected?

At present there is substantially less data on how to select patients than on the overall beneficial effects of pulmonary rehabilitation. In addition, it appears more attractive to focus training on those activities of daily living that create more problems for individual patients. This "selective training", however, has to the best of our knowledge never been critically examined and it is also not clear as to whether such "specific" training is likely to be more effective than general training programs. Although it seems likely that these specific trainings will become the way of the future for COPD patients, I will only address general rehabilitation programs.

Before admission, a number of prerequisites are considered important. For instance, it is expected that medical therapy will have been optimised and that the patient will have stopped smoking or at least enrolled in a smoking cessation program. This is important because smoking cessation is currently the only treatment known to affect the evolution of COPD (2). There is, however, no hard evidence that the beneficial effects of training programs would be less important in smokers than in non-smokers. For further selection criteria, a number of studies trying to predict outcomes after pulmonary rehabilitation may be useful to look at.

A study by ZuWallack et al. (24) was one of the first report which tried to predict an improvement in twelve minute walking distance (12-MWD), after pulmonary rehabilitation. The study was carried out in 50 severe COPD patients and the improvement was correlated to the initial 12-MWD, peak oxygen consumption, peak oxygen pulse, and ventilatory reserve at peak exercise. In multiple regression analysis only the initial 12-MWD and $FEV_1$ had power in predicting improvement of 12-MWD. It should be stressed that in this study, the relationship between improvement in 12-MWD and baseline 12-MWD posed a statistical problem and that the regression coefficient obtained is likely to have been overestimated. In subsequent studies the usefulness of $FEV_1$ as a selection criterion has also been clearly debated.

Indeed, Maltais et al. (25) demonstrated that training responses were similar in COPD patients with an $FEV_1$ above and below 40% of predicted. The effects on ventilation and heart rate at a $\dot{V}O_2$max corresponding to the pretraining maximum, peak oxygen consumption and maximal workload were all similar. Only the reduction in lactate at the pretraining maximum was slightly different between those two groups. The study also showed that workload and training time increased during the four first weeks of training, such that after four weeks, decent training loads (60% max) and times (20 minutes) could be obtained. These were perfectly capable of inducing training effects. A study by Casaburi et al (26) published in 1997 also showed that training effects were readily obtained in patients with severe COPD who were not capable of rising their lactate levels above 2 mmol/L during exercise. This is an important observation which has significant consequences for the applicability of pulmonary rehabilitation as a whole. Since patients with severe airflow obstruction appear to improve substantially with training, a rehabilitation program is an important treatment modality in end-stage COPD. It is also useful in preparing for lung transplantation or lung volume reduction surgery. It challenges the old concept that beneficial effects of exercise training were only expected in these patients who were capable of increasing their lactic acid levels substantially during exercise. At present there is no basis for this contention anymore.

In a recent study, we looked at the predictors of training effects in a group of eighty-two COPD patients entered in an outpatient rehabilitation program 6 months previously. Positive response was defined as a 15% increase in maximum workload and/or a 25% increase in six minute walking distance, 6-MWD. In general 58 (71%) out of the 82 patients had a response to treatment. Responders were characterised by lower PImax, lower 6-MWD, lower maximal workload, and lower heart rate and ventilation at peak exercise. The differences between responders and non-responders are summarised in table 21.1.

The pretraining ratio VEmax/MVV, 6-MWD and PImax, were related to the subsequent response. In discriminant analysis, only the ratio VEmax/MVV and PImax, contributed significantly to the distinction between responders and non-responders. It should be emphasised, however, that only 15% of the variance was explained by the discriminant model. This basically means that it is quite difficult to predict the response to training from the baseline functional characteristics. As a consequence, it is important to apply a trial treatment to observe whether patients indeed improve with the treatment.

In general, the following intuitive and empirical rules may be proposed with the knowledge that available studies do not really offer a sound basis to distinguish responders from non-responders. As a whole, we would select patients who have symptomatic respiratory disease resulting in reduced health status and decreased functional status. The patients need to be motivated to attend a pulmonary rehabilitation program. Although there is no

**Table 21.1  Diffrences in Functional Characteristics Between 58 Responders to a Rehabilitation Program and 24 Non-Responders**

|  | Responders | Non-responders |
|---|---|---|
| n | 58 | 24 |
| FEV$_1$ (% pred) | 39 ± 16 | 42 ± 17 |
| TL,co (% pred) | 50 ± 26 | 45 ± 23 |
| QF (% pred) | 72 ± 27 | 74 ± 13 |
| PImax (% pred) | 64 ± 20* | 78 ± 30 |
| 6-M WD (m) | 310 ± 133*** | 425 ± 105 |
| Load (Watt) | 66 ± 33* | 83 ± 27 |
| HRmax (/min) | 132 ± 21** | 148 ± 21 |
| VE/MVV (%) | 89 ± 24* | 107 ± 34 |
| CRDQtot (AU) | 74 ± 18 | 80 ± 16 |

TL,co = transfer capacity, QF = quadriceps force, PImax = maximal inspiratory pressure, HRmax = maximal heart rate, VE/MVV = ratio of maximal exercise ventilation to maximal voluntary ventilation, CRDQtot = total score on the CRDQ.

*$p<0.05$, **$p<0.01$, ***$p<0.001$.

clear data to support this requirement. Patients should be ex-smokers or are at least be enrolled in a smoking cessation program, even if there is no clear evidence that the benefits of a rehabilitation program would be smaller in smokers. Finally, they should not have comorbidities that might interfere with the rehabilitation process (e.g. rheumatoid arthritis), or that places them at an excessive risk of complications during exercise training (e.g. ischemic cardiovascular disease) (27, 28). As previously outlined, all patients with any level of airflow obstruction are candidates for rehabilitation programs. This means that patients being prepared for volume reduction surgery or transplantation are good candidates for rehabilitation.

Empirically (29), it appears that patients with moderate airflow obstruction (FEV$_1$ between 40-60% of predicted), who have severe complaints of dyspnea, impaired health status and clear peripheral muscle weakness constitute good candidates. In such patients, rehabilitation would consist primarily of endurance training, peripheral muscle training, psychosocial support, and dietary interventions if the individual is either underweight or overweight. The need for education, psychosocial support, ergotherapy or chest physiotherapy may be real, but at present it is not clearly supported from the literature.

Based on the programs used to prepare patients for lung transplantation (30) or volume reduction surgery, it also appears that patients with more severe airflow obstruction ($FEV_1$ between 20-40% of predicted), may be good candidates for pulmonary rehabilitation, if they have severe complaints of dyspnea, reduced health status, and severe peripheral muscle weakness. In these patients, the program should be directed towards peripheral muscle training, interval or endurance training and nutritional support.

## Conclusion

Although it has been shown that pulmonary rehabilitation results in beneficial effects in COPD patients, it remains relatively difficult to develop scientific criteria for the proper selection of candidates. Muscle weakness, poor functional exercise capacity and significant ventilatory reserve at peak exercise appear to be predictors of positive response although they explain a relatively small fraction of the variance in the response. The practical attitude appears to be to identify candidates for programs on the basis of simple and empirical clinical rules. This means that patients with significantly reduced quality of life and functional status of any degree of airflow obstruction, who are sufficiently motivated and who do not present contraindications are suitable candidates.

## Acknowledgments

The studies cited in the present manuscript were supported by the "Fonds voor Wetenschappelijk Onderzoek-Vlaanderen" grants # G.0175.99 and G.0237.01 and by the Research Foundation of the Katholieke Universiteit Leuven, grant # OT 98/27. They were further supported by AstraZeneca pharmaceuticals.

## References

1. Siafakas NM, Vermeire P, Pride NB et al: Optimal assessment and management of COPD. *Eur Respir J* 1995;8:1398-420.
2. Anthonisen NR, Connett JE, Kiley JP et al: Effects of smoking intervention and the use of anticholinergic bronchodilator on the rate of decline of FEV1. The lung health study. *JAMA* 1994;272:1497-1505.
3. Pauwels RA, Löfdahl CG, Laitinen LA et al: Long-term treatment with inhaled budesonide in persons with mild COPD who continue smoking. *N Eng J Med* 1999;340:1948-1953.
4. Burge PS, Calverley PMA, Jones PW, Spencer P, Anderson JA, Maslen TK: Randomized, double blind, placebo controlled study of fluticasone propionate in patients with moderate to severe chronic obstructive pulmonary disease: the ISOLDE trial. *BMJ* 2000;320:1297-1303.
5. Lertzman R, Cherniack RS: Rehabilitation of patients with chronic obstructive pulmonary disease. State of the art. *Am Rev Respir Dis* 1976;114:1145-1163.
6. O'Donnell DE, Webb KA, McGuire MA: Older patients with COPD. Benefits of exercise training. *Geriatrics* 1993;48:59-66.
7. Toshima MT, Kaplan RM, Ries AL: Experimental evaluation of rehabilitation in chronic obstructive pulmonary disease: short-term effects on exercise endurance and health status. *Health Psychology* 1990;93:237-252.
8. Goldstein RS, Gort EH, Stubbing D, Avendano MA, Gyatt GH: Randomised controlled trial of respiratory rehabilitation. *Lancet* 1994;344:1394-1397.
9. Griffiths TL, Burr ML, Campbell IA et al: Results at 1 year of outpatient multidisciplinary pulmonary rehabilitation: a randomised controlled trial. *Lancet* 2000;355:362-368.
10. Lacasse Y, Wong E, Guyatt GH, King D, Cook DJ, Goldstein RS:. Meta-analysis of respiratory rehabilitation in chronic obstructive pulmonary disease. *Lancet* 1996;348:1115-1119.
11. Simpson K, Killian K, McCartney N, Stubbing DG, Jones NL: Randomised controlled trial of weightlifting exercise in patients with chronic airflow limitation. *Thorax* 1992;47:70-75.
12. Wijkstra PJ, van Altena R, Kraan J, Otten V, Postma DS, Koëter GH: Quality of life in patients with chronic obstructive pulmonary disease after rehabilitation at home. *Eur Respir J* 1994;7:269-273.
13. Güell R, Morante F, Sangenis M, Casan P: Effects of respiratory rehabilitation on the effort capacity and on health-related quality of life of patients with chronic obstructive pulmonary disease (Abstr). *Eur Respir J* 1995;8:356.
14. Troosters T, Gosselink R, Decramer M: Short and long-term effects of outpatient rehabilita-

tion in chronic obstructive pulmonary disease: a randomised controlled trial. *Am J Med* 2000;109:207-212.

15. Ries AL, Kaplan RM, Limberg TM, Prewitt L: Effects of pulmonary rehabilitation on physiologic and psychosocial outcomes in patients with chronic obstructive pulmonary disease. *Ann Intern Med* 1995:122:823-832.

16. Wedzicha JA, Bestall JC, Garrod R, Garnham R, Paul EA, Jones PW: Randomized controlled trial of pulmonary rehabilitation in severe chronic onstructive pulmonary disease patients, stratified with the MRC dyspnoea scale. *Eur Respir J* 1998;12:363-369.

17. Criner GA, Cordova FC, Furukawa S et al: Prospective randomised trial comparing bilateral lung volume reduction surgery to pulmonary rehabilitation in severe chronic obstructive pulmonary disease. *Am J Respir Crit Care Med* 1999;160:2018-2027.

18. Make B, Tolliver R, Christensen P, Karlo S, MacIntyre N, Ries A for the NETT Research Group: Pulmonary rehabilitation improves exercise capacity and dyspnea in the National Emphysema Treatment Trial (NETT) (abstr). *Am J Crit Care Med* 2000;161:A254.

19. Reardon J, Patel K, ZuWallack RL: Improvement of quality of life is unrelated to improvement in exercise endurance after outpatient pulmonary rehabilitation. *J Cardiopulm Rehabil* 1993;13:51-54.

20. De Paepe K, Troosters T, Gosselink R, Decramer M: Comparison of endurance training and strength training in patients with severe COPD (abstr). *Am J Respir Crit Care Med* 2000; 161:A494.

21. De Paepe K, Troosters T, Gosselink R, Decramer M: Determinants of survival in patients with COPD. *Eur Respir J* 2000;16 (Suppl31):31S.

22. Strauss MJ: Cost and outcome of care for patients with chronic obstructive lung disease. *Medical Care* 1986;24:915-924.

23. Grasso ME, Weller WE, Shaffer TJ, Diette GB, Anderson GF: Capitation, managed care and chronic obstructive pulmonary disease. *Am J Respir Crit Care* 1998;158:133-138.

24. ZuWallack RL, Patel K, Reardon JZ, Clark BA, Normandin EA: Predictors of improvement in the 12-minute walking distance following a six-week outpatient pulmonary rehabilitation program. *Chest* 1991;99:805-808.

25. Maltais F, Leblanc P, Jobin J et al: Intensity of training and physiologic adaptation in patients with chronic obstructive pulmonary disease. *Am J Respir Crit Care Med* 1997;155:555-561.

26. Casaburi R, Porszasz J, Burns MB, Carithers ER, Chang RSY, Cooper CB: Physiologic benefits of exercise training in rehabilitation of patients with severe chronic obstructive pulmonary disease. *Am J Respir Crit Care Med* 1997;155:1541-1551.

27. ZuWallack RL: Selection criteria and outcome assessment in pulmonary rehabilitation. *Monaldi Arch Chest Dis* 1998;53:429-437.

28. Morgan MDL: The prediction of benefit from pulmonary rehabilitation: setting, training intensity and the effect of selection by disability. *Thorax* 1999;54(Suppl2):S3-S7.

29. Decramer M, Donner CF, Schols AMWJ: Rehabilitation. In: Management of chronic obstructive pulmonary disease. Ed. DS Postma and NM Siafakas. *Eur Respir Monograph* 1998;3:215-234.

30. Fournier M, Derenne J PH: Exercise performance in lung transplant candidates and recipients. *Eur Respir J* 1995;5:38-41.

PART VIII

# Integrating Non-Conventional Approaches In Cardiopulmonary Rehabilitation

# Chapter 22

# Peripheral Muscle Dysfunction In Chronic Obstructive Pulmonary Disease and Chronic Heart Failure: Two Diseases, One Common Consequence

François Maltais, MD, Richard Debigaré, MSc, Didier Saey, MSc, Jean Jobin, PhD, Canada

## Introduction

Peripheral muscle wasting in patients with advanced COPD or CHF has been recognized for several years by clinicians (1). However, this problem is still receiving little attention from a diagnostic and therapeutic point of view although there has been renewed interest in it, now that the negative impact of wasting on survival has been confirmed (2,3). There is intense basic research looking at the mechanisms of wasting at the molecular level which should result in the development of new therapeutic strategies specifically targeted at improving muscle mass in wasted patients. In this chapter, we will first describe the clinical manifestations and consequences of peripheral muscle dysfunction in COPD and CHF. We will then explore some possible mechanisms to explain this problem as well as the role of exercise training.

## Evidence of Peripheral Muscle Dysfunction

Peripheral muscle abnormalities described in patients with COPD or CHF are very similar and have been discussed at length in recent reviews (4-6). Reduction in muscle mass, weakness, alteration in fiber type distribution, and decreased metabolic capacity have all been reported in association with these diseases (table 22.1). The quadriceps is the most commonly studied peripheral muscle not only because it is readily accessible but also because it is a primary effector muscle of ambulation. It should however be mentioned that in general, the disease process is more obvious in the lower than in the upper extremity muscles (7-10).

**Table 22.1   Evidence of Peripheral Muscle Dysfunction in COPD and CHF**

Muscle atrophy

Weakness

Morphological changes

   ↓ proportion of type I

   ↑ proportion of type IIb fibers

   atrophy of type I and IIa fibers

   ↓ capillarisation

Altered metabolic capacity

   ↓ intramuscular pH

   ↓ ATP concentration

   ↑ muscle lactate concentration

   ↑ ionosine monophosphate

   ↓ mitochondrial enzyme activities

## Muscle Mass and Strength

Peripheral muscle wasting is common in COPD and CHF and the prevalence of this problem increases with the severity of the disease (11,12). An important observation is that the reduction in muscle mass is proportionally greater than the loss in body weight in COPD (9,11) and CHF (13). This implies that body weight measurements may be misleading in estimating muscle mass. As it will be discussed later, this observation may also have important implications in the pathophysiology of muscle wasting.

In chronic lung or heart diseases, loss of muscle mass is associated with muscle weakness (9,14), poor exercise tolerance (9,15,16,13) and is a predictor of mortality independent of lung function (2,3,17). The strength of the quadriceps is an important determinant of exercise capacity in COPD and in CHF (7,18,19). This may be related to the influence of muscle strength on the perception of leg effort during exercise, a commonly limiting symptom in patients with lung or heart diseases (18,20,21).

Some evidence supports the concept that muscle weakness is due to muscle atrophy. In patients with COPD, the quadriceps strength/mid-thigh cross-sectional area ratio is similar to that of normal subjects (9). Similar observation has been made in CHF (22). Although these observations suggest that muscle weakness is the result of atrophy, the loss in strength may be out of proportion to the loss of muscle mass in patients exposed to systemic corticosteroids (9,23), or in advanced CHF and cachexia (24).

## Muscle Fiber Type, Size, and Capillarization

The ultrastructural modifications of the peripheral skeletal muscle are strikingly similar in COPD and CHF. The fiber type profile of the vastus lateralis muscle, an important determinant of the muscle metabolic capacity (25-27), has been assessed in patients with moderate to severe COPD and CHF using both classical histochemical fiber typing and analysis of myosin heavy chain isoform expression. In both diseases, a reduction in the proportion of type I fibers with a reciprocal increase in type IIb fibers have been reported (28-34). Type I and IIa fibers are atrophic in COPD while atrophy predominates in type II fibers in CHF (31). In chronic lung and heart diseases, the capillarization of the vastus lateralis muscle, an important determinant of muscle aerobic capacity is reduced when compared to age-matched healthy subjects (30,31,34).

## Skeletal Muscle Metabolism

The metabolism of the peripheral muscles in COPD and CHF has been studied extensively over the past 10-15 years. In line with the fiber-type profile described above, low activity of two mitochondrial enzymes, citrate synthase and 3-hydroxyacyl-CoA dehydrogenase has been reported in needle biopsy specimens of the vastus lateralis muscle in COPD and CHF (31,35,36). These two enzymes, which are respectively involved in the citric acid cycle and b-oxidation of fatty acids, are good markers of muscle oxidative capacity. In keeping with these enzymatic changes, muscle energy metabolism is modified at rest and during exercise in COPD. Low intracellular pH, reduced phosphocreatine (PCr) and adenosinetriphosphate (ATP) contents, and increased lactate and ionosine monophosphate concentrations have been found in the vastus lateralis muscle (28,37-39). Using nuclear magnetic resonance spectroscopy ($^{31}$P-NMR) to study the oxidative metabolism of skeletal muscle during exercise, a greater decline in muscle intracellular pH and in phosphocreatine/inorganic phosphate (PCr/Pi) ratio was observed during exercise in patients with chronic lung disease or CHF compared to normal subjects (40-46). These findings are indicative of impaired oxidative phosphorylation and ATP resynthesis, with a high reliance on anaerobic glycolysis within the contracting muscles (40-46). Although these exercise-induced peripheral muscle metabolic abnormalities may be worsened by hypoxemia and can be partially reversed with oxygen supplementation (43,44,47), they are not necessarily related to reduction in peripheral $O_2$ delivery (26,48-50). This suggests that altered muscle metabolism during exercise in COPD and CHF is related, at least in part, to poor muscle oxidative capacity or abnormal metabolic regulation (51).

In keeping with the histochemical and enzymatic changes, the resistance to fatigue of the vastus lateralis muscle, measured during isometric contractions, is reduced in patients with COPD and CHF (22,52,53).

## Upper Extremity and Respiratory Muscles Versus Lower Limb Muscles

Interestingly, all peripheral muscles are not affected to the same extent in patients with COPD or CHF. For instance, the strength of the upper extremity muscles is relatively preserved compared to that of muscles of the lower extremity (7-9). In a preliminary study, the activity of citrate synthase of the deltoid muscle was found to be preserved and even increased in patients with severe COPD compared to subjects with normal respiratory function (10). The adaptation of the diaphragm in COPD is also different than that of the vastus lateralis (54,55). While the vastus lateralis shows a low capacity for aerobic metabolism and increased susceptibility to fatigue (30,36), the structural changes found in the diaphragm are characterized by an increased proportion of fatigue-resistant fibers (54,55). A shift from fast to slow myosin heavy chain isoforms with increased oxidative capacity has also been reported in patients with advanced CHF compared to subjects with normal cardiorespiratory function (56). The observation of a differential adaptation of the respiratory, upper and lower limb muscles is intriguing and may lead to insights into the mechanisms responsible for peripheral muscle dysfunction in patients with chronic cardiorespiratory disorders. For instance, a differential adaptive response of the different muscle groups does not support the presence of a generalized myopathic disorder, but would be consistent with local muscular events in the deterioration of the lower limb muscle function.

## Etiology of Peripheral Muscle Dysfunction in COPD and CHF

The striking resemblance in the peripheral muscle function in COPD and CHF suggest as least some similitude in the underlying mechanisms. In fact, the same factors have been evoked to explain the occurrence of muscle dysfunction in both diseases (Table 22.2). Peripheral muscle dysfunction is probably multifactorial in origin and is unlikely to be explained by a unique mechanism in all patients.

## Chronic Inactivity and Deconditioning

The most obvious potential cause of peripheral muscle dysfunction in COPD and CHF is chronic

**Table 22.2 Possible Etiologies of the Skeletal Muscle Dysfunction in COPD and CHF**

---

Chronic inactivity and disuse atrophy

Systemic inflammation

Nutritional imbalance

Systemic corticosteroids

Hypoxemia

Electrolyte disturbances

---

inactivity and muscle deconditioning. It is a common observation that patients with chronic lung or heart diseases often reduce their level of activity to avoid the dyspnea that ambulation engenders. Further, the similarity between the histochemical and enzymatic muscle changes associated with chronic inactivity in healthy humans and those reported in patients with COPD and CHF (57-60) is another indication that muscle deconditioning is likely to be involved in peripheral muscle dysfunction associated with chronic lung and heart diseases. The different degree of activation between the lower limb muscles and upper limb and diaphragmatic muscles may be responsible for the different level of abnormalities in these three muscle groups (9,54). Compared to lower limb muscles, those of the upper limb remain probably more active in daily living explaining why their function is relatively maintained (9,10). Furthermore, in COPD, the pectoralis major and the latissimus dorsi muscles may also act as accessory inspiratory muscles, another potential source of stimulation (61,62). The level of activation of the diaphragm is also greater than that of lower limb muscles in COPD and CHF and the chronic increase in work of breathing faced by the diaphragm is, in fact, a continuous training stimulus. The increased proportion in type I fibers in the diaphragm of patients with COPD or CHF is likely to represent an adaptation to training reinforcing the role of deconditioning in peripheral muscle dysfunction in these individuals (54,56).

There are however evidences in COPD and CHF supporting the idea that inactivity may not be sufficient in itself to explain all muscle changes found in these diseases. Profound alterations in MHC isoform expression in the vastus lateralis muscle are seen in patients with moderate to severe COPD or CHF compared to healthy subjects despite only modest differences in exercise capacity and, presumably, in the level of daily activity (32,33). The possible role of the low level of daily activity in explaining muscle changes in COPD has been recently addressed in an animal model of emphysema (63). In hamsters, much like in humans, the induction of emphysema is associated with a reduction in the oxidative capacity of the gastrocnemius and vastus lateralis muscles but has an opposite effect on the diaphragm (63). Interestingly, these differences could not be attributed to a reduction in physical activity levels since these were documented to be similar in emphysematous and control hamsters. After induction of heart failure in dogs, Sabbah and colleagues observed a decrease in type I muscle fiber surface area. However, these changes appeared only one month after the induction of heart failure and before any significant change in cardiac output was observed, indicating that changes in left ventricule geometry might be sufficient to trigger some skeletal muscle changes very early in the evolution of CHF (64).

## Inflammation

Peripheral muscle dysfunction is not specific to COPD and has indeed been reported in other chronic illnesses such as chronic heart failure (65), cystic fibrosis (66,67), AIDS (68) and chronic renal failure (69). In these chronic conditions, peripheral muscle wasting is also associated with adverse clinical outcome, independent of the impairment of the primary diseased organ.

The release of proinflammatory cytokines such as TNFα, IL-1, and IL-6 by neutrophils and macrophages has been implicated in cachexia associated with COPD (70-74), chronic heart failure (3,65,75,76), cystic fibrosis (66,67), and AIDS (68). In AIDS, thalidomide, a TNFα inhibitor, induces weight gain (77). These pro-inflammatory cytokines can stimulate proteolysis by activating the ubiquitin-proteasome pathway which is responsible for muscle wasting in several human diseases (78). TNFα, IL-1, and IL-6 may down-regulate the hepatic production of IGF-1 which mediates the anabolic action of GH (79). Inflammation may also induce an oxidant/antioxidant imbalance in patients with chronic disorders by providing a continuous source of oxidative stress (80) which may contribute to poor muscle performance (81). Accordingly, it is conceivable that a low grade and chronic systemic inflammatory process may participate in the development of peripheral muscle wasting and dysfunction in COPD and CHF.

Increased prevalence of low blood level of anabolic steroids and insulin growth hormone factor (IGF-1) has been reported in patients with COPD (82,83) and CHF (84-86). One emerging concept is that peripheral muscle homeostasis in chronic diseases such as COPD and CHF may be disrupted by an imbalance between anabolic (growth factors) and catabolic (cortisol, proinflammatory cytokines) factors. Such an imbalance has been previously reported in patients with CHF and was related to body weight (84). This important issue will need to be further studied as well as the relationship between circulating factors and their level and action within the muscles.

## Cachexia Versus Nutritional Imbalance

Cachexia that accompanies chronic diseases such as COPD and CHF differs markedly from reduced nutritional intake or starvation (87). The former situation is characterized by increased muscle proteolysis, preferential loss of muscle over other body compartments, systemic inflammation, and poor response to nutritional intervention. Clearly wasting in patients with COPD and CHF has much more similarities with cachexia than with poor nutritional intake. This probably explains why simple nutritional interventions have failed to produce any clinically meaningful improvement in muscle mass and strength (88).

## Other Factors

Other factors may be implicated in muscle wasting in COPD and CHF depending on the clinical situation. Hypoxemia (28,29,89,90), use of systemic corticosteroids (4,23), electrolytes disturbances (91) should be considered as potential causes depending on the clinical situations.

## Clinical Implications

### Exercise Intolerance

Exercise intolerance is a major consequence of COPD and CHF. Several observations have made it clear that exercise intolerance in these individuals cannot be explained solely on the basis of limitation in ventilation and gas exchange. For instance, the degree of impairment in lung or heart function is a poor predictor of exercise capacity (92,93). Perhaps the most striking clinical observation pointing to a peripheral component of exercise limitation in these diseases is that exercise capacity remains abnormally low in most lung transplant recipients despite normalization of lung or heart function (94-97).

Patients with COPD or CHF stop exercise because of exertional discomfort (18,92) and not necessarily because physiological constraints have been reached. Peripheral muscle weakness increases the perception of leg fatigue (18), which is a commonly limiting symptom in chronic heart or lung diseases (20,98). In turn, patients with stronger limb muscles tolerate greater exercise intensity (18). Patients are likely to have a better exercise tolerance if they feel less discomfort in the exercising muscles.

Lower capacity for muscle aerobic metabolism may influence exercise tolerance in several fashions. Increased lactic acidosis for a given exercise work rate, which is a common finding in COPD (99-102) and CHF (26,103), enhances the ventilatory needs by increasing non-aerobic $CO_2$ production (101,104, 105). This imposes an additional burden on the respiratory muscles already facing increased impedance to breathing. In addition, the resulting acidemia may act as a breathing stimulus via the carotid bodies. Lastly, premature muscle acidosis, a contributory factor to muscle fatigue and early exercise termination in healthy subjects, (106-108) may be an important mechanism contributing to exercise intolerance in COPD (48) and CHF (50). This may be exacerbated by a tendency to retain $CO_2$ (i.e. a respiratory acidosis) during exercise (101). Consistent with the alteration in muscle metabolism and with the greater proportion of fatigue susceptible fibers, evidence of contractile fatigue of the quadriceps (defined as a 15% reduction in the quadriceps twitch force after exercise) has been found following high intensity cycle exercise in COPD patients (109). In CHF, ergoreceptors or metaboreceptors located within the peripheral muscle may be sensitive to the accumulation of different metabolites during exercise. Excessive stimulation of these receptors during exercise may participate to the abnormal heart rate, blood pressure, and ventilation responses, perhaps contributing to exercise limitation (110). To our knowledge, such a phenomenon has not been reported in COPD.

## Survival and Other Consequences of Muscle Dysfunction

An important consequence of muscle wasting associated to chronic diseases may be its implication in determining survival. The relationship between low body weight and poor survival has been established both in COPD (2,17) and CHF (3). However, the mechanistic link between body weight and survival has not been elucidated. One question is whether the loss of muscle mass has more prognostic implications than the loss of other body compartment. We have recently addressed this issue in 142 patients with COPD who were followed for

29 months (111). In this cohort of patients, we have found that low muscle mass assessed by CT Scan of the mid-thigh was a strong predictor of mortality. Also when this variable was entered in a multivariate model to predict mortality, body mass index had no longer a significant impact on mortality suggesting that the loss of muscle mass is more strongly associated to survival than body weight. Other likely consequences of poor peripheral muscle function include reduction in quality of life (112,113) and greater utilization of health care resources (114).

## Treatment of Peripheral Muscle Dysfunction in COPD

As of today, there are no specific treatment available for muscle wasting associated with COPD and CHF. This reflects the fact that the etiology of this problem has not been completely elucidated. The most effective and readily available therapy is exercise training. So far, the reported effects of anabolic drugs either alone or in conjunction with exercise training on muscle function have been modest. Specific treatments for muscle wasting should become available in the near future as our understanding of how muscle homeostasis is regulated evolves.

## Exercise Training

It is now accepted that peripheral muscle adaptation to training can occur in patients with advanced COPD or CHF. Several studies have shown that patients with severe COPD or CHF can sustain the necessary training intensity and duration for a skeletal muscle adaptation to training to occur (30,101, 115-119). Improvement in the skeletal muscle oxidative capacity with endurance training has been reported in both diseases (30,117-119). As a consequence of the improvement in muscle oxidative capacity with training, changes in muscle metabolism also occur with a reduction in lactic acid efflux during exercise (49). These metabolic changes consist in reduction in exercise lactic acidosis, $CO_2$ production and ventilation for a given exercise level (101,119-122). Other investigators have reported increased quadriceps endurance during voluntary contractions after 3 weeks of endurance training (123) and less susceptibility to the development of contractile fatigue (124).

Strength training also appears to be an interesting strategy in patients with COPD (112), as this type of training has greater potential to improve muscle mass and strength than aerobic training. In addition, strength training causes less dyspnea during the exercise period, making this strategy easier to tolerate for patients with severe COPD than aerobic training (112). Simpson and colleagues studied 34 patients with severe COPD randomized to a control group or to 8 weeks of strength training consisting of 3 different exercises (one for the arms, two for the legs) (112). Muscle strength increased by 16-40%, depending on the muscle group evaluated, and this was associated with an improvement in submaximal exercise endurance time. Importantly, improvement in muscle strength after training does not necessarily imply muscle physiological adaptation since it may be due to a more efficient neuromuscular coupling as suggested by the observation that low intensity muscle exercises also improve upper and lower limb muscle endurance (125).

Whether strength training is a useful adjunct to aerobic training has been addressed recently (126). In this study, the effects of aerobic training alone or in combination with strength training on peripheral muscle function were evaluated in 36 patients with severe COPD. The combination of aerobic and strength training resulted in a greater improvement in peripheral muscle strength and in thigh muscle cross-sectional area than aerobic training alone. This study confirms that the peripheral muscles may show structural adaptation with a multimodal training regimen despite severe ventilatory impairment.

In summary, exercise training is probably the best available option to treat peripheral muscle dysfunction in COPD. More work needs to be done in order to optimize training strategies for these patients since, in most cases, muscle function is not completely normalized with training.

## Anabolic Drugs

The efficacy of anabolic steroids to improve muscle mass, especially when combined with exercise training, has been confirmed in normal men (127). Given the positive relationship between quadriceps strength and exercise tolerance in patients with COPD (7,18), the possibility that muscle mass can be increased with anabolic drugs is an interesting therapeutic option. As previously mentioned, a profound reduction in anabolic hormone levels has been has been reported in patients with COPD and CHF and may provide further rationale for the use of

anabolic drugs in these patients (82-86). However, only a few studies have evaluated this possibility. The combination of anabolic steroids, nutritional support, and exercise training was found to increase muscle mass but produced only small or absent improvement in peripheral muscle function (88,128). Similarly, 1 to 8 weeks of exercise training combined with the administration of growth hormone induces gain in muscle mass but does not provide any additional improvement in muscle strength or exercise tolerance (129,130). So far, very little is known on the effects of anabolic drug supplementation in patients with CHF. In one study, the use of growth hormone did not improve exercise tolerance in patients with CHF (131,132). In summary, modest increase in muscle mass has been demonstrated when the administration of anabolic steroids or growth hormone is combined with a training program in patients with COPD. Whether anabolic drugs will prove to be a useful adjunct to exercise training programs is uncertain and requires further study.

## Conclusion

Peripheral muscle dysfunction is a common systemic complication of COPD and CHF. This problem may contribute to disability, handicap, and premature mortality in these diseases independently of the degree of impairment in lung or heart function. In contrast to the lung or heart impairment, which is largely irreversible, peripheral muscle dysfunction is potentially remediable with exercise training and anabolic drugs. However, the therapeutic success is often incomplete and a better understanding of the mechanisms involved in the development of peripheral muscle dysfunction in these diseases needed to help develop innovative and more effective therapeutic strategies.

## References

1. Sadoul, P. 1969. Les cachexies respiratoires. *Bull Physio-patho Resp* 5:3-11.
2. Schols, A. M. W. J., J. Slangen, L. Volovics, and E. F. M. Wouters. 1998. Weight loss is a reversible factor in the prognosis of chronic obstructive pulmonary disease. *Am J Respir Crit Care Med* 157:1791-1797.
3. Anker, S. D., P. Ponikowski, S. Varney, T. Peng Chua, A. L. Clark, K. M. Webb-Peploe, D.

Harrington, W. J. Kox, P. A. Poole-Wilson, and A. J. S. Coats. 1997. Wasting as independent risk factor for mortality in chronic heart failure. *Lancet* 349:1050-1053.

4. Decramer, M., V. de Bock, and R. Dom. 1996. Functional and histologic picture of steroid-induced myopathy in chronic obstructive pulmonary disease. *Am J Respir Crit Care Med* 153:1958-1964.

5. Gosker, H. R., E. F. Wouters, G. J. van der Vusse, and A. M. Schols. 2000. Skeletal muscle dysfunction in chronic obstructive pulmonary disease and chronic heart failure: underlying mechanisms and therapy perspectives. *Am.J.Clin.Nutr.* 71:1033-1047.

6. Maltais, F., P. Leblanc, J. Jobin, and R. Casaburi. 2000. Peripheral muscle dysfunction in chronic obstructive pulmonary disease. *Clin.Chest Med.* 21:665-677.

7. Gosselink, R., T. Troosters, and M. Decramer. 1996. Peripheral muscle weakness contributes to exercise limitation in COPD. *Am J Respir Crit Care Med* 153:976-980.

8. Newell, S. Z., D. K. McKenzie, and S. C. Gandevia. 1989. Inspiratory and skeletal muscle strength and endurance and diaphragmatic activation in patients with chronic airflow limitation. *Thorax* 44:903-912.

9. Bernard, S., P. Leblanc, F. Whittom, G. Carrier, J. Jobin, R. Belleau, and F. Maltais. 1998. Peripheral muscle weakness in patients with chronic obstructive pulmonary disease. *Am J Respir Crit Care Med* 158:629-634.

10. Gea, J., Pasto, M., Blanco, L., Barreiro, E., Hernandez, N., Palacio, J., and Broquetas, J.

11. Schols, A. M. W. J., P. B. Soeters, M. C. Dingemans, R. Mostert, P. J. Frantzen, and E. F. M. Wouters. 1993. Prevalence and characteristics of nutritional depletion in patients with stable COPD eligible for pulmonary rehabilitation. *Am.Rev.Respir.Dis.* 147:1151-1156.

12. Mancini, D. M., G. Walter, N. Reichek, R. Lenkinski, K. K. McCully, J. L. Mullen, and J. R. Wilson. 1992. Contribution of skeletal muscle atrophy to exercise intolerance and altered muscle metabolism in heart failure. *Circulation* 85:1364-1373.

13. Harrington, D., S. D. Anker, T. P. Chua, K. M. Webb-Peploe, P. P. Ponikowski, P. A. Poole-Wilson, and A. J. Coats. 1997. Skeletal muscle function and its relation to exercise tolerance in chronic heart failure. *J.Am.Coll.Cardiol.* 30:1758-1764.

14. Engelen, M. P. K. J., A. M. W. J. Schols, W. C. Baken, G. J. Wesseling, and E. F. M. Wouters. 1994. Nutritional depletion in relation to respiratory and peripheral skeletal muscle function in out-patients with COPD. *Eur Respir J* 7:1793-1797.

15. Schols, A. M. W. J., R. Mostert, P. B. Soeters, and E. F. M. Wouters. 1991. Body composition and exercise performance in patients with chronic obstructive pulmonary disease. *Thorax* 46:695-699.

16. Minotti, J. R., P. Pillay, R. Oka, L. Wells, I. Christoph, and B. M. Massie. 1993. Skeletal muscle size: relationship to muscle function in heart failure. *J Appl Physiol* 75:373-381.

17. Wilson, D. O., R. M. Rogers, E. C. Wright, and N. R. Anthonisen. 1989. Body weight in chronic obstructive pulmonary disease. The National Institutes of Health Intermittent Positive-Pressure Breathing Trial. *Am.Rev.Respir.Dis.* 139:1435-1438.

18. Hamilton, A. L., K. J. Killian, E. Summers, and N. L. Jones. 1995. Muscle strength, symptom intensity and exercise capacity in patients with cardiorespiratory disorders. *Am J Respir Crit Care Med* 152:2021-2031.

19. Harrington, D., S. D. Anker, and A. J. Coats. 2001. Preservation of exercise capacity and lack of peripheral changes in asymptomatic patients with severely impaired left ventricular function. *Eur.Heart J.* 22:392-399.

20. Killian, K. J., P. Leblanc, D. H. Martin, E. Summers, N. L. Jones, and E. J. M. Campbell. 1992. Exercise capacity and ventilatory, circulatory, and symptom limitation in patients with airflow limitation. *Am.Rev.Respir.Dis.* 146:935-940.

21. Mahler, D. A. and A. Harver. 1988. Prediction of peak oxygen consumption in obstructive airway disease. *Med Sci Sports Exerc* 20:574-578.

22. Magnusson, G., B. Isberg, K. E. Karlberg, and C. Sylven. 1994. Skeletal muscle strength and endurance in chronic congestive heart failure secondary to idiopathic dilated cardiomyopathy. *Am.J.Cardiol.* 73:307-309.

23. Decramer, M., L. M. Lacquet, R. Fagard, and P. Rogiers. 1994. Corticosteroids contribute to muscle weakness in chronic airflow obstruction. *Am.Rev.Respir.Dis.* 150:11-16.

24. Anker, S. D., J. W. Swan, M. Volterrani, T. P. Chua, A. L. Clark, P. A. Poole-Wilson, and A. J. Coats. 1997. The influence of muscle mass, strength, fatigability and blood flow on exercise capacity in cachectic and non-cachectic

patients with chronic heart failure. *Eur.Heart J.* 18:259-269.

25. Holloszy, J. O. and E. F. Coyle. 1984. Adaptations of skeletal muscle to endurance exercise and their metabolic consequences. *J.Appl.Physiol.* 56:831-838.

26. Sullivan, M. J., H. J. Green, and F. R. Cobb. 1991. Altered skeletal muscle metabolic response to exercise in chronic heart failure. Relation to skeletal muscle aerobic enzyme activity. *Circulation* 84:1597-1607.

27. Ivy, J. L., R. T. Withers, P. J. Van Handel, D. H. Elger, and D. L. Costill. 1980. Muscle respiratory capacity and fiber type as determinants of the lactate threshold. *J.Appl.Physiol.* 48:523-527.

28. Jakobsson, P., L. Jorfeldt, and A. Brundin. 1990. Skeletal muscle metabolites and fibre types in patients with advanced chronic obstructive pulmonary disease (COPD), with and without chronic respiratory failure. *Eur Respir J* 3:192-196.

29. Hildebrand, I. L., C. Sylvén, M. Esbjornsson, K. Hellstrom, and E. Jansson. 1991. Does hypoxaemia induce transformations of fiber types? *Acta Physiol Scand* 141:435-439.

30. Whittom, F., J. Jobin, P. M. Simard, P. Leblanc, C. Simard, S. Bernard, R. Belleau, and F. Maltais. 1998. Histochemical and morphological characteristics of the vastus lateralis muscle in COPD patients. Comparison with normal subjects and effects of exercise training. *Med Sci Sports Exerc* 30:1467-1474.

31. Sullivan, M. J., H. J. Green, and F. R. Cobb. 1990. Skeletal muscle biochemistry and histology in ambulatory patients with long-term heart failure. *Circulation* 81:518-527.

32. Maltais, F., M. J. Sullivan, P. Leblanc, B. D. Duscha, F. H. Schachat, C. Simard, J. M. Blank, and J. Jobin. 1999. Altered expression of myosin heavy chain in the vastus lateralis muscle in patients with COPD. *Eur Respir J* 13:850-854.

33. Sullivan, M. J., B. D. Duscha, H. Klitgaard, W. E. Kraus, F. R. Cobb, and B. Saltin. 1997. Altered expression of myosin heavy chain in human skeletal muscle in chronic heart failure. *Med Sci Sports Exerc* 29:860-866.

34. Drexler, H., U. Riede, T. Munzel, H. Konig, E. Funke, and H. Just. 1992. Alterations of skeletal muscle in chronic heart failure. *Circulation* 85:1751-1759.

35. Jakobsson, P., L. Jorfeldt, and J. Henriksson. 1995. Metabolic enzyme activity in the quadriceps femoris muscle in patients with severe chronic obstructive pulmonary disease. *Am J Respir Crit Care Med* 151:374-377.

36. Maltais, F., A. A. Simard, C. Simard, J. Jobin, P. Desgagnés, and P. Leblanc. 1996. Oxidative capacity of the skeletal muscle and lactic acid kinetics during exercise in normal subjects and in patients with COPD. *Am J Respir Crit Care Med* 153:288-293.

37. Gertz, I., G. Hedenstierna, G. Hellers, and J. Wahren. 1977. Muscle metabolism in patients with chronic obstructive lung disease and acute respiratory failure. *Clin Sci Mol Med* 52:395-403.

38. Fiaccadori, E., S. Del Canale, P. Vitali, E. Coffrini, N. Ronda, and A. Guariglia. 1987. Skeletal muscle energetics, acid-base equilibrium and lactate metabolism in patients with severe hypercapnia and hypoxia. *Chest* 92:883-887.

39. Pouw, E. M., A. M. W. J. Schols, G. J. van der Vusse, and E. F. M. Wouters. 1998. Elevated inosine monophosphate levels in resting muscle of patients with stable chronic obstructive pulmonary disease. *Am J Respir Crit Care Med* 157:453-457.

40. Wuyam, B., J. F. Payen, P. Levy, H. Bensaidane, H. Reutenauer, J. F. Le Bas, and A. L. Benabid. 1992. Metabolism and aerobic capacity of skeletal muscle in chronic respiratory failure related to chronic obstructive pulmonary disease. *Eur Respir J* 5:157-162.

41. Tada, H., H. Kato, T. Misawa, F. Sasaki, S. Hayashi, H. Takahashi, Y. Kutsumi, T. Ishizaki, T. Nakai, and S. Miyabo. 1992. [31]P-nuclear magnetic resonance evidence of abnormal skeletal muscle metabolism in patients with chronic lung disease and congestive heart failure. *Eur Respir J* 5:163-169.

42. Kutsuzawa, T., S. Shioya, D. Kurita, M. Haida, Y. Ohta, and H. Yamabayashi. 1992. [31]P-NMR study of skeletal muscle metabolism in patients with chronic respiratory impairment. *Am.Rev. Respir.Dis.* 146:1019-1024.

43. Payen, J. F., B. Wuyam, P. Levy, H. Reutenauer, P. Stieglitz, B. Paramelle, and J. F. Le Bas. 1993. Muscular metabolism during oxygen supplementation in patients with chronic hypoxia. *Am.Rev.Respir.Dis.* 147:592-598.

44. Lévy, P., B. Wuyam, J. L. Pépin, H. Reutenauer, and J. F. Payen. 1996. Anomalies des muscles squelettiques des BPCO en insuffisance respiratoire. Apport de la spectroscopie RMN [31]P. *Rev Mal Resp* 13:183-191.

45. Wilson, J. R., J. Fink, J. Maris, N. Ferraro, J. Power-Vanwart, S. Eleff, and B. Chance. 1985. Evaluation of energy metabolism in skeletal muscle of patients with heart failure with gated phosphorus-31 nuclear magnetic resonance. *Circulation* 71:57-62.

46. Massie, B. M., M. Conway, R. Yonge, and et al. 1987. 31P nuclear magnetic resonance evidence of abnormal skeletal muscle metabolism in patients with congestive heart failure. *Am J Cardiol* 60:309-315.

47. Mannix, E. T., M. D. Boska, P. Galassetti, G. Burton, F. Manfredi, and M. O. Farber. 1995. Modulation of ATP production by oxygen in obstructive lung disease as assessed by $^{31}$P-MRS. *J.Appl.Physiol.* 78:2218-2227.

48. Maltais, F., J. Jobin, M. J. Sullivan, S. Bernard, F. Whittom, K. J. Killian, M. Desmeules, M. Bélanger, and P. Leblanc. 1998. Metabolic and hemodynamic responses of the lower limb during exercise in patients with COPD. *J.Appl. Physiol.* 84:1573-1580.

49. Sala, E., J. Roca, R. M. Marrades, J. Alonso, J. M. Gonzalez de Suso, A. Moreno, J. A. Barbera, J. Nadal, L. de Jover, R. Rodriguez-Roisin, and P. D. Wagner. 1999. Effects of endurance training on skeletal muscle bioenergetics in chronic obstructive pulmonary disease. *Am J Respir Crit Care Med* 159:1726-1734.

50. Massie, B., M. Conway, R. Yonge, S. Frostick, J. Ledingham, P. Sleight, G. Radda, and B. Rajagopalan. 1987. Skeletal muscle metabolism in patients with congestive heart failure: Relation to clinical severity and blood flow. *Circulation* 76:1009-1019.

51. Putman, C. T., N. L. Jones, L. C. Lands, T. M. Bragg, M. G. Hollidge-Horvat, and G. J. F. Heigenhauser. 1995. Skeletal muscle pyruvate dehydrogenase activity during maximal exercise in humans. *Am J Physiol* 269:E458-E468.

55. Serres, I., Gautier V., A. L. Varray, and C. G. Préfaut. 1998. Impaired skeletal muscle endurance related to physical inactivity and altered lung function in COPD patients. *Chest* 113:900-905.

56. Minotti, J. R., I. Christoph, R. Oka, M. W. Weiner, L. Wells, and B. M. Massie. 1991. Impaired skeletal muscle function in patients with congestive heart failure. Relationship to systemic exercise performance. *J.Clin.Invest* 88:2077-2082.

57. Levine, S., L. Kaiser, J. Leferovich, and B. Tikunov. 1997. Cellular adaptation in the diaphragm in chronic osbtructive pulmonary disease. *N Engl J Med* 337:1799-1806.

58. Mercadier, J. J., K. Schwartz, S. Schiaffino, C. Wisnewsky, S. Ausoni, M. Heimburger, R. Marrash, R. Pariente, and M. Aubier. 1998. Myosin heavy chain gene expression changes in the diaphragm of patients with chronic lung hyperinflation. *Am J Physiol* 274:L527-L534.

59. Tikunov, B., S. Levine, and D. Mancini. 1997. Chronic congestive heart failure elicits adaptations of endurance exercise in diaphragmatic muscle. *Circulation* 95:910-916.

60. Booth, F. W. and P. D. Gollnick. 1983. Effects of disuse on the structure and function of skeletal muscle. *Med Sci Sports Exer* 15:415-420.

61. Larsson, L. and T. Ansved. 1985. Effects of long-term physical training and detraining on enzyme histochemical and functional skeletal muscle characteristics in man. *Muscle & nerve* 8:714-722.

62. Coyle, E. F., W. H. Martin, S. A. Bloomfield, O. H. Lowry, and J. O. Holloszy. 1985. Effects of detraining on responses to submaximal exercise. *J.Appl.Physiol.* 59:853-859.

63. Casaburi, R. 1996. Deconditioning. In A. P. Fishman, editor Pulmonary rehabilitation Marcel Dekker, New York. 213-230.

64. Orozco-Levi, M., J. Gea, J. Sauleda, J. M. Corominas, J. Minguella, X. Aran, and J. Broquetas. 1995. Structure of the latissimus dorsi muscle and respiratory function. *J.Appl.Physiol.* 78:1132-1139.

65. Muza, S. R., G. Criner, and S. G. Kelsen. 1991. Pectoralis muscle recruitment during weaning in patients with chronic respiratory failure. *Am Rev Respir Dis* 143:A163.

66. Mattson, J. P. and D. C. Poole. 1998. Pulmonary emphysema decreases hamster skeletal muscle oxidative enzyme capacity. *J Appl Physiol* 85:210-214.

67. Sabbah, H. N., F. Hansen-Smith, V. G. Sharov, T. Kono, M. Lesch, P. J. Gengo, R. P. Steffen, T. B. Levine, and S. Goldstein. 1993. Decreased proportion of type I myofibers in skeletal muscle of dogs with chronic heart failure. *Circulation* 87:1729-1737.

68. Levine, B., J. Kalman, L. Mayer, H. M. Fillit, and M. Packer. 1990. Elevated circulating levels of tumor necrosis factor in severe chronic heart failure. *N Engl J Med* 323:236-241.

69. Norman, D., J. S. Elborn, S. M. Cordon, R. J. Rayner, M. S. Wiseman, E. J. Hiller, and D. J. Shale. 1991. Plasma tumour necrosis factor alpha in cystic fibrosis. *Thorax* 46:91-95.

70. Ionescu, A. A., L. S. Nixon, W. D. Evans, M. D. Stone, V. Lewis-Jenkins, K. Chatham, and D. J.

Shale. 2000. Bone density, body composition, and inflammatory status in cystic fibrosis. *Am.J.Respir.Crit Care Med.* 162:789-794.

71. Moldawer, L. L. and F. R. Sattler. 1998. Human immunodeficiency virus-associated wasting and mechanism of cachexia associated with inflammation. *Semin Oncol* 25 (suppl 1):73-81.

72. Casaburi, R. 1996. Rehabilitative exercise training in chronic renal failure. In J. D. Koople and S. G. Massry, editors Nutritional management of renal disease Williams & Wilkins, Philadelphia. 817-841.

73. Schols, A. M. W. J., W. A. Buurman, A. J. Staal-van den Brekel, M. A. Dentener, and E. F. M. Wouters. 1996. Evidence for a relation between metabolic derangements and increased levels of inflammatory mediators in a subgroup of patients with chronic obstructive pulmonary disease. *Thorax* 51:819-824.

74. Di Francia, M., D. Barbier, J. L. Mege, and J. Orehek. 1994. Tumor necrosis factor-alpha levels and weight loss in chronic obstructive pulmonary disease. *Am J Respir Crit Care Med* 150:1453-1455.

75. de Godoy, I., M. Donahoe, W. J. Calhoun, J. Mancino, and R. M. Rogers. 1996. Elevated TNF-a production by peripheral blood monocytes of weight-losing COPD patients. *Am J Respir Crit Care Med* 153:633-637.

76. Sridhar, M. K. 1995. Why do patients with emphysema lose weight? *Lancet*.

77. Eid, A. A., A. A. Ionescu, L. S. Nixon, V. Lewis-Jenkins, S. B. Mathews, T. L. Griffiths, and D. J. Shale. 2001. The inflammatory response and body composition in chronic obstructive pulmonary disease. *Am J Respir Crit Care Med* (In press).

78. Ceconi, C., S. Curello, T. Bachetti, A. Corti, and R. Ferrari. 1998. Tumor necrosis factor in congestive heart failure: a mechanism of disease for the new millennium? *Prog Cardiovasc Dis* 41:25-30.

79. Deswal, A., N. J. Petersen, A. M. Feldman, J. B. Young, B. G. White, and D. L. Mann. 2001. Cytokines and cytokine receptors in advanced heart failure. An analysis of the cytokine database from the vesnarinone trial (VEST). *Circulation* 103:2055-2059.

80. Haslett, P. A. J. 1998. Anticytokine approaches to the treatment of anorexia and cachexia. *Semin Oncol* 25 (suppl 6):53-57.

81. Mitch, W. E. and A. L. Goldberg. 1996. Mechanism of muscle wasting. *N Engl J Med* 335:1897-1905.

82. Lazarus, D. D., L. L. Moldawer, and S. F. Lowry. 1993. Insulin-like growth factor-1 activity is inhibited by interleukin-1 alpha, tumor necrosis factor-alpha, and interleukin-6. *Cytokine Res* 12:219-223.

83. Repine, J. E. and A. L. I. Bast. 1999. Oxidative stress in chronic obstructive pulmonary disease. *Am J Respir Crit Care Med* 156:341-357.

84. Lands, L. C., V. L. Grey, and A. A. Smountas. 1999. The effect of supplementation with a cysteine donor on muscular performance. *J Appl Physiol* 87:1381-1385.

85. Kamischke, A., D. E. Kemper, M. A. Castel, M. Lüthke, C. Rolf, H. M. Behre, H. Magnussen, and E. Nieschlag. 1998. Testosterone levels in men with chronic obstructive pulmonary disease with or without glucocorticoid therapy. *Eur Respir J* 11:41-45.

86. Casaburi, R., Goren, S., and Bhasin, S. 1996. Substantial prevalence of low anabolic hormone levels in COPD patients undergoing rehabilitation. *Am J Respir Crit Care Med* 153: A128.

87. Anker, S. D., A. L. Clark, M. Kemp, C. Salsbury, M. M. Teixeira, P. G. Hellewell, and A. J. Coats. 1997. Tumor necrosis factor and steroid metabolism in chronic heart failure: possible relation to muscle wasting. *J Am Coll Cardiol* 30:997-1001.

88. Anker, S. D., T. P. Chua, P. Ponikowski, D. Harrington, J. W. Swan, W. J. Kox, P. A. Poole-Wilson, and A. J. Coats. 1997. Hormonal changes and catabolic/anabolic imbalance in chronic heart failure and their importance for cardiac cachexia. *Circulation* 96:526-534.

89. Niebauer, J., C. D. Pflaum, A. L. Clark, C. J. Strasburger, J. Hooper, P. A. Poole-Wilson, A. J. Coats, and S. D. Anker. 1998. Deficient insulin-like growth factor I in chronic heart failure predicts altered body composition, anabolic deficiency, cytokine and neurohormonal activation. *J Am Coll Cardiol* 32:393-397.

90. Kotler, D. P. 2000. Cachexia. *Ann Intern Med* 133:622-634.

91. Schols, A. M. W. J., P. B. Soeters, R. Mostert, R. J. Pluymers, and E. F. M. Wouters. 1995. Physiologic effects of nutritional support and anabolic steroids in patients with chronic obstructive pulmonary disease. A placebo-controlled randomized trial. *Am J Respir Crit Care Med* 152:1268-1274.

92. Green, H. J., J. R. Sutton, A. Cymerman, P. M. Young, and C. S. Houston. 1989. Operation

Everest II: adaptations in human skeletal muscle. *J Appl Physiol* 66:2454-2461.

93. Kayser, B., H. Hoppeler, H. Claassen, and P. Cerretelli. 1991. Muscle structure and performance capacity of Himalayan Shepas. *J Appl Physiol* 70:1938-1942.

94. Aubier, M., D. Murciano, Y. Lecocguic, N. Viires, Y. Jacquens, P. Squara, and R. Pariente. 1985. Effect of hypophosphatemia on diaphragmatic contractility in patients with acute respiratory failure. *N Engl J Med* 313:420-424.

95. Jones, N. L. and K. J. Killian 1991. Limitation of exercise in chronic airway obstruction. In N. S. Cherniack, editor Chronic obstructive pulmonary disease,1 ed. W.B. Saunders, Philadelphia. 196-206.

96. Gulec, S., F. Ertas, E. Tutar, N. Caglar, G. Akgun, A. Alpman, and D. Oral. 1998. Exercise performance in patients with dilated cardiomyopathy: relationship to resting left ventricular function. *Int J Cardiol* 65:247-253.

97. Williams, T. J., G. A. Patterson, P. A. Mcclean, N. Zamel, and J. R. Maurer. 1992. Maximal exercise testing in single and double lung transplant recipients. *Am Rev Respir Dis* 145:101-105.

98. Evans, A. B., A. J. Al-Himyary, M. I. Hrovat, P. Pappagianopoulos, J. C. Wain, L. C. Ginns, and S. M. Systrom. 1997. Abnormal skeletal muscle oxidative capacity after lung transplantation by $^{31}$P-MRS. *Am J Respir Crit Care Med* 155:615-621.

99. Wang, X. N., T. J. Williams, M. J. McKenna, J. L. Li, S. F. Fraser, E. A. Side, G. I. Snell, E. H. Walters, and M. F. Carey. 1999. Skeletal muscle oxidative capacity, fiber type, and metabolites after lung transplantation. *Am J Respir Crit Care Med* 160:57-63.

100. Schaufelberger, M., B. O. Eriksson, R. Lonn, B. Rundqvist, K. S. Sunnerhagen, and K. Swedberg. 2001. Skeletal muscle characteristics, muscle strength and thigh muscle area in patients before and after cardiac transplantation. *Eur J Heart Fail* 3:59-67.

101. Coats, A. J., A. L. Clark, M. Piepoli, M. Volterrani, and P. A. Poole-Wilson. 1994. Symptoms and quality of life in heart failure: the muscle hypothesis. *Br Heart J* 72:S36-S39.

102. Shuey, C. B., A. K. Peirce, and R. L. Johnson. 1969. An evaluation of exercise tests in chronic obstructive lung disease. *J Appl Physiol* 27:256-261.

103. Jones, N. L., G. L. Jones, and R. H. T. Edwards. 1971. Exercise tolerance in chronic airway obstruction. *Am Rev Respir Dis* 103:477-491.

104. Casaburi, R., A. Patessio, F. Ioli, S. Zanaboni, C. F. Donner, and K. Wasserman. 1991. Reductions in exercise lactic acidosis and ventilation as a result of exercise training in patients with obstructive lung disease. *Am Rev Respir Dis* 143:9-18.

105. Maltais, F., S. Bernard, J. Jobin, R. Belleau, and P. Leblanc. 1997. Lactate kinetics during exercise in chronic obstructive pulmonary disease. *Can Respir J* 4:251-257.

106. Weber, K. T. and J. S. Janicki. 1985. Lactate production during maximal and submaximal exercise in patients with chronic heart failure. *J Am Coll Cardiol* 6:717-724.

107. Beaver, W. L., K. Wasserman, and B. J. Whipp. 1986. Bicarbonate buffering of lactic acid generated during exercise. *J Appl Physiol* 60:472-486.

108. Jones, N. L. and G. J. F. Heigenhauser. 1996. Getting rid of carbon dioxide during exercise. *Clin Sci* 90:323-335.

109. Mainwood, G. W. and J. M. Renaud. 1985. The effect of acid-base balance on fatigue of skeletal muscle. *Can J Physiol Pharmacol* 63:403-416.

110. Hultman, E., S. Carale, and H. Sjoholm. 1985. Effect of induced metabolic acidosis on intracellular pH, buffer capacity and contraction force of human skeletal muscle. *Clin Sci* 69:505-510.

111. Westerblad, H., J. A. Lee, J. Lannergren, and D. G. Allen. 1991. Cellular mechanisms of fatigue in skeletal muscle. *Am J Physiol* 261:C195-C209.

112. Mador, M. J., T. J. Kufel, and L. Pineda. 2000. Quadriceps fatigue following cycle exercise in patients with COPD. *Am J Respir Crit Care Med* 161:447-453.

113. Grieve, D. A., A. L. Clark, G. P. McCann, and W. S. Hillis. 1999. The ergoreflex in patients with chronic stable heart failure. *Int J Cardiol* 68:157-164.

114. Marquis, K., Debigaré, R., LeBlanc, P, Lacasse, Y., Jobin, J., and Maltais, F. 2001. Mid-thigh muscle cross-sectional area is a better predictor of mortality than body mass index in patients with COPD. *Am J Respir Crit Care Med* 163: A75.

115. Simpson, K., K. Killian, N. McCartney, D. G. Stubbing, and N. L. Jones. 1992. Randomised controlled trial of weightlifting exercise in patients with chronic airflow limitation. *Thorax* 47:70-75.

116. Mostert, R., A. Goris, C. Weling-Scheepers, E. F. M. Wouters, and A. M. W. Schols. 2000.

Tissue depletion and health related quality of life in patients with chronic obstructive pulmonary disease. *Respir Med* 94:859-867.

117. Decramer, M., R. Gosselink, T. Troosters, M. Verschueren, and G. Evers. 1997. Muscle weakness is related to utilization of health care resources in COPD patients. *Eur Respir J* 10:417-423.

118. Maltais, F., P. Leblanc, J. Jobin, C. Bérubé, J. Bruneau, L. Carrier, M. J. Breton, G. Falardeau, and R. Belleau. 1997. Intensity of training and physiologic adaptation in patients with chronic obstructive pulmonary disease. *Am J Respir Crit Care Med* 155:555-561.

119. Casaburi, R., J. Porszasz, M. R. Burns, E. Carithers, R. S. Y. Chang, and C. B. Cooper. 1997. Physiologic benefits of exercise training in rehabilitation of patients with severe chronic obstructive pulmonary disease. *Am J Respir Crit Care Med* 155:1541-1551.

120. Maltais, F., P. Leblanc, C. Simard, J. Jobin, C. Bérubé, J. Bruneau, L. Carrier, and R. Belleau. 1996. Skeletal muscle adaptation to endurance training in patients with chronic obstructive pulmonary disease. *Am J Respir Crit Care Med* 154:442-447.

121. Hambrecht, R., J. Niebauer, E. Fiehn, B. Kalberer, B. Offner, K. Hauer, U. Riede, G. Schlierf, W. Kubler, and G. Schuler. 1995. Physical training in patients with stable chronic heart failure: effects on cardiorespiratory fitness and ultrastructural abnormalities of leg muscles. *J Am Coll Cardiol* 25:1239-1249.

122. Hambrecht, R., E. Fiehn, J. Yu, J. Niebauer, C. Weigl, L. Hillbrich, V. Adams, U. Riede, and G. Schuler. 1997. Effects of endurance training on mitochondrial ultrastructure and fiber type distribution in skeletal muscle in patients with stable chronic heart failure. *J Am Coll Cardiol* 29:1067-1073.

123. Vyas, M. N., E. W. Banister, J. W. Morton, and S. Grzybowski. 1971. Response to exercise in patients with chronic airway obstruction. I. Effects of exercise training. *Am Rev Respir Dis* 103:390-400.

124. Mohsenifar, Z., D. Horak, H. V. Brown, and S. K. Koerner. 1983. Sensitive indices of improvement in a pulmonary rehabilitation program. *Chest* 83:189-192.

125. Sullivan, M. J., M. B. Higginbotham, and F. R. Cobb. 1988. Exercise training in patients with severe left ventricular dysfunction. Hemodynamic and metabolic effects. *Circulation* 78:506-515.

126. Serres, I., A. Varray, G. Vallet, J. P. Micallef, and C. Préfaut. 1997. Improved skeletal muscle performance after individualized exercise training in patients with chronic obstructive pulmonary disease. *J Cardiopulmonary Rehab* 17:232-238.

127. Mador, M. J., T. J. Kufel, L. A. Pineda, A. Steinwald, A. Aggarwal, A. M. Upadhyay, and M. A. Khan. 2001. Effect of pulmonary rehabilitation on quadriceps fatiguability during exercise. *Am J Respir Crit Care Med* 163:930-935.

128. Clark, A. L., P. A. Poole-Wilson, and A. J. Coats. 1996. Exercise limitation in chronic heart failure: central role of the periphery. *J Am Coll Cardiol* 28:1092-1102.

129. Bernard, S., F. Whittom, P. Leblanc, J. Jobin, R. Belleau, C. Bérubé, G. Carrier, and F. Maltais. 1999. Aerobic and strength training in patients with COPD. *Am J Respir Crit Care Med* 159:896-901.

130. Bhasin, S., T. W. Storer, N. Berman, C. Callegari, B. Clevenger, J. Phillips, T. J. Bunnell, R. Tricker, A. Shirazi, and R. Casaburi. 1996. The effects of supraphysiologic doses of testosterone on muscle size and strength in normal men. *N Engl J Med* 335:1-7.

131. Martins Ferreira, I., I. T. Verreschi, L. E. Nery, R. S. Goldstein, N. Zamel, D. Brooks, and J. R. Jardim. 1998. The influence of 6 months of oral anabolic steroids on body mass and respiratory muscles in undernourished COPD patients. *Chest* 114:19-28.

132. Burdet, L., B. de Muralt, Y. Schutz, C. Pichard, and J. W. Fitting. 1997. Administration of growth hormone to underweight patients with chronic obstructive pulmonary disease. A prospective, randomized, controlled study. *Am J Respir Crit Care Med* 156:1800-1806.

133. Casaburi, R., Carithers, E., Tosolini, J., Phillips, J., and Bhasin, S. 1997. Randomized placebo controlled trial of growth hormone in severe COPD patients undergoing endurance exercise training *Am J Respir Crit Care Med* 155: A498.

134. Isgaard, J., C. H. Bergh, K. Caidahl, M. Lomsky, A. Hjalmarson, and B. A. Bengtsson. 1998. A placebo-controlled study of growth hormone in patients with congestive heart failure. *Eur Heart J* 19:1704-1711.

135. Fazio, S., D. Sabatini, B. Capaldo, C. Vigorito, A. Giordano, R. Guida, F. Pardo, B. Biondi, and L. Sacca. 1996. A preliminary study of growth hormone in the treatment of dilated cardiomyopathy. *N Engl J Med* 334:809-814.

# Chapter 23

# Upper Extremity Exercise In Rehabilitation of COPD

Bartolome R. Celli, MD, USA

Homo Sapiens is best described by three characteristics; brain size, upright biped position and its highly developed use of the upper extremities and hands. The change from the quadruped stance of most mammals to the biped one, which then allows full expression of dexterity, is associated with important adaptations of the osteomuscular system. Much has been learned about the physiologic response to activities that involve the lower extremities. In contrast, surprisingly little is known about arm exercise, even though the accomplishment of manual tasks (an activity known to characterize high brain development), requires the use of not only of the hand muscles but also the concerted action of other muscle groups that participate in upper torso and arm positioning. This monograph reviews what is known about arm exercise, its complex interaction with the rest of the respiratory system and very importantly, its use as a therapeutic modality to improve activities of daily living in patients limited by chronic obstructive pulmonary disease (COPD).

## Anatomic and Mechanical Considerations

To fully understand the relationship between arm exercise and respiration a minimal understanding of the respiratory muscles is necessary. The diaphragm is the best studied respiratory muscle. It is thought to exert its inflating action on the ribcage by three mechanisms: 1) by using the abdomen as a fulcrum against which it leans exerting an expanding action on the ribcage, 2) by the vertical and downward orientation of its fibers and the curvature of its shape and 3) the transmission of the increase in abdominal pressure during contraction to the ribcage through its zone of apposition (1-3) It is thought that with the hyperinflation of chronic airflow obstruction as the fibers become more horizontal, the curvature of the diaphragm decreases and this impairs its capacity to generate pressures (4,5). Recent evidence obtained from animal (6,7) and human studies (8) suggest that the diaphragm adapts to the chronic changes of CAO by shortening the optimal length of its fibers, so that each bundle generates its maximal tension for that new length. If this is correct, the decreased diaphragmatic pressure generating capacity of patients with COPD is due to mechanical derangement or to contractile dysfunction, and not to simple length tension changes.

The external intercostals, the parasternal part of internal intercostal and scalene are essential muscles of respiration since they are active even during quiet breathing in normals (9,10). Their functional importance increases with the hyperinflation of COPD, because they undergo less marked shortening and are at less of a mechanical disadvantage than the diaphragm (11).

Other muscles are called "accessory" inspiratory muscles because they are inactive during quiet breathing in normal subjects, but because of their anatomic arrangement they may be inspiratory in action under certain circumstances (2,12,13). The sternomastoid, subclavian, pectoralis minor and major, serratus anterior, upper and lower trapezius and latissimus dorsi share a common anatomical arrangement. They hold an extra thoracic anchoring point and a ribcage insertion. If they are fixed on their extra thoracic anchoring point, they may exert a pulling force on the ribcage. Except for the sternomastoid and pectoralis, the respiratory function of these muscles has not been fully studied (12,14). They are probably inactive during quiet breathing in normal subjects, but may be called to partake in ventilation during strenuous circumstances. This may explain the common observation that normal subjects after a fatiguing exercise will brace their arms, thereby anchoring the shoulder girdle accessory muscles and allowing them to pull the rib cage during inspiration. Three studies confirm this observation. Banzett et al. showed that normal volunteers could sustain a higher ventilatory target if their arms were braced on a table than if they were unsupported at the sides (15). Maestro et al., and from the same group Dolmage and coworkers, showed that normal volunteers would manifest higher minute ventilation at similar work loads when cycling with the arms elevated vs. supported on the ergometer handle (16,17). We have shown that unsupported arm exercise may be more limiting than leg exercise, and have hypothesized that this is due to derecruitment of the shoulder girdle muscles from their ventilatory contribution during unsupported arm activity (18,19). As we shall discuss later, these muscles become most important in patients with poorly functioning diaphragms, as is the case in severe COPD. The understanding of their function opens new therapeutic avenues. Techniques aimed at either decreasing ventilatory requirements during arm exercise or at improving the function of these muscles, should prove beneficial to patients suffering from ventilatory limitations specifically when performing upper extremity activities.

The abdominal muscles are considered muscles of expiration (2,20). In as much as they oppose diaphragmatic contraction by helping generate abdominal pressure, they are also inspiratory (21). It is also thought that by contracting during expiration, they tend to decrease end expiratory lung volume, a position in which the chest wall stores elastic energy that assists in the subsequent inspiratory effort (22). We have recently shown that with worsening of airflow obstruction, there is progressive recruitment of the abdominal muscles of exhalation (5). This finding was confirmed by Ninane et al., who showed EMG evidence of transverse abdominal contraction during tidal breathing in patients with COPD. They also showed that this contraction increases as airflow obstruction worsens (23). It is unclear why patients with the most severe COPD would choose a breathing strategy that tends to close even more the already compromised airways. The best explanation is that by recruiting accessory muscles during inspiration and the abdominal muscles during expiration, the patients may shift work away from an overworked and inefficient diaphragm. This seems to be the case during pursed

lip breathing whereby using this strategy, the patients are capable of breathing larger inspiratory volumes at similar transdiaphragmatic pressures (24).

## Composition, Metabolism, Blood Flow and Coordination of the Respiratory Muscles

The diaphragm and other respiratory muscles are composed of striated muscle fibers (6,25). The actual composition of most of the accessory respiratory muscles and muscles of the shoulder girdle remain unknown. Regardless of their specific composition, what is known for all muscles may apply to arm muscles. With progressive efforts (loads) more fibers are recruited so that muscle loading will induce hypertrophy (strength), or change its composition to one that is more fatigue resistant (endurance).

Very important in training is the state of blood flow and energy supply since it is believed that imbalances in energy supply and demand may result in fatigue. Most of what is known about blood supply and energetics concerns the diaphragm and more recently muscles of the ribcage. Like the heart, diaphragmatic perfusion occurs preferentially during relaxation and decreases during contraction, even though the diaphragm is supplied by a well developed system that is arranged to minimize the decrease in blood flow during inspiration (26,27). Two factors determine the contracting compromise of the diaphragm during breathing. The duration of contraction or duty cycle, which can be expressed as the ratio of inspiratory time to total cycle time ($T_I/T_{TOT}$) and the load which can be inferred by relating the pressure needed to perform the ventilatory effort, as a function of the maximal pressure that the muscle can generate. The latter relationship has been defined as $Pdi/Pdi_{max}$ for the diaphragm or $P_I/Pi_{max}$ for the sum of the inspiratory pressure measured at the mouth. The product of both ratios has been termed tension time index (TTi) and has been shown to relate to electromyographic and other signals of muscle fatigue both in normal individuals (28) and patients with COPD (29). It follows that arm exercise testing and training should take this into account, in order to maximize our results. This is most important in patients with COPD where it has been shown that increased ventilation could be the limiting factor during exercise (30-32).

The best theoretical training would be one that combines enough load over a long enough period of time where the muscle is loaded but not fatigued.

## Neural Control, Coordination

The diaphragm and other respiratory muscles are innervated by a wide array of motor neurons that range from cranial nerve 11 (C-11) to lumbar roots L2-L3. The respiratory cycle is regulated by a complex series of centrally organized neurons. This complex arrangement maintains rhythmic breathing that goes usually unnoticed, but can be voluntarily overridden by cortical connections. Since we use primarily the diaphragm, the scalene and some intercostals to quiet breath, the system is capable of functioning at a low cost of energy and very efficiently, making respiration an unnoticed physiologic function. Some of the respiratory muscles serve other purposes. Upper torso and shoulder girdle muscles partake in positioning of the upper chest and upper extremity, while the diaphragm and muscles of the abdomen partake in the generation of sound (speech, singing) cough, defecation and parturition. It has been postulated that the autonomic and voluntary ventilatory pathways are different (33). Along the same line, studies in humans and animals show that the respiratory and tonic functions of these muscles are driven from different central nervous areas and integrated at the spinal level (34). In patients in whom some of these muscles are partaking in respiration, to be able to perform non-ventilatory work they must maintain a high degree of coordination. Either because of the load, or because of competing central integration, muscle function may become dyscoordinated and result in their dysfunction and perception of dyspnea. From this review, it is clear that a simplistic approach to arm exercise in terms of testing and training is impossible. The rest of the monograph will summarize our knowledge specifically insight into the practical approach that may help clinicians better test and treat patients with COPD.

## Arm Exercise Testing

Lower extremity testing is performed in a rhythmical continuous motion usually walking, using a treadmill or a cycle ergometer (31-35). Of these modalities, ergometry offered the best alternative to test the upper extremities since it was an already validated form of exercise for the lower extremities. In consequence it seemed logical to exercise the arms in a similar way as the legs. Unfortunately, leg ergometry bears little resemblance to the way in which upper extremity are normally utilized by humans. Nevertheless, since it is widely used and has been validated, it remains the gold standard for upper extremity testing.

## Arm Cycle Ergometry (Arm Cranking)

Testing is performed with an arm ergometer, mounted on an adjustable table so that the axis of the crank can be kept in line with the glenohumeral joint (36). Subjects or patients, crank at a fixed rate (60-80 rpm) and resistance is added at regular intervals (2-3 minutes). Most laboratories start with no load and then increase the resistance at increments of 7 to 30 watts. When studying normal subjects the upper range is preferred, while patients seldom tolerate these loads and increases are limited to 10 watts. The exercise may be terminated by symptoms (maximal), by a defined end point (inability to maintain cranking rate), or targeted for a sub maximal load (60-80% of maximal). The measurements obtained are the same as those described for leg exercise and are summarized in table 23.1. In patients, we strongly recommend the evaluation of dyspnea utilizing either the Visual Analog Scale or a modified Borg Scale, since this may help guide subsequent training or more important provide us with an important outcome which then allows us to evaluate the response to training.

Table 23.1  Methodology of Arm Cranking Testing

| Testing method | Measurements |
| --- | --- |
| Arm ergometer | Endurance time (seconds or minutes) |
| Cycle at 60-80 rpm | Minute ventilation |
|  | Oxygen uptake ($\dot{V}O_2$) |
| Increase resistance | $CO_2$ production ($\dot{V}CO_2$) |
| 7-30 Watts every 2-3 minutes | Respiratory frequency (R) |
|  | Oxygen saturation |
|  | Blood gases |
|  | Cyspnea rating |

## Respiratory, Cardiac and Metabolic Response

In contrast to leg exercise, information regarding the response to arm cranking is more limited. Fortunately, the published results are uniform and there is agreement in their overall interpretation (37,52).

Maximal $\dot{V}O_2$, $\dot{V}CO_2$ and $V_E$ is lower for arm than for leg exercise (45,51,53-57). Stated differently, maximal arm cranking represents a submaximal cardiopulmonary exercise test. Table 23.2 shows the results from several selected series, all of which have found maximal values to range between 65 and 80% of those observed for leg ergometry (45,57). On the other hand, at similar $\dot{V}O_2$ (normalized work), $\dot{V}CO_2$, $V_E$ and lactate production is higher during arm work. Where it has been measured, anaerobic threshold occurs earlier during arm cranking (57). These overall changes are best explained by the smaller muscle mass involved in arm cranking, which have to "work" more in order to achieve the same $\dot{V}O_2$. More insight about the effects of arm ergometry on ventilation was provided by Alison et al. in a study of the ventilatory response in normals and patients with cystic fibrosis (59). These authors showed that arm exercise induced similar degrees of dynamic hyperinflation as leg ergometry. This did not occur in the normal controls. Dynamic hyperinflation is known to be closely related to development of exercise dyspnea and respiratory muscle dysfunction.

The response of the cardiovascular system is also different with arm vs. leg cycling and the changes described, parallel those seen in the metabolic parameters. At similar $\dot{V}O_2$ (normalized work), heart rate, blood pressure and peripheral vascular resistance is higher during arm cranking, but overall cardiac output and stroke volume is lower for this exercise (55,58). It is from such findings that it has been said, that upper extremity exercise is of some danger to patients with heart disease. The practical experience on these patients is different, perhaps because peak exercise for them occurs at much lower loads than that achieved by normal individuals with leg exercise (45,46,61,62). With appropriate monitoring, there is very little danger in evaluating exercise performance with the use of arm ergometry, and arm cranking remains a very good option for the testing of cardiopulmonary reserve in patients who cannot complete leg exercise.

## Gas Exchange Response

Arm cranking also modifies gas exchange. Martin et al. have shown that arm cranking induces a higher $PaO_2$, $O_2$ Sat, VD/VT and a lower $P(A-a)O_2$ at the same $\dot{V}O_2$ compared to leg cycling (45). The explanation for these changes remain elusive and may include differences in alveolar ventilation, $CO_2$ production, ventilation-perfusion inequality, diffusion and control of breathing. Studying patients with dyspnea (46), the same authors have established criteria for normal gas exchange response to maximal arm cranking. The criteria are: 1) $P(A-a)O_2$ should be equal to or less than 13 torr, 2) $PaO_2$ should be equal to or greater than 85 torr, 3) VD/VT equal to or less than 0.26. The explanation for these changes remain elusive. Interestingly, the finding in patients with COPD is similar, although not as well characterized. It has been shown that with arm exercise $O_2$ saturation falls, but the drop is of a

**Table 23.2   Effect of Arm Cranking on Cardiopulmonary and Metabolic Function in Normal Individuals**

|  | Max $\dot{V}O_2$ L/min | | Max HR | | Max VE L/min | |
|---|---|---|---|---|---|---|
|  | LC | AC | LC | AC | LC | AL |
| Astrand et al. | 4.7 | 3.3 | 190 | 177 | 173 | 122 |
| Reybrock et al. | 3.7 | 2.4 | 168 | 15 | 178 | 73 |
| Martin et al. | 3.3 | 2.2 | 189 | 168 | 144 | 101 |
| Mean | 3.9 | 2.6 | 182 | 165 | 165 | 99 |

Data obtained from 3 series. VO = oxygen uptake, HR = heart rate, VE = minute ventilation, LC = leg cycling, AC = arm cycling.

lesser magnitude than that observed during leg exercise (18). Although not proven for arm exercise the data from lower extremity exercise indicate that with increased age, there is worsening in gas exchange, with an increase in A-a $O_2$ gradient and a decrease in "efficiency" (less power at same $\dot{V}O_2$) (35). Since testing is very often performed in elder individuals, the values mentioned above should be extrapolated with caution.

## Training Upper Extremities With Arm Cranking

Multiple groups have included arm cranking as a therapeutic tool that may improve upper extremity function. The most important concept that has promoted its inclusion is the one of specificity of training, that is to say that only those muscles that are trained, will manifest the response to the training. The best example of this is the study of Belman and Kendregan. They studied 15 patients with COPD before and after 6 weeks of training. The patients were divided in two groups; 8 underwent training of upper extremities using arm cranking while 7 exercised with leg ergometry. The sessions lasted 20 minutes four times weekly. The study demonstrated significant increase in arm cycle endurance for the arm trained group and leg cycle endurance for the leg trained group, without cross-over effect (62). Since then, several other studies have shown beneficial effects when arm cranking is added to leg exercise as part of comprehensive programs of rehabilitation (47,63).

The training protocols vary significantly from group to group. We train at 60% of maximal $\dot{V}O_2$, determined by a baseline test, as shown in Table 23.3. In many patients who stop exercising even without added resistance (patients on ventilators, severe COPD) we progressively increase exercise time until reaching a total of 20 minutes daily. In those patients that are capable of completing 20 minutes, we proceed to increase resistance on a regular basis (every 3 sessions). The results of several reports of training lower extremity indicate that a minimum of 12 sessions may be required to obtain improvement in endurance (64). It also must be emphasized that once started, regular exercise must be maintained since deconditioning occurs rather quickly. Arm cranking is well tolerated and liked, but requires an ergometer, which may not be available in sufficient numbers even in large centers, and is rarely available at home. As I shall review later, unsupported arm exercise is another form of training, requires no apparatus, is easy to complete and offers a valid alternative to arm ergometry.

**Table 23.3   Arm Cranking Training**

1. Train at 60% of maximal work capacity*
2. Increase load every 3rd-5th session as tolerated
3. Monitor: heart, dyspnea
4. Train for as long as tolerated, up to 30 minutes
5. Aim to 24 sessions

*Work capacity as determined by an arm ergometer test and not necessarily by heart rate.

## Unsupported Arm Exercise

The arms are used much differently than the legs. While the latter are used to support us (posture and locomotion), the former require significant action against gravity (without support). The unsupported activities of the arms ranges from work (typing, painting) to sports (karate, baseball) but most importantly involve our daily care (eating, grooming, cleaning). It is surprising that we have persisted in testing the upper extremities with the same tool utilized to test lower extremities when in humans the arm function is so different. As a matter of fact, it was not until 1973 that it was reported, that patients with COPD complained of severe dyspnea while performing simple activities of daily living with upper extremities. Using a pneumobelt, Tangri and Wolf studied the breathing pattern of 7 patients while they tied their shoes or combed their hair. The patients developed an irregular, shallow, rapid pattern of breathing while performing the activity. After the exercise, the patients breathed faster and deeper. The authors postulated that this pattern was best explained by rapid ineffective shallow breathing during arm exercise with compensatory hyperventilation after the task was completed (65).

We have explored the respiratory and metabolic response to unsupported arm exercise (UAE) and compared it to the response seen with leg and arm ergometry in normal subjects and in patient with chronic obstructive lung disease (18,19,66,67). We showed that unsupported arm exercise results in dyssynchronous thoracoabdominal excursion and dyspnea at an earlier time and at lower $\dot{V}O_2$, than the more metabolically demanding leg exercise (18). In that study, the thoracoabdominal dyssynchrony was not solely due to diaphragmatic fatigue since the post exercise maximal transdiaphragmatic pressure decreased by the same magnitude in both groups. We postulated that UAE shifts work to the diaphragm, as some of the shoulder girdle muscles decrease their participation in ventilation and have to increase their participation in arm positioning (68). These changes may have led to earlier fatigue of the involved muscles. To test this hypothesis, we have used gastric-pleural pressures (Pg-Ppl) plots (using gastric and esophageal balloons) while patients and normal subjects perform unsupported arm exercise, arm and leg cycle ergometry. We documented lower peak $\dot{V}O_2$, $\dot{V}CO_2$, heart rate during UAE vs. the other forms of exercise. Nevertheless, during UAE there is increased gastric pressure swings which can be summarized as more contribution to ventilatory pressure generation by the diaphragm and abdominal muscles, and less contribution by the inspiratory muscles of the ribcage (19,66). To test for unsupported arm exercise, we use a pegboard with pegs separated 10 cms vertically. The patient seats with a straight back and has to shift rings with the extended arms at the shoulder level. Our experience with patients show that exercise time is a good indicator of exercise endurance. In normal subjects, we have added weights to the arms. The test has been validated by using an electrical device, both in normal subjects as well as in patients with COPD. That study showed that whether the testing is done with a rotating drum, with the rings shifting at a constant rate or spontaneously by the patient at his/her own pace, the results are the same in terms of peak $\dot{V}O_2$, VE, respiratory rate, and exercise endurance.

We have evaluated a very simple test that is useful in patients with severe COPD. The test consists in simple anterior elevation of the arms. We studied 22 normal subjects and noted that arm elevation significantly increased $\dot{V}O_2$, $\dot{V}CO_2$, VE, VT and Pg without changes in respiratory rate. The change in Pg with arm elevation, and the sudden drop immediately after lowering the arms, indicates a mechanical rather than metabolic or ventilatory need as the best explanation for the changes in respiratory muscle recruitment (69). The changes observed may be of limited significance in normals, but they become more important in patient with COPD. To test this hypothesis, we evaluated the same parameters in 20 patients with CAO. Arm elevation re-

sulted in significant increases in $\dot{V}O_2$, and $\dot{V}CO_2$. In contrast to normals, and very likely due to the inability to increase tidal volume at a low mechanical cost, patients increased VE by increasing the respiratory rate with lesser increases in the tidal volume. The respiratory muscle recruitment pattern indicate that arm elevation not only increased diaphragmatic recruitment during inspiration, but that it also generates a more vigorous recruitment of the abdominal muscles (5,70). This data supports the hypothesis that simple arm elevation can be used as a submaximal arm exercise test, especially in patients with COPD since it is simple and well tolerated (70).

Barrends et al compared the effect of arm elevations on metabolic and ventilatory response in patients with COPD and age matched normals (71). There was a difference between the groups. Patients had a faster but sluggish rise in all variables compared with normals, but both groups manifested a significant increase in all parameters. We have recently also shown that arm elevation in the most severe patients with COPD can be used as a test of diaphragmatic reserve (70). As I shall explain later, it may be used as a test of intervention outcome, since a lower rise in $\dot{V}O_2$, VE or $\dot{V}CO_2$ after therapy would support a beneficial effect from the exercise.

## Unsupported Arm Training

There are few studies of the effect of unsupported arm training in the rehabilitation of patients with COPD. They are summarized in Table 23.4. Perhaps the oldest one is by Keens and coworkers who studied of group of patients with cystic fibrosis before and after a training period of 6 weeks. Arm training consisted of swimming and canoeing for 1.5 hours daily. After training the authors observed an increase in upper extremity endurance, but perhaps more importantly, there was an increase in maximal sustainable ventilatory capacity, that was similar in magnitude to the increase observed in another group of patients treated with ventilatory muscle training (72). Ries and coworkers studied the effect of two forms of arm exercise on a group of patients with COPD; gravity resistance and modified proprioceptive neuromuscular facilitation. They compared the results with those obtained in another group who did not complete arm exercise (73). All of the 45 COPD patients were involved in a comprehensive, multidisciplinary pulmonary rehabilitation program. Even though only 20 patients completed the program, they showed improved

**Table 23.4   Controlled Studies of Arm Exercise in Patients With Chronic Obstructive Lung Disease**

| Authors | # patients | Duration | Course | Type | Results |
|---|---|---|---|---|---|
| Keens | 7 arms | 1.5 hr qd | 4 wks | Swimming Canoeing | ↑ VME (56%) |
| | 4 VMT | 15 min qd | 4 wks | VMT | ↑ VME (52%) |
| | 4 control | — | — | VMT | ↑ VME (22%) |
| Ries | 8 gravity resistance arms | 15 min qd | 6 wks | Low resistance/ high repetition | ↑ arm endurance Dyspnea |
| | 9 neuromuscular facilitation arms | 15 min qd | 6 wks | Weight lifting | ↑ arm endurance Dyspnea |
| | 11 controls | — | 6wks | Walking | No change |
| Epstein | 13 arm | 30 min qd | 8 wks | UAE | ↓ $\dot{V}O_2$ and VE for arm elevation ↑ $PI_{max}$ |
| | 10 VMT | 30 min qd | 8 wks | VMT | ↑ $Pi_{max}$ and VME |

↑ = increase, ↓ = decrease, VMT = ventilatory muscle training, VME = ventilatory muscle endurance, $PI_{max}$ = maximal inspiratory pressure.

performance on the tests that were specific for the training. In that study, the patients reported a decrease in fatigue in all tests performed.

Because we had shown that simple arm elevation results in a significant increase in VE and $\dot{V}O_2$, we reasoned that if we trained the arms to perform more work or we decreased the ventilatory requirement for the same work, we should improve the capacity of the patient to perform arm activity. We first studied 14 patients with COPD before and after 8 weeks of 3 times weekly, 30 minutes sessions of unsupported arm exercise, as part of a comprehensive rehabilitation program that included leg exercise (74). The arm exercise consisted of intermittent vertical and oblique lifting of a dowel as described in Table 23.5. After training, there was a 35% decrease in the pretreatment rise in $\dot{V}O_2$ and $\dot{V}CO_2$ seen with arm elevation. There was a small but significant drop in the rise of VE during arm elevation. We have completed a study of 26 patients with COPD, randomized to either unsupported arm training (11 patients) or threshold resistance breath-

**Table 23.5 Method for Unsupported Arm Training**

1. Dowl (weight 500-750 grams)

2. Lift to shoulder level for 2 minutes. Frequency gated to breathing rate

3. Rest for 2 minutes

4. Repeat sequence as tolerated up to 7-8 times (28-32 minutes)

5. Monitor: dyspnea, heart rate

6. Increase weight (250 gr) every 5th session, as tolerated

7. Aim for 24 sessions

ing training (14 patients) (75,76). Arm training increased arm exercise endurance and decreased the VE, $\dot{V}O_2$ and $\dot{V}CO_2$ during arm elevation, whereas ventilatory muscle trainees did not show any change in those values. Interestingly, maximal inspiratory pressure increased significantly for both groups, indicating that arm training may induce increases in force generation by those muscles of the ribcage that hinge on the shoulder girdle.

Martinez et al compared training using arm ergometry, with training using unsupported arm exercise as part of a rehabilitation program for patients with COPD. They found that unsupported arm training decreased the metabolic requirement for an exercise that more closely resemble that performed during daily living activities, concluding that simple repeated arm elevation may help more than arm ergometry (77). More work is needed to select those patients who may benefit more from arm training. We should also develop training programs for the different muscles of the shoulder girdle that may exert ventilatory force. This concept has already been explored for the pectoralis muscle (78). Estenne et al trained the pectoralis muscle of six tetraplegic patients with negative isometric exercise and evaluated their strength and pulmonary function after 6 weeks. The results were compared with those obtained in six patients who underwent conventional pulmonary rehabilitation. Trained patients significantly increased their expiratory muscle strength and expiratory reserve volume. Taken together, these results indicate a possible role for the training of shoulder girdle muscles, as a way to improve respiratory muscle function.

Certainly, arm exercise training results in improved performance for arm activities, and in a drop in the ventilatory requirement for upper extremity activity, such as elevating the arms. Whether this results in less symptoms for similar work remains to be determined. Likewise, we are not sure as to the impact of arm training on other outcomes of importance to patients limited by pulmonary disease. As more studies address this important area, it will be possible to help select those patients more likely to benefit from arm training.

## Conclusion

There has been recent revival and interest in the interaction between arm exercise and ventilation. Although arm ergometry continues to be the gold standard for the testing and training of upper extremities, an increasingly larger body of evidence indicates a more important role for the testing and training of upper extremities in forms that more closely resemble their physiologic adaptation in humans. As our knowledge of the functional anatomy of shoulder girdle muscles improves, so will our capacity to apply this knowledge in more rational and effective exercise regimens.

## References

1. Sharp JT. Therapeutic considerations in respiratory muscle function. *Chest,* 88(2):118-23, 1985.
2. Epstein SK, An overview of respiratory muscle function. *Clin Chest Med,* 4:619-639, 1994.
3. Roussos CH, Macklem PT. The respiratory muscles. *N Engl J Med,* 307:786-97, 1982.
4. Tobin M. Respiratory muscles in disease. *Clin Chest Med,* 9:263-86, 1979.
5. Martinez FJ, Couser JI, Celli BR. Factors influencing ventilatory muscle recruitment in patients with chronic airflow obstruction. *Am Rev Respir Dis,* 142:276-82, 1990.
6. Farkas G, Roussos CH. Adaptability of the hamster's diaphragm to emphysema and/or exercise. *J Appl Physiol,* 53:1263-71, 1982.
7. Supinsky GS, Kelsen SG. Effects of elastase-induced emphysema on the force generating ability of the diaphragm. *J Clin Invest,* 70:978-80, 1982.
8. Simolowski T, Yan S, Gautheir AP, Macklem PT, Bellemare F. Contractile properties of the human diaphragm during chronic hyperinflation. *N Engl J Med,* 325:917-23, 1991.
9. DeTroyer A, Estenne M. Coordination between ribcage muscles and diaphragm during quiet breathing in humans. *J Appl Physiol,* 57:899-906, 1984.
10. Farkas GA, Decramer M, Rochester DF, et al. Contractile properties of intercostal muscles and their functional significance. *J Appl Physiol,* 59:528-35, 1985.
11. Raper AJ, Tagliaferro-Thompson W, Shapiro W, et al. Scalene and sternomastoid muscle function. *J Appl Physiol,* 21:497-502, 1966.
12. Druz WS, Sharp JT. Activity of the respiratory muscles in upright and recumbent humans. *J Appl Phsiol,* 51:1552-61, 1981.
13. Moxham J, Wiles CM, Newham D, et al. Sternomastoid function and fatigue in man. *Clin Sci and Molec Med,* 59:463-8, 1980.
14. Reid DC, Bowden J, Lynne-Davies P. Role of selected muscles of respiration as influenced by position and tidal volume. *Chest,* 70: 636-40, 1976.

15. Banzett R, Topulos G, Leith D, Natzios C. Bracing arms increases the capacity for sustained hyperpnea. *Am Rev Respir Dis*, 133:106-9, 1983.
16. Dolmage TE, Maestro L, Avendano MA, Goldstein RS. The ventilatory response to arm elevation of patients with chronic obstructive pulmonary disease. *Chest*, 104:1097-1100, 1993.
17. Maestro L, Dolmage T, Avendano MA, Goldstein R. Influence of arm position in ventilation during incremental exercise in healthy individuals. *Chest*, 98:113(S), 1990.
18. Celli BR, Rassulo J, Make BJ. Dyssynchronous breathing during arm but not leg exercise in patients with chronic airflow obstruction. *N Engl J Med*, 314:1486-90, 1986.
19. Criner GJ, Celli BR. Effect of unsupported arm exercise on ventilatory muscle recruitment in patients with sever chronic airflow obstruction. *Am Rev Respir Dis*, 138:856-61, 1988.
20. Campbell EJM, Agostoni E, Newsom Davis J. The respiratory muscles. Mechanics and neural control. 2nd ed. London. Lloyd-Luke. 246. 1970.
21. Celli BR, Rassulo J, Berman JS, Make B. Respiratory consequence of abdominal hernia in a patient with severe chronic obstructive pulmonary disease. *Am Rev Respir Dis*, 131:178-80, 1985.
22. Dodd DS, Brancatisano T, Engle LA. Chest wall mechanics during exercise in patients with severe chronic airflow obstruction. *Am Rev Respir Dis*, 129:33-8, 1984.
23. Ninane V, Rypens F, Yernault JC, DeTroyer A. Abdominal muslce use during breathig in patients with chronic airflow obstruction. *Am Rev Respir Dis*, 146:16-21, 1992.
24. Breslin E. The pattern of respiratory muscle recruitment during pursed lip breathing. *Chest*, 101:75-8, 1992.
25. Sieck G. Physiological effects of diaphragm muscle denervation and disuse. *Clin Chest Med* 15; 641-659. 1994.
26. Comtois A, Gorczyca A, Grassino A. Anatomy of diaphragmatic circulation. *J Appl Physiol*, 58:238-44, 1987.
27. Rochester DF. Measurement of diaphragmatic blood flow and oxygen consumption in the dog by the Key-Schmidt technique. *J Clin Invest*, 53:1216-25, 1974.
28. Bellemare F, Grassino A. Evaluation of diaphragmatic fatigue. *J Appl Physiol*, 53:1196-206, 1982.
29. Bellemare F, Grassino A. Force reserve of the diaphragm in patients with chronic obstructive pulmonary disease. *J Appl Physiol*, 35:8-15, 1983.
30. Dillard T. Ventilatory limitation of exercise: Prediction in COPD. *Chest*, 92:195-6, 1987.
31. Spiro SG. Exercise testing in clinical medicine. *Bri J Dis of the Chest*, 71:145-72, 1977.
32. Stubbing DG, Pengelly LD, Morse JL, Jones NL. Pulmonary mechanics during exercise in subjects with chronic airflow obstruction. *J Appl Physiol*, 49:511-5, 1980.
33. Euler von C. On the central pattern generator for the basic breathing rhythmicity. *J Appl Physiol*, 55:1647-59, 1983.
34. Moltke E, Skouby AP. The influence of tonic neck reflexes on the activity of some muscles of the trunk in patient with asthma. *Acta Medica Scandinavica*, 173:299-305, 1963.
35. Wasserman K. Priniciples of exercise testing and interpretation. 3rd Edition, Lea and Febiger, Philadelphia, 1987.
36. Bohannon RW. Adapting a bicycle ergometer for arm crank ergometry. Suggestion from the field. *Phys Ther*, 66:362-3, 1986.
37. Astrand I. ST depression, heart rate, and blood pressure during arm and leg work. *Scand J Clin Lab Invest*, 30:411-4, 1972.
38. Balady GJ, Weiner DA, Rose L, Ryan TJ. Physiologic responses to arm ergometry exercise relative to age and gender. *J Am Coll Cardiol*, 16:130-5, 1990.
39. Blomqvist CG. Upper extremity exercise testing and training. Cardiovasc Clin, 15:175-83, 1985.
40. Eston RG, Brodie DA. Responses to arm and leg ergometry. *Br J Sports Med*, 20:4-6, 1986.
41. Louhevaara V, Sovijarvi A, Llmarinen J, Teraslinna P. Differences in cardiorespiratory responses during and after arm crank and cycle exercise. *Acta Physiol Scand*, 138:133-43, 1990.
42. Ishii M, Ogawa T, Ushiyama K, Tomizawa T, Noguchi Y, Sugishita Y, Ito I. Cardiorespiratory responses to standing arm ergometry in patients with ischemic heart disease. Comparison with the results of treadmill exercise. *Jpn Heart J*, 32:425-33, 1991.
43. Jensen JI. Neural ventilatory drive during arm and leg exercise. *Scand J Clin Lab Invest*, 29:177-84, 1972.
44. Lamont LS, Finkelhor RS, Rupert SJ, Swierad PS, Alexander J. Combined arm-leg ergometry exercise test. *Am Heart J*, 124:1102-4, 1992.
45. Martin TW, Zeballos RJ, Weisman IM. Gas exchange during maximal upper extremity exercise. *Chest*, 99:420-425, 1991.
46. Martin TW, Zeballos RJ, Weisman IM. Use of arm crank exercise in the detection of abnormal

pulmonary gas exchange in patients at low altitude. *Chest,* 102:169-75, 1992.

47. Owens GR, Thompson FE, Sciurba FC, Robertson R, Metz KF, Volmer RR. Comparison of arm and leg ergometry in patients with moderate chronic obstructive lung disease. *Thorax,* 43:911-5, 1988.

48. Moldover JR, Downey JA. Cardiac response to exercise: comparison of 3 ergometers. *Arch Phys Med Rehabil,* 64:155-9, 1983.

49. Sawka MN. Physiology of upper body exercise. *Exerc Sport Sci Rev,* 14:175-211, 1986.

50. Nagle FJ, Richie JP, Giese MD. $\dot{V}O_2$max responses in separate and combined arm and leg air-braked erogmeter exercise. *Med Sci Sports Exerc,* 16:563-6, 1984.

51. Stenberg J, Astrand PO, Ekblom B, Royce J, Saltin B. Hemodynamic response to work with different muscle groups, sitting and supine. *J Appl Physiol,* 22:61-70, 1967.

52. Wetherbee S, Franklin BA, Hollingsworth V, Gordon S, Timmis GC. Relationship between arm and leg training work loads in men with heart disease. Implications for exercise prescription. *Chest,* 99:1271-3, 1991.

53. Williams JR, Armstrong N, Kirby BJ. The influence of the site of sampling and assay medium upon the measurement and interpretationof blood lactate responses to exercise. *J Sports Sci,* 10:95-107, 1992.

54. Osmundson PJ. Noninvasive tests in the diagnosis of peripheral vascular disease. *Cardiovasc Clin,* 10:271-7, 1980.

55. Astrand I, Guharay A, Wahren J. Circulatory responses to arm exercise with different arm positions. *J Appl Physiol,* 25:528-32, 1968.

56. Bobbert AC. Physiological comparison of three types of ergometry. *J Appl Physiol,* 15:1007-14, 1960.

57. Davis JA, Vodak P, Wilmore JH, Vodak J, Kurtz P. Anaerobic threshold and maximal aerobic power for three modes of exercise. *J Appl Physiol,* 41:544-50, 1976.

58. Balady GJ, Weiner DA, McCabe CH, Ryan TJ. Value of arm exercise testing in detecting coronary artery disease. *Am J Cardiol,* 55:37-9, 1985.

59. Alison J, Requis J, Donnelly P, Adams R, Sullivan C, Bye PT. End-expiratory lung volume during arm and leg exercise in normal subjects and patients cystic fibrosis. *Am J Respir Crit Care Med* 1998;158:1450-1458.

60. Balady GJ, Weiner DA, Rothendler JA, Ryan TJ. Arm exercise-thallium imaging testing for the detection of coronary artery disease. *J Am Coll Cardiol,* 9:84-8, 1987.

61. Reybronck T, Heigenhouser GF, Faulkner JA. Limitations to maximum oxygen uptake in arms, leg and combined arm-leg ergometry. *J Appl Physiol,* 38:774-779, 1975.

62. Belman M, Kendregan BA. Exercise training fails to increase skeletal muscle enzymes in patients with chronic obstructive pulmonary disease. *Am Rev Respir Dis,* 36:256-61, 1981.

63. Lake FR, Hendersen K, Briffa T, et al. Upper limb and lower limb exercise training in patients with chronic airflow obstruction. *Chest,* 97:1077-82, 1990.

64. Make BJ, Buckolz J. Exercise training in COPD patients improves cardiac function. *Am Rev Respir Dis,* 143;80A, 1991.

65. Tangri S, Wolf CR. The breathing pattern in chronic obstructive lung diseas during the performance of the some common daily activities. *Chest,* 63:126-7, 1973.

66. Celli B, Criner G, Rassulo J. Ventilatory muscle recruitment during unsupported arm exercise in normal subjects. *J Appl Physiol,* 64:1936-41, 1988.

67. Celli B, Martinez F, Couser J, Rassulo J. Factors determining the pattern of ventilatory muscle recruitment (VMR) in patients with chronic obstructive pulmonary disease (COPD). *Chest,* 97:68S, 1990.

68. Celli BR. Arm exercise and ventilation (editorial). *Chest,* 93:673-4, 1988.

69. Martinez FJ, Couser JI, Celli BR. Respiratory response to arm elevation in patients with chronic airflow obstruction. *Am Rev Respir Dis,* 143:476-80, 1991.

70. Epstein S, Celli B, Williams J, Tarpy S, Roa J, Shannon T. Ventilatory response to arm elevation . Its determinant and use in patients with COPD. *Am J Respir Crit Care Med* 152:211-216, 1995.

71. Barrends EM, Schols AM, Slebos DJ, Mostert R, Jansen P, Woters E. Metabolic and ventilatory response pattern to arm elevation in patients with COPD and healthy age-matched subjects. *Eur Respir J,* 8:1345-1351, 1995.

72. Keens T, Krastins I, Wannamaker E, Levinson H, Crozier D, Bryan A. Ventilatory muscle endurance training in normal subjects and patients with cystic fibrosis. *Am Rev Respir Dis,* 116:853-860, 1977.

73. Ries AL, Ellis B, Hawkins RW. Upper extremity exercise training in chronic obstructive pulmonary disease. *Chest,* 93:688-92, 1988.

74. Couser J, Martinez F, Celli B. Pulmonary rehabilitation that includes arm exercise reduces metabolic and ventilatory requirements

for simple arm elevation. *Chest,* 103:37-41, 1993.

75. Epstein S, Breslin E, Roa J, Celli B. Impact of unsupported arm training (AT) and ventilatory muscle training (VMT) on the metabolic and ventilatory muscle training (VMT) on the metabolic and ventilatory consequences of unsupported arm elevation (UAE) and exercise (UAEX) in patients with chronic airflow obstruction (CAO). *Am Rev Respir Dis,* 143(4):A-81, 1991.

76. Epstein SK, Celli BR, Martinez FJ, Couser J, Roa J, Pollock M, Benditt JO. Arm training reduces the $\dot{V}O_2$ and VE cost of unsupported arm exercise and elevation in chronic obstructive pulmonary disease. *J Cardiopulmonary Rehabil* 1997; 17: 171-177.

77. Martinez FJ, Vogel PD, Dupont DN, Stanopoulos I, Gray A, Beamis J. Supported arm exercise vs. unsupported arm exercise in the rehabilitation of patients with chronic airflow obstruction. *Chest,* 103:1397-1402, 1993.

78. Estenne M, Knoop C, Janvaerenbergh J, Heilporn A, DeTroyer A. The effect of pectoralis muscle training in tetraplegic subjects. *Am Rev Respir Dis,* 139:1218-22, 1989

## Chapter 24

# Ambulatory Chronic Heart Failure Patients In Rehabilitation: Cardiopulmonary Approaches

Dany Michel Marcadet, MD, France

## Introduction

In the past, bed rest was recommended for patients in chronic heart failure and physical exercise was considered contraindicated. This strategy was aimed at reducing oxygen demand and peripheral arterial resistance, therefore reducing cardiac work. Similar results can now be obtained through the judicious use of new drugs, thus avoiding potential complications of bed rest such as decubitus ulcers, muscle atrophy, venous thrombosis with pulmonary embolism, which can all significantly increase morbidity.

Lowering the level of physical activity is not only done because the physician prescribes it but also because patients with chronic heart failure have a natural tendency to reduce their physical activity, both as a result of psychosocial pressure from friends and family as well as their own desire to avoid the physical discomfort resulting from exercise.

In the early 1980s, several clinical studies showed that regular physical activity in a monitored environment was not only possible, but also functionally beneficial. As a result, patients were encouraged to engage in physical activities in order to avoid muscular atrophy and decubitus ulcers. Since those early publications, a number of other studies have also confirmed the efficacy of physical exercise, and currently most of the world's heart associations recommend it (1,2).

There are several differences between the rehabilitation of a patient with chronic heart failure and that of a patient with coronary artery disease (CAD). Reconditioning exercises should not begin immediately after an acute event, but rather after a three to four week interval during which the stability of the disease is ensured. It is also important to note that heart failure is a chronic pathology which will require long-term care, and where associated significant costs are generally related to repeated hospitalizations.

For those reasons, long-term cardiac rehabilitation exercise training for patients with chronic heart failure should be carried out on an ambulatory basis or at home rather than in the hospital. A similar approach is recommended for the management of chronic obstructive pulmonary disease (COPD), which is often present concurrently with cardiovascular disease.

## Cardiopulmonary Approach

When managing a patient with heart failure, one has to consider the respiratory system not only because the primary symptom limiting functional capacity is dyspnea but also because most patients are smokers who may have associated COPD (16% of cases, in our experience).

## Pulmonary Effects of Cardiovascular Diseases

In patients with congestive heart failure, exercise tolerance is most frequently limited by dyspnea and it is generally thought that hyperventilation and reduction in pulmonary compliance contribute to this symptom. Ventilation and ratio of minute ventilation to carbon dioxide production ($VE/\dot{V}CO_2$) are increased in patients with heart failure when these individuals are compared to controls both at rest and during exercise with any workload and oxygen consumption (3,4). By itself, $VE/\dot{V}CO_2$ is considered to be an independent prognostic marker of survival (5).

Several factors can explain the hyperventilation (6) observed in heart failure. These include increase in dead-space ventilation, relationship between dead-space ventilation and tidal volume (7), premature attainment of the anaerobic threshold, and pulmonary ventilation/perfusion mismatches (8). Chemoreceptor stimulation and hypoxia can also contribute to hyperventilation (9), as does cardiomegaly which can cause compressive atelectasis of the lung with shunt effect. To that list, one can add secondary pulmonary hypzertension and the restrictive syndrome related to the alteration of respiratory muscles, whose strength decreases along with pulmonary compliance (10,11,12,13).

These factors alone, however, do not explain the decrease in performance noted in these dyspneic patients. Indeed, ventilatory reserve in heart failure patients who do not have concurrent pulmonary disease is generally normal, even when they experience dyspnea (14). Moreover, performance does not correlate with dyspnea indices, hypoxemia, or altered carbon dioxide tension (15).

Dyspneic heart failure patients usually feel fatigued and this perception is partly due to the psychosocial factors often associated with this pathology. The reduction in physical activity is not solely linked to hemodynamic or pulmonary disturbances but often to pressures exerted by the patient's entourage, including the physician. Depression, which is commonly associated to cardiovascular diseases, further decreases the patient's motivation to adhere to an exercise program, thereby resulting in a more sedentary and dependent lifestyle (16,17,18).

The rehabilitation of patients with chronic pulmonary disorders is very similar to that of patients with heart failure. The same tools, physical exercises, educational programs and psychosocial supports are used (19). More individualized components should however be added and these include bronchial drainage, secretion color monitoring, abdominal breathing training, aerosol and assisted ventilation (with positive pressure), and sometimes oxygen therapy during exercise for patients who experience desaturation.

Patients with a dual pathology—cardiac and lung—also have exercise limitations due to their lowered or absent ventilatory reserve (20). In patients with CAD, a reduction in the ischemia threshold can be linked to oxygen desaturation. In addition, hypercarbia, hypoxia, and bronchodilator therapy can be the cause of arrhythmias (21). It is therefore important that adequate consideration be given to the patient's pulmonary status while beginning cardiovascular disease rehabilitation exercise training programs, so that unrecognized respiratory deficiencies can be identified and properly managed.

## Patient Classification

Before beginning an ambulatory physical rehabilitation program for patients with chronic heart failure, one has to confirm the stability of the disease as well as making sure that no other contraindication for physical activity is present (table 24.1).

**Table 24.1   Contraindications to Exercise in Chronic Heart Failure**

Absolute

  Acute myocardial infarction

  Myocarditis, pericarditis or active endocarditis

  Pulmonary oedema, embolism, or phlebitis

  Severe aortic stenosis

  Severe obstructive cardiomyopathy

  Dissecting aneurysm

  Arrhythmia, unstable angina

  Intercurrent febrile illness

Relative

  Left main coronary artery obstruction

  Moderate aortic stenosis

  Hypertrophic cardiomyopathy with rest gradient

  Hight degree atrioventricular block

  Electrolytic abnormalities

  Unmonitored arterial hypertension

  Unmonitored metabolic disease

  Advanced pregnancy

  Physical or mental difficulties resulting in inability to exercise

  Tachy or brady arrhythmia

Not a contraindication

  Age

  Abollute ejection fraction

  Presence of pacemaker or cardioverter/defibrillator

Patients should be classified into one of three categories based on clinical evaluation and results of relevant non-invasive tests. Their pulmonary and cardiac functions, functional capacity, ischemia threshold, and risk of arrhythmia should be determined. The classification is based on the severity of the pathology as well as the potential risks of engaging in physical exercise, these risks being characterized as low, medium, or high. Based on this information, it then becomes possible to design an appropriate cardiac rehabilitation exercise training program.

Functional capacity should be determined clinically through dyspnea assessment, NYHA classification, Borg scale during stress test, and quality of life analysis. In addition, symptoms suggestive of ventricular dysfunction, pleural effusion, pulmonary obstruction, or of other comorbidities which may limit exercise capacity, should be investigated further. The patient's psychological and social status should also be evaluated, and neuro-muscular, osteo-articular, metabolic, or hormonal anomalies should be ruled out.

The prognosis of the underlying cardiac disease can be determined through left ventricular ejection fraction measured by echocardiography, technetium 99m isotopic ventriculography, or angiography.

The stress test performed on a treadmill or cycle ergometer is a key examination because it evaluates the functional repercussion of the variously related pathologies as well as being able to identify potential complications that could result from exertion. The six-minute walk test can also be used (22) for the same purposes. Measurements of gas exchange during the stress test gives a more accurate evaluation of patients' functional capacity in relation to their maximum oxygen uptake ($\dot{V}O_2$max) or anaerobic threshold (Weber classification) (23). In addition, this examination identifies the dyspneic patient and helps to document if the dyspnea is cardiac or pulmonary in origin. Deconditioning can by itself be the cause of dyspnea and of decreased $\dot{V}O_2$max during exertion. In such cases, the cardiopulmonary response is usually normal. When exercise limitation is related to the cardio-vascular system, ventilatory reserve is between 20% and 50% of predicted , ventilatory reserve being determined by the ratio MVV – VE max/MVV where MVV is the maximum recorded ventilation at the end of exertion (L/min). In patients where exercise limitation is cardiac in origin, the anaerobic threshold is lower than normal, as is the maximum $\dot{V}O_2$. When exercise limitation is pulmonary in origin, ventilatory reserve is low or nonexistent, ventilation is el-

evated and MVV is decreased. In the more severe cases, oxygen desaturation may only occur during exertion, or it may be present at rest and worsening during exercise.

If the patient has an associated pulmonary pathology, a more complete assessment must be obviously carried out. This should include basic pulmonary function tests, blood gas analysis at rest and during exercise, chest radiographs, and CT-scan. Potential nocturnal desaturation or sleep apnea should also be documented if present. In patients with COPD, exercise testing gives an evaluation of the ischemia threshold. In such cases, stress echocardiography, myocardial perfusion imaging, and angiography are sometimes needed to assess the severity of the disease.

A proper evaluation of the risk for arrhythmias is finally indispensable, specially when home rehabilitation is planned. This evaluation involves documentation of the onset of arrythmia during exercise, 24-hour ECG recording, dispersion of QT and sinus variability, and signal-averaged electrocardiography. New technology involving the detection of micro-alternans of the T wave during exertion, [defined as variation in amplitude from one interval to another (1/2) of the T wave] can also be used. The presence of alternans during exercise is a very strong indicator of the risk of developing serious arrhythmias. In fact the results of this test are comparable to those of endocavitary electrophysiology (24,25,26).

By judiciously using this information, one can categorize patients according to the severity of their pathology and possible risks of problems during exercise (table 24.2). Selected patients at medium risk can benefit from ambulatory rehabilitation, while only those with low risk can benefit from both ambulatory and home rehabilitation.

## Treatment

An ambulatory rehabilitation exercise training program can be conducted at a rehabilitation center, at home, or, even better, in both settings concurrently. A most important difference between these programs is that the exercise program is not medically supervised during home rehabilitation and consequently resuscitation cannot be immediately started in the event of a complication. Specific restrictions in the selection of patient for home rehabilitation must therefore be followed. The planning and development of the exercise program must consider the setting, and

**Table 24.2   Patient Classification**

| Risk | Low | Medium | High |
|---|---|---|---|
| Functional capacity | | | |
| NYHA | I | II and III | III and IV |
| Weber | A | B and C | D and E |
| $\dot{V}O_2$ max (ml/mn/kg) | > 22 | 15 – 21 | < 14 |
| Ischemia | | | |
| Rest | 0 | 0 | + |
| Exercise | 0 | moderate | severe |
| Arrhythmia | | | |
| Rest | 0 | 0 | + |
| Exercise | 0 | moderate | severe |
| T wave alternans | 0 | 0 | + |
| Respiratory | | | |
| $PaCO_2$ | N | N | Hypercarbia |
| $PaO_2$ | N | hypoxia (exercise) | Hypoxia *(rest, exercise)* |
| $SaO_2$ | > 90% | < 90% effort | < 90% *(rest, exercise)* |
| VE | > 50 | < 50 | < 30 |
| VEMS | > 70% | 40-70% | < 40% |

for a home rehabilitation patient, instructions regarding potential difficulties and ways in which they should be handled must be given. Although home rehabilitation is an indispensable complement to ambulatory rehabilitation, liability and reimbursement issues for this type of treatment are still unclear.

## Approach

### Activity

The specific contents of a physical reconditioning exercise program are based on the pathology involved. The suggested exercises should always be simple and easy to perform by the patient alone since they will need to be performed consistently and sometimes for the rest of the patient's life.

An exercise training session should begin with a warm-up period consisting of simple physical exercises, respiratory exercises, stretching, and segmentary isotonic exercises on a Koch bench (27) or with low resistance. The warm-up should be followed by walking and bicycling, which are the two types of exercise easiest to implement.

### Intensity

Although the recommended target level of physical activity should be between 50% and 70% of the patient's $\dot{V}O_2$max as determined initially, it is sometimes preferable to target 50% in order to ensure that the anaerobic threshold is never reached (28). By doing so, the duration of the patient's cardiac exercise training program can be extended, thereby reinforcing and further encouraging the patient's adherence to the rehabilitation program. The use of oxygen during exercise sessions is indispensable for patients with combined cardiovascular and pulmonary diseases who experience oxygen desaturation during physical activity.

In order to assess the patient's subjective state of dyspnea (29), several tools including the Borg scale of perceived exertion should be used to determine the level of physical exercise being reached. Heart rate should be monitored, the target heart rate having been established during the initial stress test. It is important to recognize that the target heart rate approach has limitations in patients with cardiovascular disease receiving medications such as betablockers, amiodarone, and digitaline, in those with a pacemaker, and in those with chronotropic incompetence and even tachycardia.

## Duration

The duration of an exercise session should be of thirty minutes for warm-up and respiratory exercises followed by twenty to thirty minutes of walking and/or bicycling. Ideally, a patient should have three to five sessions per week, though most patients only attend two sessions. Patients should be encouraged to perform their exercises at home between ambulatory rehabilitation sessions. Any patient pursuing physical activity at home should have telephone assistance nearby. On occasion, the option of telephone monitoring of the patient's electrocardiogram should also be considered.

## Results

In the past, one of the reasons why physical exercise was not encouraged in cardiovascular patients was because it was thought that it could deteriorate ventricular function and induce ventricular remodeling (30). Recent studies have however shown that this is not the case by documenting that moderate physical exercise does not have a deleterious effect on cardiac function (31).

Contrary to earlier thinking, regular physical activity has significant beneficial effects such as improving exercise capacity and increasing maximum oxygen uptake, ejection fraction, and cardiac output. Patients with pulmonary limitations experience an improvement in dyspnea and quality of life, undoubtedly related to the lowering of minute ventilation and $VE/\dot{V}CO_2$ ratio generated by regular physical activity.

Clearly, these results are very positive and encouraging, though the long-term effects of physical activity on survival are not yet known (32).

## Conclusion

In future years, cardiac rehabilitation exercise training in an ambulatory setting for patients with cardiovascular diseases will continue to evolve. Combined with home rehabilitation and management of associated respiratory problems, it could become the ideal solution for this significant health problem. Hopefully, we will continue to improve rehabilitation results, exercise capacity, and—ultimately—survival of patients with cardiovascular diseases.

## References

1. Konstam MA, Dracup K, Baker DW, et al. *Heart failure: evaluation and care of patients with left-ventricular dysfonction.* Clinical Practice Guideline N.11.Rockville MD:US Departement of Heart and Human Services, Public Health Service, Agency for Health Care Policy and Research. AHCPR Publication #94-0612, June 1994.

2. Wenger NK, Froelicher ES, Smith LK, et al. *Cardiac rehabilitation as secondary prevention.* Clinical Practice Guideline N. 17. Rockeville, MD: US Department of Health and Human Services, Public Health Service, Agency for Health Care Policy and Research and the National Heart, Lung, and Blood Institute. AHCPR Publication #96-0673, October 1995.

3. Sullivan MJ, Higginbotham MB, Cobb FR. Increased exercise ventilation in patients with chronic heart failure: intact ventilatory control despite hemodynamic and pulmonary abnormalities. *Circulation* 1988;77:552-559.

4. Davies SW, Emery TM, Watling MI, et al. A critical threshold of exercise capacity in the ventilatory response to exercise in heart failure. *Br Heart J* 1991;65:179-183.

5. Chua TP, Ponikowski P, Harrington D, et al. Clinical correlates and pronostic significance of the ventilatory response to exercise in chronic heart failure. *J Am Coll Cardiol* 1997;29:1585-1590.

6. Metra M, Raddino R, Dei Cas L, et al. Assessment of peak oxygen consumption, lactate and ventilatory threshold and correlation with the resting and exercise hemodynamic data in chronic congestive heart failure. *Am J Cardiol* 1990;65:1127-1133.

7. Al-Rawas OA, Carter R, Richens D. Ventilatory and gas exchange abnormalities on exercise in chronic heart failure. *Eur Respir* 1995;8:2022-2028.

8. Davies SW, Emery TM, Watling MI et al. A critical threshold of exercise capacity in the ventilatory response to exercise in heart failure. *Br Heart J* 1991;65:179-183.

9. Chua TP, Clark AL, Amadi AA, et al. Relation between chemosensitivity and the ventilatory response to exercise in chronic heart failure. *J Am Coll Cardiol* 1996;27:650-657.

10. Hammond MD, Bauer KA, Sharp JT, et al. Respiratory muscle strength in congestive heart failure. *Chest* 1990;98:1091-1094.

11. McParland C, Krishnan B, Wang Y, et al. Inspiratory muscle weakness and dyspnea in heart failure. *Am Rev Respir Dis* 1992;146:467-472.

12. Mancini DM, Henson D, LaManca J, et al. Respiratory muscle function and dyspnea in patients with congestive heart failure. *Circulation* 1992;86:909-918.

13. Lindsay D, Lovegrove C, Dunn M, et al. Histological abnormalities of diaphragmatic muscle may contribute to dyspnoea in heart failure (Abstract). *Circulation* 1997;95:910-916.

14. Wasserman K. Dyspnea on exertion: is it the heart or the lungs? *JAMA* 1982.248:2039-2043.

15. Franciosa JA, Leddy CL, Wilen M, et al. Relation between hemodynamic and ventilatory responses in determining execise capacity in severe congestive heart failure. *Am J Cardiol* 1984;53:127-134.

16. Freedland KE, Carney RM, Rich MW, et al. Depression in elderly patients with heart failure. *J Geriatr Psych* 1991; 24: 59-71.

17. Steinhart MJ. Depression and chronic fatigue in the patients with heart disease. *Prim Care* 1991; 18: 309-25.

18. Rengo F, Acafora D, Trojano L, Furgi G. Congestive heart failure and cognitive impairment in the ederly. *Arch Gerontol Geriatr* 1995; 20: 63-8.

19. Reardon JZ, Levine S, Peske G, et al. A comparaison of outpatient cardiac and pulmonary rehabilitation patients. *J Cardpulm Rehabil* 1995;15:277-282.

20. Casaburi R, Porszasz J, Burns MR, et al. Physiologic benefits of exercise training in rehabilitation of patients with severe chronic obstructive pulmonary disease. *Am J Respir Crit Care Med* 1997;155:1541-1551.

21. Shih HT, Webb CR, Conway WA, et al. Frequency and significance of cardiac arrythmias in chronic obstructive lung disease. *Chest* 1988;94:44-88.

22. Guyatt G, Thompson P, Berman L, et al. How should we measure function in patients with chronic heart and lung disease. *J Chronic Dis* 1985;38:517-524.

23. Weber KT, Janicki JS, Fishman AP. Respiratory gas exchange during exercise in the non-invasive evaluation of the severity of chronic cardiac failure, in Braunwald E, Mock MB, Watson JT (eds). *Congestive Heart Failure.* Grune & Stratton, New York, 1982, pp 221-235.

24. Klingenheben T, Zabel M, D'Agostino RB, Cohen RJ, Hohnloser SH. Predictive Value of T-wave alternans for Arrhythmic Events in Patients with Congestive Heart Failure. *Lancet* 2000; 356:651-52.

25. Adachi K, Ohnishi Y, Shima T, Yamashiro K, Takei A, Tamura N, Yokoyama M. Determinant of Microvolt T-wave Alternans in Patients with Dilated Cardiomyopathy. *J Am Coll Cardiol* 1999; 34: 374-80.

26. Hennersdorf MG, Perings C, Niebch V, Vester EG, Strauer B. T Wave Alternans as a Risk Predictor in Patients with Cardiomyopathy and Mild-to-Moderate Heart Failure. *PACE* 2000; 23: 1386-1391.

27. Koch M., Douard H., Broustet J.P. The benefit of graded physical exercise in chronic heart failure. *Chest,* 1992; 13 (suppl. H): 59-69.

28. Belardinelli R, Georgiou D, Scocco V, et al. Low intensity exercise training in patients with chronic heart failure. *J Am Coll Cardiol* 1995;26:975-982.

29. Borg GA. Psycho-physical bases of perceived exertion. *Med Sci Sports Exerc* 1982; 14 : 377-387.

30. Jugdutt BI, Michororski BL, Kappagoda CT. Exercise training after anterior Q wave myocardial infarction: importance of regional left ventricular function and topography. *J Am Coll Cardiol* 1988;12:362-372.

31. Dubach P, Myers J, Dzickan G, et al. Effect of exercise training on myocardial remodeling in patients with reduced left ventricular function after myocardial infarction. *Circulation* 1997;95:2060-2067.

32. Coats AJ, Adamopoulos S, Meyer TE, et al. Effects of physical training in chronic heart failure. *Lancet* 1990;335:63-66.

# PART IX

# Integrating Psychosocial Factors Into Rehabilitation

# Chapter 25

# Involvement of the Partner In Rehabilitation

David R. Thompson, PhD, United Kingdom

Coronary artery disease and pulmonary disorders are major causes of mortality and morbidity in the western world. Because some forms of these diseases are potentially life-threatening, it is hardly surprising that they cause distress and impairment of quality of life for the patients and their relatives, especially their partners. This is the reason why the partner must play a major role in any patient's recovery and readjustment.

Although there is increasing evidence to support involvement of partners in rehabilitation, it is important to note that most studies of reactions to illnesses and of rehabilitation have focused on men with coronary artery disease (usually myocardial infarction patients) and most studies of partners have been of women (usually wives). It should, however, be recognized that women may also experience cardiac events and that in such cases, the most likely partner will be a man.

## Reactions to Illness

Any potentially life-threatening illness affects family members, so their attitude may have a profound effect on the patients' reactions and emotional adjustment to the illness and rehabilitation (1-3). Partners have the ability to influence recovery but this will depend on the demands placed upon them as well as their own level of stress and means of coping and adjustment.

Approximately 30 years ago a number of studies showed that families, particularly partners, of coronary patients experienced significant distress, poor understanding of advice and information and that they suffered consequences that were often as important as those of the patient (4-11). Many of these problems are still present today (12-15).

Most of these studies have brought attention to the important role of partners in patients convalescence and their influence on recovery. Many have recommended that one should help and advise the whole family (especially partners) during the acute phase of disease and throughout the convalescence. Even when support, advice and information are provided to partners by health professionals, many are dissatisfied and they would rather go to relatives and close friends (16-18) for these services.

Apart from the feeling of guilt, the partner may experience various fears, including loss of loved ones, changes in life objectives and financial status, a new role within the family and possibly a recurrence of the event (10,19-23). The perceived needs of family members during the acute illness include information, reassurance, relief of anxiety, hope, comfort, support and acceptance (3,16,17,24-27).

A patient's ability to adapt to his or her illness is largely dependent on the partner's ability to cope with emotional stress (28). Said differently, the extent to which partners experience difficulties to adjust limits the amount of support that they are able and willing to provide. As a consequence, it influences the whole rehabilitation process and ultimately the outcome. There is some research and a great deal of anecdotal evidence indicating that family members, particularly the wives of patients with myocardial infarction often become overprotective or too demanding (4,5,29). For these reasons, family tensions are common during the recovery period (19). Some couples report having too little support and experience conflict in their relationships with others. Helping efforts are misinterpreted in some partner relationships (14). In addition, some partners note the detrimental impact of the illness on the amount of time available for their other roles (14). However, high levels of involvement and protectiveness for their loved one may sometimes be necessary on the part of the partner (30).

In one large study (31) of over 1700 partners of myocardial infarction patients, 97% reported moderate or severe distress immediately after the event. After their partner was discharged from hospital, 69% reported similar levels of distress. There were no differences between men and women, although older partners were less distressed than younger ones (31). A more recent study (15) suggests that many partners of patients undergoing cardiac rehabilitation experience significant levels of psychological distress, and two-thirds of partners who elected to participate in a spousal support group were significantly distressed. These findings are similar to those of earlier studies (3,32).

Some researchers (33) have shown that greater use of protective buffering by wives of male patients with myocardial infarction was associated with increased distress for the wife. "Relationship-focused coping" may be as important, if not more than "emotion-focused" (involving reducing any negative emotional consequences without addressing the initial cause) and "problem-focused" (involving managing the source of stress) coping.

Return to normal social and sexual activities may also be impaired by emotional distress. Over the first few months of recovery from an illness, many patients fear to resume sexual activities and, unless this is dealt with, some will never resume them. Partners share the same worries and their fear is often the most significant factor in overall reduced sexual activity and diminished enjoyment. There is no evidence that sex is deleterious and patients and partners should be told so in an unequivocal fashion.

Often, the partner will have higher levels of emotional distress than the patient, particularly during the early stages of the illness. Although this phenomenon is normal, it may contribute to a less satisfactory rehabilitation than may otherwise have been achieved by the patient (4,34).

There is some evidence that overprotectiveness may be seen in couples that are getting closer, while hostility is associated with couples that are becoming more distant and that have fewer useful discussions about coping (35).

## Assessment

In order to minimize the impact of stress upon the family, and particularly the partner, health professionals must assess in a comprehensive, systematic, and sensitive manner the needs of family members, recognizing that there will always be individual differences and that those may vary over time.

This individual assessment should begin as soon as possible after admission to hospital. In 1990, Doherty and Power (36) described three facets to this assessment: (a) needs of the partner, (b) partner's level of skill, and (c) degree of burden that the illness represents for the partner. Thus, health professionals must assess the partner's awareness of his or her own needs, and determine if he or she is able to seek help and support. They must also evaluate the extent and adequacy of the support network, as well as the ability to access that support system.

Over two decades ago Frank and colleagues (37) concluded that early intervention was desirable, that partners should usually be included and that supportive-educative and behavioural interventions were likely to be the most effective. At the same time, Stern and Pascale (29) specifically suggested that in-hospital education or psychological therapy group for couples might prove beneficial. Despite these recommendations, it was not until about a decade later that systematic studies of this type of intervention were carried out (38-39). Interventions after hospital discharge have also been shown to be effective (40).

## Education

Advice given to patients should be realistic, practical and very specific about what should be done. Vague advice such as 'listen to your body' or 'do what you can manage' are less likely to be helpful. Patients and their relatives should be warned about common physical and psychological sequelae, such as moodiness, tearfulness, disturbed sleep, irritability, acute awareness of minor somatic sensations, and poor concentration and memory (41). It should be further explained that these symptoms are normal, and universal, and that they are part of the natural course of recovery after a potentially life threatening event. Partners should be told to alter family routines as little as possible except maybe for lifestyle. They must tactfully be advised against overprotecting the patient and in the case of a female patient, be told not to expect the patient to resume all of the housework immediately. In order to make sure they understand this advice, they should be asked to summarize it.

Clear information about the illness, its treatment and rehabilitation must be given in an easy to understand language. Sometimes, it is also helpful to have written or tape recorded advice (41).

Some degree of coordination is required if one is to avoid giving conflicting advice. For instance, written and taped information should complement the verbal communication and if required be available in appropriate languages. The educational impact can also be increased by using various formats such as education classes or group discussions. Treatment plans should be discussed with the patient and partner and a copy of the plan given to them.

## Support

It has been shown that sustained family support has a positive effect on long-term recovery (3,8). Unfortunately, family members, including partners, often receive little counseling from health care professionals either initially or during the early stages of recovery and convalescence. A support package tailored to the particular needs, skills and resources of the couple should be discussed and implemented.

Partners should be screened using validated instruments, and those with psychological distress should be offered interventions to assist them in dealing with specific stressors. These interventions can use stress-management techniques, such as relaxation training and assertiveness training, and engagement-coping strategies. In addition, marital and family concerns must be primarily and directly addressed (15). In some instances, patients and partners may require sexual counseling, which can be initiated while the patient is still in hospital. This can then be continued throughout the patient's recovery period.

Couples should be given ample opportunity to express their feelings because patients who feel that they cannot talk to their partners often have a worse recovery (43). Given the tendency of partners to avoid disclosing their feelings for fear of distressing the patient (44,45) and given also that prevalent stressors include patients' moodiness, helplessness or apathy and worries about treatment, recovery and progress, partners may benefit from engaging in more relationship-focused coping strategies, such as open communication, mutual problem solving, cognitive restructuring and expressing emotions (15,18).

There should always be regular follow-ups and re-assessments The support must be concrete, with clearly defined and measurable goals. It must also take into account the individual's own beliefs. Continued support should be provided or modified as the support network is identified and re-evaluated.

Support may be provided in a variety of formats. On occasion, it may only consist of brief meetings or even telephone calls to reemphasize the goals, look at progress, or help solve any difficulties that may have arisen.

With co-habiting couples, recovery may be better understood as a dyadic rather than individual response (12). In 1991, Coyne & Smith (33) pointed out that partners dealing with a serious illness are required not only to manage their own individual distress and attend to instrumental tasks but also to adopt strategies to grapple with each other's emotional needs. In their study, wives' distress was increased by the patients' use of avoidant-coping strategies such as hiding concerns or denying worries (protective buffering) and was decreased by active involvement with their husband through discussion and constructive problem solving.

One other approach involves both the patient and his or her partner working together to come to terms with the impact of the illness. This can be a relatively simple and inexpensive form of intervention. Brief and early nurse-led interventions have also been shown to be highly effective in reducing anxiety and depression and improving knowledge and satisfaction in patients with myocardial infarction (38) and their partners (39). These interventions are also relatively inexpensive. A recent study of extended nurse-led cardiac counseling for in-hospital patients and their partners showed that these interventions resulted in significant and enduring benefits of clinical value (46).

## Discharge and Aftercare

Patient's discharge from the hospital can be particularly stressful for the partner, who often feels vulnerable, unsupported and over-protective. It has also been shown that wives tend to have more conservative opinions of their husband's ability to engage in physical activity than the husbands themselves (47). There may further be a honeymoon period of increased cooperation and suppressed conflict soon after the patient has returned home. Unfortunately, this is often not indicative of the patterns of later adjustments (20). Appropriate and timely discharge planning and aftercare are therefore essential and require preparing the partner for the stress associated with care giving (30). It has been suggested that, for some families, the need for and ability to benefit from education may not be apparent until the patient has been discharged from hospital (21).

It is important that partners are offered access to, and encouraged to take up and adhere to, cardiac rehabilitation programs. Not only will they benefit from such programs but their partner might benefit just as much. Usually both partners and patients highly rate rehabilitation programs (48). In the event that a partner does not wish to participate in rehabilitation, alternative means of support, such as telephone follow-up and home visits should be offered. These will allow progress reviews based on objectives and identification of further problems.

Increased flexibility in rehabilitation and aftercare follow-up will enable health professionals to provide extra help for those who have identified problems.

## Conclusion

Cardiopulmonary rehabilitation can have a significant impact on the quality of life of partners. It can influence patient outcome and it is crucial that partners be involved appropriately at all stages of the rehabilitation process. Arguments for including the partner in the rehabilitation process are both practical and therapeutic. The partner can be incorporated in the patient's program with little additional effort or cost and his or her presence alone can improve confidence and morale in the patient. It is commonly the partner who has the most important role in the patient's readjustment during convalescence, and his or her behavior is an important determinant of the rate and extent of the patient's recovery. Partners' perceptions of patients' physical capabilities can either help or impede the rehabilitation process. In the worse case scenario, it may create dependency, while in the best it may enhance recovery through influencing successful adaptation to the illness. The inclusion of partners in rehabilitation programmes seems essential and they should be offered, as a matter of routine, participation in all aspects of the rehabilitation process.

## References

1. Bedsworth J, Molen M: Psychological stress in spouses of patients with myocardial infarction. *Heart Lung* 1982;11:450-456.
2. Riegel J, Dracup K: Does overprotection cause cardiac invalidism after acute myocardial infarction? *Heart Lung* 1992;21:529-535.
3. Moser D, Dracup K, Marsden C: Needs of recovering cardiac patients and their spouses: compared views. *Int J Nurs Stud* 1993;30:105-114.
4. Wishnie HA, Hackett TP, Cassem NH: Psychological hazards of convalescence following infarction. *JAMA* 1971;215:1292-1296.
5. Skelton M, Dominian J: Psychological distress in wives of patients with myocardial infarction. *Br Med J* 1973;2:101-103.
6. Mayou R, Williamson B, Foster A: Attitudes and advice after myocardial infarction. *Br Med J* 1976;1:1577-1579.
7. Finlayson A: Social networks as coping resources. Lay help and consultation patterns used by women in husband's post-infarction career. *Soc Sci Med* 1976;10:97-103.
8. Croog S, Levine S: *The Heart Patient Recovers: Social and Psychological Factors.* New York: Human Sciences Press, 1977.
9. Finlayson A, McEwan J: *Coronary Heart Disease and Patterns of Living.* London: Croom Helm, 1977.
10. Mayou R, Foster A, Williamson B: The psychological and social effects of myocardial infarction in wives. *Br Med J* 1978;1:699-701.
11. Davidson D: The family and cardiac rehabilitation. *J Fam Pract* 1979;8:253-261.
12. Bennett P, Connell H: Dyadic processes in response to myocardial infarction. *Psychol Health Med* 1999;4:45-55.
13. Kettunen S, Solovieva S, Laamanen R, Santavirta N: Myocardial infarction, spouses' reactions and their need of support. *J Adv Nurs* 1999;30:479-488.
14. Stewart M, Davidson K, Meade D, Hirth A, Makrider L: Myocardial infarction: survivors' and spouses' stress, coping, and support. *J Adv Nurs* 2000;31:1351-1360.
15. O'Farrell P, Murray J, Hotz SB: Psychologic distress among spouses of patients undergoing cardiac rehabilitation. *Heart Lung* 2000;29:97-104.
16. Hentinen M: Need for instruction and support of the wives of patients with myocardial infarction. *J Adv Nurs* 1983;8:519-524.
17. Thompson DR, Cordle CJ: Support of wives of myocardial infarction patients. *J Adv Nurs* 1988;13:223-228.
18. Thompson DR, Ersser SJ, Webster RA: The experiences of patients and their partners one month after a heart attack. *J Adv Nurs* 1995;22:707-714.

19. Doehrman SR: Psycho-social aspects of recovery from coronary heart disease: a review. *Soc Sci Med* 1977;11:199-218.

20. Speedling EJ: *Heart Attack: The Family's Response at Home and in the Hospital*. London: Tavistock, 1982.

21. Dhooper S: Social networks and support during the crisis of heart attack. *Health Soc Work* 1983;9:294-303.

22. Nyamathi A: The coping responses of female spouses of patients with myocardial infarction. *Heart Lung* 1987;16:86-92.

23. Orzeck SA, Staniloff HM: Comparison of patients' and spouses' needs during the posthospital convalescence phase of a myocardial infarction. *J Cardiopulmon Rehabil* 1987;7:59-67.

24. Molter NC: Needs of critically ill patients: a descriptive study. *Heart Lung* 1979;8:332-339.

25. Bramwell L: Wives' experiences in the support role after husbands' first myocardial infarction. *Heart Lung* 1986;15:578-584.

26. Thoebald K: The experiences of spouses whose partners have suffered a myocardial infarction: phenomenological study. *J Adv Nurs* 1997;26:595-601.

27. Turton J: Importance of information following myocardial infarction: a study of the self-perceived information needs of patients and their spouse/partner compared with the perceptions of nursing staff. *J Adv Nurs* 1998;27:770-778.

28. Beach EK, Maloney BH, Plocica AR, Sherry SE, Weaver M, Luthringer L, Utz S: The spouse: a factor in recovery after acute myocardial infarction. *Heart Lung* 1992;21:30-38.

29. Stern M, Pascale L: Psychosocial adaptation post-myocardial infarction: the spouse's dilemma. *J Psychosom Res* 1979;23:83-87.

30. Gilliss CL: Reducing family stress during and after coronary artery bypass surgery. *Nurs Clin North Am* 1984;19:1103-1111.

31. Jones D: Influence on spouses and influence of spouses. In: Jones D, West R eds *Cardiac Rehabilitation*. London: BMJ Publishing Group, 1995:227-243.

32. Hilbert G: Family satisfaction and affect of men and their wives after myocardial infarction. *Heart Lung* 1993;22:200-205.

33. Coyne JC, Smith DAF: Couples coping with myocardial infarction: a contextual perspective on wives' distress. *J Person Soc Psychol* 1991;61:404-412.

34. Waltz M: Martial context and postinfarction quality of life: is it social support or something more? *Soc Sci Med* 1986;22:791-805.

35. Fiske V, Coyne JC, Smith DA: Couples coping with myocardial infarction: an empirical reconsideration of the role of overprotectiveness. *J Fam Psychol* 1991;5:4-20.

36. Doherty ES, Power PW: Identifying the needs of coronary patient wife-caregivers: implications for social workers. *Health Soc Work* 1990;15:291-299.

37. Frank KA, Heller SS, Kornfeld DS: Psychological intervention in coronary heart disease: a review. *Gen Hosp Psychiat* 1979;1:18-23.

38. Thompson DR, Meddis R: A propsective evaluation of in-hospital counseling for first time myocardial infarction men. *J Psychosom Res* 1990;34:237-248.

39. Thompson DR, Meddis R: Wive's responses to counseling early after myocardial infarction. *J Psychosom Res* 1990;34:249-258.

40. Dracup K: A controlled trial of couples group counseling in cardiac rehabilitation. *J Cardiopulmon Rehabil* 1985;5:436-442.

41. Thompson DR, Lewin RJP: Management of the post-myocardial patient: rehabilitation and cardiac neurosis. *Heart* 2000;84:101-105.

42. Thompson DR Bowman GS, Kitson AL, de Bono DP, Hopkins A: Cardiac rehabilitation in the United Kingdom: guidelines and audit standards. *Heart* 1996;75:89-93.

43. Helgerson VS: The effects of masculinity and social support on recovery from myocardial infarction. *Psychosom Med* 1991;53:621-633.

44. Adsett C, Bruhn J: Short-term group psychotherapy for post-myocardial infarction patients and their wives. *Can Med Assoc J* 1968;99:577-584.

45. Harding A, Morefield M: Group intervention for wives of myocardial infarction patients. *Nurs Clin North Am* 1976;11:339-347.

46. Johnston M, Foulkes J, Johnston D, Pollard B, Gudmundsdottir H: Impact on patients and partners of inpatient and extended cardiac counseling and rehabilitation: a controlled trial. *Psychosom Med* 1999;61:225-233.

47. Taylor CB, Bandura A, Ewart CK, Miller NH, DeBusk RF: Exercise testing to enhance wives' confidence in their husband's cardiac capacity soon after clinically uncomplicated acute myocardial infarction. *Am J Cardiol* 1985;55:635-638.

48. Jones DA, West RR: Psychological rehabilitation after myocardial infarction: multicentre randomised controlled trial. *BMJ* 1996;313:1517-1521.

# Chapter 26

# Smoking Cessation
# In Pulmonary Rehabilitation:
# Goal or Prerequisite?

Yves Lacasse, MD, MSc, Canada

It has now been more than 35 years since the Surgeon General of the United States released the first report of the Advisory Committee on Smoking and Health (1). Cigarette smoking has been identified as the most important source of preventable morbidity and premature mortality in North America (2). During the 1990s, tobacco was the largest single cause of premature death in the developed world (3). Smoking cessation has immediate and substantial health benefits, both on symptoms and organ functions (4), and dramatically reduces the risk of most smoking-related diseases (5), including chronic obstructive pulmonary disease.

Respiratory rehabilitation is now defined as "a multidimensional continuum of services directed to persons with pulmonary disease and their families, usually by an interdisciplinary team of specialists, with the goal of achieving and maintaining the individual's maximum level of independence and functioning in the community" (6). Accordingly, an European Respiratory Society task force on rehabilitation recently commented that a comprehensive respiratory rehabilitation program should be able to address the need for medical management, reinforcement of smoking cessation, education of the patient and family, exercise reconditioning, physical, and occupational therapy, nutritional support, long term oxygen therapy and home mechanical ventilation (7).

Most patients have quit smoking by the time they initiate pulmonary rehabilitation (8). Nevertheless, the inclusion of smokers in respiratory rehabilitation programs remains controversial (9). Among the 14 trials included in a meta-analysis of respiratory rehabilitation in COPD (10), the smoking status of the patients was reported in nine. Patients had to be non-smokers in only two of them (11,12). Some investigators have used a trial of smoking cessation as an index of the patient's motivation to participate in pulmonary rehabilitation (13). This paper is a reflection on the effect of smoking on the course of COPD and on the opportunity to deal with smoking within the frame of comprehensive rehabilitation.

## Smoking Causes COPD

In 1960, the British Medical Research Council commissioned a prospective study of respiratory symptoms and changes in ventilatory function over a period of eight years in a large group of working men (14). From an initial stratified sample of 1136 men aged 30-59 working in West London (mostly as skilled manual and clerical), 792 were seen every 6 months over the next eight years. From the 9190 measurements that were made of the changes in $FEV_1$ between successive six-monthly surveys, the investigators concluded that 1) $FEV_1$ declines continuously and smoothly over an individual's life; 2) non-smokers lose $FEV_1$ slowly and almost never developed clinically significant airflow obstruction; 3) most smokers lose $FEV_1$ almost as slowly as non-smokers and never develop clinically severe airflow limitation; 4) only a relatively small proportion of smokers (probably 10-15%) show a rate of decline that is fast enough to result in clinical disease; and 5) a susceptible smoker who stops smoking will not recover lost $FEV_1$, but the subsequent rate of loss of $FEV_1$ will revert to normal (figure 26.1).

A prospective study of Canadian women over a five-year period agreed with the conclusions of Fletcher and Peto's study (15). Also, data obtained by Tager et al. (16) on younger individuals suggested that a major effect of cigarette smoking on lung function decline involves the premature onset of a "normal" rate of decline in function and, to a lesser extent, more rapid rates of decline later in life, underlying the importance of early intervention.

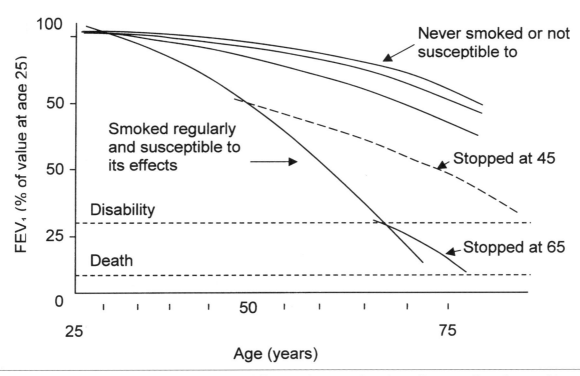

**Figure 26.1**   Risks for various men if they smoke: differences between these lines illustrate effects that smoking, and stopping smoking, can have on $FEV_1$ of man who is liable to develop chronic obstructive lung disease if he smokes. Although this shows rate of loss of $FEV_1$ for one particular susceptible smoker, other susceptible smokers will have different rates of loss, thus reaching "disability" at different ages.

Reprinted, by permission, from C Fletcher and R Peto, "The natural history of chronic airflow obstruction," *British Medical Journal* i:1645-1648.

## The Effect of Smoking Cessation

Evidence is continuing to accumulate that there is less rapid decline in lung function upon smoking cessation (17-20). In this regard, the latest and most informative data in support to those of the British Medical Council's study are from the *Lung Health Study* (21). The primary objective of this large multicenter randomized controlled trial conducted in the United States and in Canada was to determine whether a program incorporating smoking intervention and use of an inhaled bronchodilator can slow the rate of decline in $FEV_1$ over a 5-year period in smokers aged 35 to 60 years who had mild obstructive disease. The 5887 participants were allocated to one of the following three groups: 1) smoking intervention plus bronchodilator; 2) smoking intervention plus placebo; or 3) no intervention. The $FEV_1$ rates of decline after the first annual visit were similar in the three groups. This apparently disappointing result stemmed from the fact that smoking cessation rates were rather small, approxi-

mating 22% at the fifth annual visit in the smoking cessation groups as compared with about 5% in the usual care group. The beneficial effect of smoking cessation was therefore diluted within each group. However, sustained quitters (whatever the group they were allocated in at study entry) had a rate of decline in $FEV_1$ that was considerably less than the one in continuous smokers. The *Lung Health Study* was useful in emphasizing that smoking cessation is challenging even in patients who have a smoking-related disease, and that, in average, smokers with airflow obstruction benefit from quitting despite previous heavy smoking.

## Further Deleterious Effects of Smoking in COPD

COPD is now considered as a systemic disease. The respiratory syndrome is often accompanied by osteoporosis, depression and peripheral muscle dysfunction that determines exercise intolerance, poor quality of life and reduced survival (22). Accordingly, exercise training is a mandatory component of any successful rehabilitation program (23).

A comprehensive review of the physiological basis of rehabilitation is beyond the scope of the current reflection. However, a brief discussion on the basic mechanisms of oxygen transportation and oxidative capacity of the peripheral muscles is useful to underline some of the pathophysiological effects of smoking on the rehabilitation process.

The affinity of hemoglobin for carbon monoxide is 200 times its affinity for oxygen. In addition to reducing the oxygen-carrying capacity of the blood, carbon monoxide directly increases the oxygen-binding affinity of hemoglobin and impairs oxygen extraction (24). There is sparse but convincing evidence that cigarette smoking determines the severity of secondary polycythemia in patients with hypoxemic COPD and that it prevents its correction by long-term oxygen therapy (25). In this study, Calverley et al. related the red cell mass in 47 hypoxemic patients (including 31 current smokers) with COPD to their smoking habits and carboxyhemoglobin concentrations. From these 31 smokers, fifteen were available at 12-month follow-up; 7 of them were still smoking whereas 8 stopped smoking during the 12 months of long-term oxygen treatment. Despite receiving 12 months of long-term oxygen therapy (given 15 hours/day), there was no significant change in red cell mass, pulmonary artery pressure and carboxyhemoglobin concentration in the 7 patients who continued to smoke.

Smoking may have a deleterious effect on skeletal muscle function that is independent from that of COPD. In a study that antedated the recent resurgence of interest on muscle dysfunction in COPD, Orlander et al. (26) compared smokers and nonsmokers of a homogeneous population of apparently healthy but sedentary men with respect to skeletal muscle (vastus lateralis) morphological, metabolic and functional characteristics. The percentage type I fibers was lower and that of type IIB fibers higher in the smokers. Fiber areas were almost equal in the two groups. Muscle oxidative capacity was lowered in the smokers, as judged from decreased mitochondrial enzyme activities and a lowered fibrillar space mitochondrial volume fraction. The authors suggested that the lowered muscle oxidative capacity and strength in the smokers may be partly a consequence of the different fibre type distribution. A possibly lower physical activity level, and tobacco smoke constituents may also be instrumental. Interestingly, the changes observed in the group of smokers were similar to those recently observed in COPD patients engaged in respiratory rehabilitation (22).

These effects of smoking on the oxygen transportation and the oxidative capacity of the skeletal muscle must be added to the direct relation between initial $FEV_1$ level and the slope of $FEV_1$ decline that is known as the "horse race effect" (to describe the observation that the horse leading in the middle of the race is most likely to win the race) (27).

## Smoking Cessation Interventions in COPD

Standards for a comprehensive smoking cessation intervention have been proposed (28). The evidence for the effectiveness of the available intervention's components have recently been summarized by the *Cochrane Tobacco Addiction Review* group (29). Advice from physicians, structured intervention from nurses, as well as individual and group counseling are effective. All forms of nicotine replacement therapy are also effective. The antidepressant bupropion increased quit rates in a small number of trials. These available interventions are usually integrated in comprehensive programs that are tailored to models that assume that smoking involves both physiologic addiction to nicotine and psychological dependence on other aspects of smoking (30-31).

The results of the *Lung Health Study* (21) have demonstrated that an aggressive smoking cessation behavioral intervention including nicotine replacement therapy may be effective in increasing the cessation rate of patients with mild obstructive disease. However, as COPD is a disease of the elderly, whether these results can be generalized to patients with symptomatic COPD eligible to rehabilitation is uncertain. In average, the patients enrolled in the *Lung Health Study* were aged 48, which is short of the typical 65 years of age of those patients with moderate to severe COPD usually engaged in respiratory rehabilitation (10).

In one hand, it is reassuring to learn that most smoking cessation interventions that have been shown to be effective in the general population also have been shown to be effective with older smokers (28): counseling interventions, physician advice, buddy support programs, age-tailored self-help materials, telephone counseling, and the nicotine patches have all been shown to be effective in treating tobacco use in adults aged 50 and older.

On the other hand, few controlled trials have specifically addressed the effectiveness of smoking cessation interventions in patients with COPD. In fact, the ACCP/AACVPR Pulmonary Rehabilitation Guidelines Panel (8) could identify only one randomized trial of a smoking cessation intervention in COPD patients (32). This trial was conducted in patients who were hospitalized for acute exacerbations of their disease. The rationale for such an intervention in hospitalized patients is that hospitalization may be seen as "window of opportunity" (33), that is a time when perceived vulnerability to dangers of smoking, quitting motivation and receptivity to smoking cessation intervention may be at their peak, especially for those smokers hospitalized for a condition that is caused or complicated by smoking (34). Despite the apparent optimal conditions in which the study was conducted, the investigators reported only modest success with smoking cessation, suggesting that COPD does not facilitate the cessation process.

## Smoking as a Predictor of Adherence to and Success of Rehabilitation

Do non-smokers really fare better than smokers in rehabilitation? This question lies at the heart of this reflection and involves two different important outcomes of respiratory rehabilitation: the adherence to rehabilitation and its actual results.

Young and al. (35) published the results of an interesting study in which they sought to determine whether patients with COPD who decline participation in, or fail to complete a rehabilitation program differ from those who complete the program. Fifty-five patients completed their 4-week program and composed the "adherent group". Thirty patients declined to take part in the program and 6 failed to complete it. These 36 patients composed the "non-adherent group". Patients in the non-adherent group were more likely to be current smokers (28% vs. 8%, p < 0.02) and were more likely to be dissatisfied with disease-specific social support (51% vs. 2%, p < 0.001). There was no difference in terms of physiological impairment between the two groups. Also, the non-adherent group was not significantly likely to be depressed or anxious. This study showed that smokers are less likely to participate in rehabilitation. The interpretation of this study is limited by its nonadherent group being composed of a minority of patients who began the program but failed to complete it. Another study suggested that the high-rate of non-compliance in

smokers (35% vs. 13% in non-smokers) may be an indication for a review of the cost-effectiveness of programs which enroll smokers (36).

The question of actual results was recently addressed by Singh et al. (37). In their study, 31 ex-smokers were matched with 31 current smokers recruited to a pulmonary rehabilitation program. Both groups underwent assessment of exercise tolerance and quality of life before and after a 7-week course of rehabilitation. There was no significant difference in $FEV_1$, shuttle walk distance, treadmill endurance time and quality of life (measured by the Chronic Respiratory Questionnaire) between the two groups at baseline. On reassessment, there was a significant improvement in exercise tolerance and quality of life scores in both groups. The degree of improvement obtained by the non-smokers was not significantly better than those seen in current smokers. The authors concluded that current smokers benefit from rehabilitation as much as non-smokers and should not be denied rehabilitation. Whether this improvement can be sustained over time in both groups remains unknown.

## Smoking Cessation in Respiratory Rehabilitation: Goal or Prerequisite?

### The Case of Transplantation, Lung Volume Reduction Surgery and Oxygen Therapy

Candidates for lung transplantation must have been free of substance addiction (including tobacco) for at least 6 months. Appropriate preoperative biochemical monitoring is even recommended in selected patients (38). Pathophysiological considerations as well as philosophical reasons are the usual arguments put forward in order to exclude smokers from the candidate selection process. Similarly, patients who continue to smoke are usually denied lung volume reduction surgery (39). Although qualified of "rather arbitrary", the condition of smoking cessation usually serves as an index of motivation in the selection of patients (40).

The prescription of long-term oxygen therapy in COPD patients who are still smoking is more controversial. Although high carboxyhemoglobin concentrations resulting from smoking are likely to inhibit the beneficial effect of supplemental oxygen (25), around 20% of the patients registered in some respiratory home care services are active smokers

(41). This situation might be influenced by the British Medical Research Council's trial of oxygen therapy (42) in which 43% of the 87 patients enrolled in the study were current smokers.

Are there really two sets of standards as to how we select patients for surgical and non-surgical interventions? The answer may pertain more to past history of medical practice and philosophy than to science. The concept of risks and benefits is certainly more tangible in surgical than in medical interventions, whereas cost-effectiveness has yet to be assimilated by most patients, health care providers and, often, third-party payers.

## Guidelines

What do guidelines issued by official organizations say about the selection of smokers in respiratory rehabilitation programs? (7,43,44). Most are nondirective as to how to deal with COPD patients still actively smoking (Table 26.1). However, the guidelines all emphasize the opportunity of smoking cessation interventions in smokers accepted for pulmonary rehabilitation.

## Results of Surveys

From our survey of pulmonary rehabilitation programs in Canada conducted in 1998 (45), we found that the majority of the programs (80%) accepted current smokers. However, only one third of the programs offered smoking cessation interventions as part of the rehabilitation. The situation was similar in the United States in 1993 (46): 83% of the pulmonary rehabilitation programs allowed patients who were still smoking at the time of entry to participate in the program. 52 percent of the programs stated that a smoking cessation program was offered by the pulmonary rehabilitation team. From both surveys, it appears that there is a discrepancy between the means offered to many patients involved in rehabilitation and its goals. Smoking cessation is certainly an objective of early prevention (table 26.2). If smoking cessation is not a pre-requisite to full rehabilitation, smoking cessation interventions should, at least, be offered as part of the program.

## Conclusions

Those who fund and provide health care should be challenged to identify and implement the best approaches to the prevention as well as the management of COPD. These strategies include continuing antismoking campaigns (primary prevention), early detection and intervention on those individuals at risk for the late consequences of COPD (secondary prevention), and the widespread application of effective therapeutic modalities in reducing the complications of the disease (tertiary prevention). Respiratory rehabilitation clearly falls in the latter category of interventions whereas smoking cessation falls in the second one. Smoking cessation interventions should logically be offered before respiratory rehabilitation. Those programs

**Table 26.1  Guidelines for Patients Selection for Pulmonary Rehabilitation Regarding Active Smokers**

| | |
|---|---|
| American Thoracic Society (43) | Although including current cigarette smokers in a pulmonary rehabilitation program remains a subject of debate, it is reasonable to consider enrolling these individuals, particularly if they are participating actively in a smoking cessation program. (page 1670) |
| European Respiratory Society (7) | Well-organized criteria of rehabilitation will provide a multidisciplinary team with a medical supervisor. Usually, their recommendation for electing patients is that optimal therapy is already conducted on nonsmoking patients or patients actively involved in a smoking cessation programme. (page 744) |
| American Association of Cardiopulmonary Rehabilitation (44) | Current smoking status has been used by some programs as a consideration in accepting or denying patients' participation. Some programs exclude active cigarette smokers from participating in pulmonary rehabilitation, believing that they are less motivated and committed than the non- or ex-smokers. If active smokers are accepted, smoking cessation is a major goal of the rehabilitation process. (page 15) |

**Table 26.2    Levels of Prevention and Associated Health Interventions in COPD**

| Level of prevention | Objective | Intervention |
|---|---|---|
| Primary | Removal of risk factors | Anti-smoking campaigns |
| Secondary | Early detection and treatment of COPD | Population-based screening of COPD |
| | | Smoking cessation programs |
| Tertiary | Decrease in complications of COPD | Education |
| | | Vaccination |
| | | Long-term oxygen therapy |
| | | Respiratory rehabilitation |

who accept current smokers should at least provide smoking cessation interventions as a routine and even mandatory component of rehabilitation. Otherwise, they should review the cost-effectiveness of their intervention.

# References

1. US Public Health Service: US Public Health Service, Smoking and Health. Report of the Advisory Committee to Surgeon General of the Public Health Services. Washington, DC, US Department of Health, Education and Welfare, Public Health Service, Center for Disease Control. PHS Publication No. 1103, 1964.
2. Bartecchi CE, MacKenzie TD, Schrier RW. The human cost of tobacco use. *N Engl J Med* 1994; 330: 907-12 (part 1); 330: 975-80 (part 2).
3. Peto R, Lopez AD, Boreham J, et al. Mortality from tobacco in developed countries: indirect estimation from national vital statistics. *Lancet* 1992; 339: 1268-78.
4. Samet JM. Health benefits of smoking cessation. *Clin Chest Med* 1991; 12: 669-79.
5. Department of Health and Human Services. Reducing the health consequences of smoking: 25 years of progress. A report of the Surgeon General. Office of Smoking and Health, Washington D.C.: U.S. Government Printing Office, 1989; DHHS Publication No. (CDC) 89-8411.
6. Fishman AP. Pulmonary rehabilitation research. *Am J Respir Crit Care Med* 1994; 149: 825-33.
7. Donner CF, Muir JF, Rehabilitation and Chronic Care Scientific Group of the European Respiratory Society. Selection criteria and

programmes for pulmonary rehabilitation in COPD patients. *Eur Respir J* 1997; 10: 744-57.
8. ACCP/AACVPR Pulmonary Rehabilitation Guidelines Panel. Pulmonary rehabilitation: Joint ACCP/AACVPR evidence-based guidelines. *Chest* 1997; 112: 1363-96.
9. Lacasse Y, Goldstein RS. Smoking cessation in comprehensive pulmonary rehabilitation (letter). *Lancet* 1997; 349: 285.
10. Lacasse Y, Wong E, Guyatt GH, King D. Cook DJ, Goldstein RS. Meta-analysis of respiratory rehabilitation in chronic obstructive pulmonary disease. *Lancet* 1996; 348: 1115-9.
11. Goldstein RS, Gort EH, Stubbing D, Avendano MA, Guyatt GH. Randomised controlled trial of respiratory rehabilitation. *Lancet* 1994; 344: 1394-7.
12. Vallet G, Varray A, Fontaine JL, et al. Interest of individualized training program at the ventilatory threshold in mild to moderate COPD patients. *Rev Mal Resp* 1994; 11: 493-501.
13. Make BJ. Pulmonary rehabilitation: myth or reality? *Clin Chest Med* 1986; 7: 519-40.
14. Fletcher C, Peto R. The natural history of chronic airflow obstruction. *Br Med J* 1977; i: 1645-8.
15. Woolf CR, Zamel N. The respiratory effects of regular cigarette smoking in women: a five-year prospective study. *Chest* 1980; 78: 707-13.
16. Tager IB, Segal MR, Speizer FE, Weiss ST. The natural history of forced expiratory volumes: effect of cigarette smoking and respiratory symptoms. *Am Rev Respir Dis* 1988; 138: 837-49.
17. Buist AS, Nagy JM, Sexton GJ. The effect of smoking cessation on pulmonary function: a 30-month follow-up of two smoking cessation clinics. *Am Rev Respir Dis* 1979; 120: 953-7.

18. Lange P, Groth S, Nyboe J, Mortensen J, Appleyard M, Jensen G, Schnohr P. Effects of smoking and changes in smoking habits on the decline of FEV1. *Eur Respir J* 1989; 2: 811-6.

19. Tashkin DP, Clark VA, Coulson AH, Simmons M, Bourque LB, Reems C, Detels R, Sayre JW, Rokaw SN. The UCLA population studies of chronic obstructive pulmonary disease. VIII. Effects of smoking cessation on lung function: a prospective study of a free-living population. *Am Rev Respir Dis* 1984; 130: 707-15.

20. Camilli AE, Burrows B, Knudson RJ, Lyle SK, Lebowitz MD. Longitudinal changes in forced expiratory volume in one second in adults: effects of smoking and smoking cessation. *Am Rev Respir Dis* 1987; 135: 794-9.

21. Anthonisen NR, Connett JE, Kiley JP, Altose MD, Bailey WC, Buist AS, Conway WA, Enright PL, Kanner RE, O'Hara P, Owens GR, Scanlon PD, Tashkin DP, Wise RA, for the *Lung Health Study* Research Group. Effects of smoking intervention and the use of an inhaled anticholinergic bronchodilator on the rate of decline of FEV1: the *Lung Health Study. JAMA* 1994; 272: 1497-505.

22. Maltais F, LeBlanc P, Jobin J, Casaburi R. Peripheral muscle dysfunction in chronic obstructive pulmonary disease. *Clin Chest Med* 2000; 21: 665-77.

23. Lacasse Y, Guyatt GH, Goldstein RS. The components of a respiratory rehabilitation program: a systematic overview. *Chest* 1997; 110: 1077-88.

24. Hsia CCW. Respiratory function of hemoglobin. *N Engl J Med* 1998; 338: 239-47.

25. Calverley PM, Leggett RJ, McElderry L, Flenley DC. Cigarette smoking and secondary polycythemia in hypoxemic cor pulmonale. *Am Rev Respir Dis* 1982; 125: 507-10.

26. Orlander J, Kiessling KH, Larsson L. Skeletal muscle metabolism, morphology and function in sedentary smokers and nonsmokers. *Acta Physiol Scand J* 1979; 107: 39-46.

27. Fletcher CM, Peto R, Tinker C, Speizer FE. The natural history of chronic bronchitis and emphysema: an eight-year study of early chronic obstructive lung disease in working men in London. New York. Oxford University Press; 1976: 272.

28. Fiore MC, Bailey WC, Cohen SJ, et al. Treating tobacco use and dependence. Clinical practice guideline. Rockville, MD: US Department of Health and Human Services. Public Health Service. June 2000.

29. Lancaster T, Stead L, Silagy C, Sowden A, for the Cochrane Tobacco Addiction Review group. Effectiveness of interventions to help people stop smoking: findings from the Cochrane Library. *Brit Med J* 2000; 321: 355-8.

30. The Smoking Cessation Clinical Practice Guideline Panel and Staff. The Agency for Health Care Policy and Research smoking cessation clinical practice guideline. *JAMA* 1996; 275: 1270-80.

31. Smith SS, Jorenby DE, Fiore MC, et al. Smoking cessation: what's new since the AHCPR guideline? *J Respir Dis* 1998; 19: 412-26.

32. Pederson LL, Wanklin JM, Lefcoe NM. The effects of counseling on smoking cessation among patients hospitalized with chronic obstructive pulmonary disease: a randomized clinical trial. *Int J Addictions* 1991; 26: 107-19.

33. Emmons KM, Goldstein MG. Smokers who are hospitalized: a window of opportunity for cessation interventions. *Prev Med* 1992; 21: 262-9.

34. Orleans CT, Kristeller JL, Gritz ER. Helping hospitalized smokers quit: new directions for treatment and research. *J Consult Clin Psychol* 1993: 61: 778-89.

35. Young P, Dewse M, Fergusson W, Kolbe J. Respiratory rehabilitation in chronic obstructive pulmonary disease: predictors of nonadherence. *Eur Respir J* 1999; 13: 855-9.

36. Connor MC, O'Driscoll MF, McDonnell TJ. Should patients with chronic obstructive pulmonary disease (COPD) who express a desire to stop smoking be enrolled in pulmonary rehabilitation? *Eur Respir J* 1999; 14 (suppl.): 263S.

37. Singh SJ, Vora VA, Morgan MDL. Does pulmonary rehabilitation benefit current and nonsmokers? *Am J Respir Crit Care Med* 1999; 159: A764.

38. American Society for Translplant Physicians, American Thoracic Society, European Respiratory Society, International Society for Heart and Lung Transplantation. International guidelines for the selection of lung transplant candidates. *Am J Respir Crit Care Med* 1998; 158: 335-9.

39. American Thoracic Society. Lung volume reduction surgery. *Am J Respir Crit Care Med* 1996; 154: 11541-2.

40. Russi EW, Stammberger U, Weder W. Lung volume reduction surgery for emphysema. *Eur Respir J* 1997; 10: 208-18.

41. Cornette A, Petitdemange I, Briancon S, Burlet C, Polu JM. Assessment of smoking in patients with severe chronic respiratory failure treated with oxygen for long periods at home (French). *Rev Mal Respir* 1996; 13: 405-11.

42. Medical Research Council Party. Long-term domiciliary oxygen therapy in chronic hypoxic cor pulmonale complicating chronic bronchitis and emphysema. *Lancet* 1981; i: 681-6.

43. American Thoracic Society. Pulmonary rehabilitation—1999. *Am J Respir Crit Care Med* 1999: 159: 1666-82.

44. American Association of Cardiovascular and Pulmonary Rehabilitation. Guidelines for pulmonary rehabilitation programs. 1998; Champaign, Human Kinetics.

45. Brooks D, Lacasse Y, Goldstein RS. Pulmonary rehabilitation programs in Canada: national survey. *Can Respir J* 1999; 6: 55-63.

46. Bickford LS, Hodgkin JE, McInturff SL. National pulmonary rehabilitation survey: update. *J Cardiopulmonary Rehabil* 1995; 15: 406-11.

PART X

# Exercise Prescription: Special Considerations

# Chapter 27

# Exercise Training Above the Ischemic Threshold in Stable Coronary Patients

Martin Juneau, MD, Canada

Current recommendations for exercise training in coronary patients state that if exercise-induced ischemia is present, the heart rate during exercise training should be 10 beats/minute lower than that associated with significant ischemia (1). Unfortunately, this recommendation does not allow a sufficient training stimulus for some patients with a relatively low ischemic threshold.

Although there is limited information on exercise training above the ischemic threshold in coronary patients (2), we have conducted two clinical trials looking at the safety of exercise training in this setting. In the first study, troponin T levels were measured to document the possibility of myocardial damage before and after exercise training above the ischemic threshold while the second study is a retrospective analysis of all coronary events that occurred in our institution since 1991 according to the exercise training intensity.

## Exercise Training Above the Ischemic Threshold: Measurement of Troponin T

### Material and Methods

Elevated plasma troponin T is the most sensitive and specific marker of myocardial damage (3). Troponin T levels increase rapidly after acute coronary events but not after marathon running (4). In this first tudy, the cohort consisted of 21 patients with documented coronary artery disease defined as coronary stenosis of 70% or more of the lumen diameter at coronary angioplasty, previously documented myocardial infarction, or reversible perfusion defect on thallium or 99Tc Sestamibi scintigraphic exercise testing.

All patients demonstrated exercise-induced ST depression greater or equal to1 mm during standard exercise testing using a RAMP protocol. Excluded from study were patients with recent myocardial infarction, unstable angina, coronary artery bypass surgery or percutaneous transluminal coronary angiography in the prior 3 months, heart failure, hypertension with or without left ventricular hypertrophy on resting ECG, serious arrhythmias or baseline electrocardiographic abnormalities that could interfere with the interpretation of the ST segment. Patients requiring digitalis were also excluded.

The ischemic threshold was defined as the heart rate at which a 1 mm ST depression appeared on a baseline treadmill symptom-limited exercise test. ECG leads CM5, CC5 and CL were continuously monitored and a complete ECG was recorded every 30 seconds to determine as precisely as possible the onset of 1 mm or more ST segment depression. The ST segment was measured 0.08 seconds after the J point in three consecutive QRS complex with a flat baseline and R waves of equal amplitude.

Two exercise training sessions of 20 minutes each were scheduled at least 48 hours apart and both sessions were performed on the same treadmill used for the exercise test. The intensity of the first exercise training session was fixed at a heart rate below the ischemic threshold, i.e., approximately 10 beats/minute lower than the heart rate associated with the appearance of 1 mm ST depression.

The intensity of the second exercise session was fixed at a heart rate above the ischemic threshold, i.e., at a heart rate associated with a ST segment depression of 1 mm or more. The speeding grades of the treadmill were constantly adjusted to maintain the required exercise training heart rate and ST segment response at all times during both exercise training sessions. Blood samples for creatine kinase (CK), CK-MB, and troponin T were collected before, 6 hours and 24 hours after each training session. CK (N <195 IU/L ) and CK-MB (N <30 IU/L) levels were determined with reagents of Boehringer. Troponin T was measured with an enzyme-linked immunosorbent assay of Boehringer Mannheim using polyclonal antibodies (normal <0.1 ng/mL).

## Results

During the symptom-limited exercise test, the heart rate and systolic blood pressure at the ischemic threshold were 115±14 beats/minute and 176±20 mmHg (table 27.1) respectively.

The mean heart rate during the exercise session below the ischemic threshold was 91±13 beats/minute which corresponds to 65% of the mean maximal heart rate achieved during baseline symptom-limited exercise testing (table 27.2). This heart rate was 24 beats/minute lower than the heart rate at the onset of ischemia. The mean level of ST segment

depression was 0.5±0.2 mm. Total CK, CK-MB and troponin T did not increase 6 and 24 hours after the exercise session (table 27.3).

The mean heart rate recorded during the exercise session above the ischemic threshold was 120±20 beats/minute corresponding to 85% of the maximal heart rate and was 5 beats/minute above the heart rate at the onset of ischemia. The mean level of ST segment depression during this exercise session was 1.4±0.5 mm and constant ECG monitoring confirmed that ST depression equalled or was more than 1 mm at all times.

No clinical events or symptoms occurred during these sessions and no arrhythmias were recorded. Blood measurements at 6 and 24 hours after exercise did not show any increase in total CK, CK-MB and troponin T. In fact, these values remained well under the lower limit associated with myocardial damage.

We concluded that in this group of stable coronary patients, exercise training above the ischemic threshold for 20 minutes did not result in myocardial damage.

## Coronary Events Associated With Exercise Training Above or Below the Ischemic Threshold: A Retrospective Analysis

According to a 1995 review by Fletcher et al., the risk of sudden cardiac arrest during exercise training in patients with known coronary disease ranges from 1 in 6000 patient-hours of training (5) to 1 in 121,955 (6) patient-hours with an average of 1 in 59,142 patient-hours of training. Since 1991, we have been prescribing exercise training in coronary patients regardless of the occurrence of ischemia at 65

**Table 27.1   Baseline Exercise Test Results**

| | |
|---|---|
| Heart rate at ischemic threshold (bpm) | 115 ± 14 |
| Systolic blood pressure at ischemic threshold (mmHg) | 176 ± 20 |
| Maximal heart rate (bpm) | 140 ± 18 |
| Maximal systolic blood pressure (mmHg) | 197 ± 21 |
| Maximal exercise tolerance (mets) | 8.7 ± 1.5 |

Values are mean ±SD.

**Table 27.2   Exercise Test Parameters Below and Above the Ischemic Threshold**

| | Below ischemic threshold | Above ischemic threshold | P value |
|---|---|---|---|
| Heart rate (bpm) | 91.0 ± 13.0 | 120.0 ± 20.0 | <0.0001 |
| Systolic blood pressure (mmHg) | 155.0 ± 15.0 | 185.0 ± 16.0 | <0.0001 |
| METS | 3.4 ± 0.7 | 5.1 ±1.2 | <0.001 |
| ST depression (mm) | 0.5 ± 0.2 | 1.4 ± 0.5 | <0.001 |

Values are mean ± SD.

**Table 27.3  Troponin T Measurements**

|  | Below ischemic threshold | Above ischemic threshold |
|---|---|---|
| Before training (ng/mL) | 0.009 ± 0.009 | 0.014 ± 0.011 |
| 6 hours post-training (ng/mL) | 0.015 ± 0.008 | 0.014 ± 0.012 |
| 24 hours post-training (ng/mL) | 0.011 ± 0.008 | 0.011 ± 0.007 |

Values are means ± SD.

to 85% of the maximal heart rate achieved on a symptom-limited exercise test. We reviewed the charts of 605 patients with documented coronary disease. One hundred and fifty patients trained above the ischemic threshold for a period of 3 months to 10 years with a total of 55,000 patient-hours of training. Only one coronary event was documented and this event consisted of sudden cardiac arrest. Fortunately, the patient was successfully resuscitated. In this patient, significant ST segment depression had occurred at a heart rate of 112 bpm on the previous treadmill test and the target heart rates for training were between 86 and 113 bpm (maximal heart rate on the previous symptom-limited treadmill test was 133 bpm). It is therefore reasonable to assume that in this individual, exercise training occurred mostly without significant ischemia.

One hundred and thirty patients trained under the ischemic threshold for a total of 45,000 patient-hours and one of them experienced a brutal syncope with spontaneous recovery.

Three hundred and twenty-five patients with coronary disease but without exercise-induced ischemia trained for a total of 100,000 patient-hours. Two coronary events were noted and these consisted of one sudden cardiac arrest which was successfully managed, and one sudden death. In this group, the risk of sudden death was therefore 1 per 50,000 patient-hours of training.

In this preliminary analysis, exercise training above the ischemic threshold did not result in more documented coronary events than exercise training without exercise-induced ischemia.

## Conclusion

The measurement of troponin T after training above the ischemic threshold and our clinical experience suggest that exercise training above the ischemic threshold appears to be safe and allows for optimal training stimulus for coronary patients. Further studies however will be needed before modifying the current recommendations for exercise training in coronary patients with exercise-induced ischemia.

## References

1. Fletcher GF, Balady G, Froelicher VF, Hartley LH, Haskell WL, Pollock ML: Exercise standards: A statement for healthcare professionals from the American Heart Association. *Circulation* 1995;91:580-615.
2. Ades PA, Grunvald MH, Weiss RM, Hanson JS: Usefulness of myocardial ischemia as predictor of training effect in cardiac rehabilitation after acute myocardial infarction or coronary artery bypass grafting. *Am J Cardiol* 1989; 63:1032-1036.
3. Antman ME, Braunwald E: Acute myocardial infarction. In: Braunwald E, ed. *Heart Disease— A Textbook of Cardiovascular Medicine*, ed 5. Philadelphia: Saunders, 1997:1184-1288.
4. Cummins P, Young A, Auckland ML, Michie CA, Stone PCW, Shepstone BJ: Comparison of serum cardiac specific troponin-I with creatine kinase, creatine kinase-MB isoenzyme, tropomyosin, myoglobin and C-reactive protein release in marathon runners: Cardiac or skeletal muscle trauma? *Eur J Clin Invest* 1987; 17:317-324.
5. Fletcher GF, Cantwell JD: Ventricular fibrillation in a medically supervised cardiac exercise program: Clinical, angiographic and surgical correlations. *JAMA* 1977;238:2627-2629.
6. Van Camp SP, Peterson RA: Cardiovascular complications of outpatient cardiac rehabilitation programs. *JAMA* 1986;256:1160-1163.

# Chapter 28

# Resistance Training for Health, Chronic Disease and Rehabilitation: An Update

Barry A. Franklin, PhD, Adam de Jong, MA, USA

In 1995, an expert panel examined the scientific literature regarding the effects of multifactorial cardiac rehabilitation services, including medical evaluation, prescribed exercise, coronary risk reduction, and education, counseling and behavioral interventions (1). Twelve of the 334 studies that were reviewed pertained to the application of resistance testing and training in the rehabilitation of patients with coronary artery disease (CAD). Seven of the 12 studies involved strength training regimens, including four randomized controlled trials (2-5) and three nonrandomized controlled studies (6-8), whereas the remaining five were reports of cross-sectional comparisons of the electrocardiographic and hemodynamic responses to strength testing versus treadmill exercise testing (9-13). Although these studies involved a relatively small number of selected, clinically stable patients (n = 242), results suggested that strength testing and training was safe and effective for this population.

In most of the strength-training studies, circuit weight training was generally added to the physical conditioning regimens of middle-aged and older men with CAD who had already been aerobically trained, generally for 3 months or more. Three 30-60-minute strength-training sessions were typically undertaken each week, and programs varied from 6 to 26 weeks. All studies reported significant improvements in weight-carrying tolerance (time), increases in skeletal muscle strength and endurance, or both, with comparable benefits for high (80% of one-repetition maximum [1-RM]) versus moderate (40-50% 1-RM) training intensities (8). Moreover, two of three randomized controlled trials found that aerobic exercise tolerance was improved to a greater extent with combined aerobic and resistance training as compared with aerobic training alone (2,5), whereas the other study reported no significant difference (4).

The five strength testing studies demonstrated that resistance exercise resulted in significantly lower rate-pressure products than did maximal treadmill testing. Moreover, the former was also associated with a lesser frequency of angina pectoris, ischemic ST segment depression, and threatening ventricular arrhythmias (10,11,13). Increased subendocardial perfusion, secondary to elevated diastolic blood pressure, may contribute to the lower incidence of ischemic responses during resistance training as compared with dynamic exercise testing (13-15). Others have previously demonstrated that the myocardial oxygen supply/demand relationship appears to be favorably altered by superimposing static on dynamic effort, so that ischemic electrocardiographic responses are attenuated at rate pressure product values that elicit significant ST segment depression during dynamic exercise (16,17).

Although the above-referenced studies were important in changing the cautious attitude toward strength training for coronary patients, particularly in regard to vocational counseling and exercise prescription, most involved small numbers of low-risk male patients, 70 years or younger, with normal or near normal aerobic fitness and left ventricular function. Consequently, the generalizability of these results to other populations of coronary or cardiac patients (e.g., women, older patients of both genders with low aerobic fitness, and patients with left ventricular dysfunction) remained unclear. Since publication of the Clinical Practice Guideline (Cardiac Rehabilitation) (1), several studies have addressed these populations and expanded our knowledge regarding the application of resistance testing or training in patients with and without cardiovascular disease. This chapter largely emphasizes new information (i.e., since 1995) on the benefits, rationale, safety, and prescription of resistance training in men and women, with specific reference to varied patient populations.

## Benefits of Resistance Training

Traditionally, resistance exercise has been primarily viewed as a means of improving muscular strength and endurance. However, increasing evidence now suggests that weight training, like aerobic endurance exercise, can promote substantial benefits in physical fitness and health-related factors. The American College of Sports Medicine (18), American Heart Association (19), American Association of Cardiovascular and Pulmonary Rehabilitation (20), and the Surgeon General's Report on Physical Activity and Health (21) all include resistance training and complementary stretching as integral components of a comprehensive physical conditioning program.

The rationale to support resistance training in fitness programs for healthy adults and clinically stable patients with CAD stems from several lines of evidence. Resistance training is highly effective in developing and maintaining muscle strength and endurance, muscle mass, and physical function, which may be helpful in reducing the susceptibility to falls in elderly persons (21,22). It is also of value in the prevention and treatment of obesity, expending calories via an increase in lean body mass and basal metabolism, and in the management of other chronic conditions (e.g., low back pain, osteoporosis, sarcopenia, diabetes). Moreover, regular resistance training may have favorable effects on metabolism and coronary risk factors, including glucose tolerance, insulin sensitivity, serum lipids/lipoproteins, and resting blood pressure (23-26).

Although it is widely believed that resistance training programs offer little or no benefit to cardiovascular function, this notion has now been dispelled. Because the pressor response to static exertion is proportionate to the relative intensity (percent of maximal voluntary contraction [MVC]) (figure 28.1) (27), duration, and muscle mass involved (28-30), increased muscular strength should

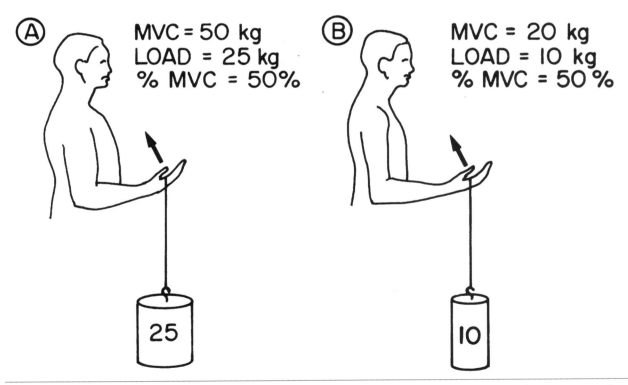

**Figure 28.1**   The hemodynamic response to resistance exercise is proportional, at least in part, to the percentage of maximal voluntary contraction (% MVC) of the muscle group involved. The heart rate and blood pressure response depends on the tension exerted relative to the greatest tension possible in the muscle group (MVC). A high degree of tension exerted by a stronger person (A) will produce approximately the same rate-pressure product as a low tension representing an equivalent relative tension (% MVC) developed by a weaker person (B), if all other factors are equal.

**Table 28.1 Hemodynamic Responses at Identical Loads\* Before and After Weight Training⁺**

| Variables | Pre | Post |
|---|---|---|
| Heart rate (beats/min) | 108 ± 4 | 94 ± 2** |
| Systolic blood pressure (Torr) | 247 ± 14 | 206 ± 9** |
| Diastolic blood pressure (Torr) | 156 ± 9 | 116 ± 5** |
| Rate-pressure product (mm Hg × beats/min × $10^{-2}$) | 268 ± 22 | 196 ± 12** |

\* = Following 10 reps of the double leg press at 80% of the pretraining one-repetition maximum. \*\* = Significantly lower ($p < 0.05$) than pretraining. ⁺ = Adapted from McCartney N, et al. (31).

result in an attenuated heart rate and systolic blood pressure response to any given load because the load now represents a lower percentage of the MVC. One 12-week strength training study of 15 healthy, older men (X ± SE age = 66.3 ± 0.8 years) demonstrated a marked attenuation of the hemodynamic responses after training during repeated lifting of identical loads (table 28.1) (31). These findings suggest that resistance training can decrease cardiac demands during daily activities like carrying groceries or lifting moderate to heavy objects.

Resistance training can also increase muscular endurance capacity without an accompanying increase in maximal oxygen consumption ($\dot{V}O_2max$). In one study, $\dot{V}O_2max$ during treadmill and cycle ergometer testing remained essentially unchanged after a heavy resistance training program (5 days a week for 10 weeks), despite a 40% increase in muscular strength; however, submaximal endurance time to exhaustion increased with both testing modalities, 12% and 47%, respectively (32). Similarly, Ades et al. (33) reported that 12 weeks of resistance-training in 24 healthy, older men and women increased submaximal walking endurance time by 38%. These studies suggest that endurance is not a function of aerobic exercise alone, but can be significantly enhanced by increased muscle strength and/or girth.

## Special Patient Populations

Although the safety and effectiveness of resistance training has, for the most part, been demonstrated in young and middle-aged men and low risk patients with CAD, several recent studies suggest that these benefits may be extrapolated to other populations, including middle-aged and older men and women, post-myocardial infarction (MI) patients, those who have undergone coronary revascularization, and individuals with left ventricular dysfunction. A more comprehensive description of resistance exercise testing and prescription protocols for these patient subsets, and the associated training outcomes, is available elsewhere (34).

## Middle-Aged and Older Men and Women

The role of resistance training in women's health/fitness and rehabilitation programs has been the subject of several recent investigations. To clarify the chronic musculoskeletal adaptations to varied resistance training protocols, Marx et al. (35) randomized 34 healthy, untrained women to one of the following groups: a low-volume, single-set circuit resistance training group (n = 12); a high-volume, periodized multiple-set resistance training group (n = 12); and, a nonexercising control group (n = 10). The training groups performed one set of 8-12 repetitions to volitional fatigue 3 days/week, or two to four sets of 3-15 repetitions with periodized volume and intensity, 4 days/week. Body composition and muscular performance testing was conducted at baseline and after 12 and 24 weeks of training. Although significant improvements in muscular performance were noted in both training groups over the short-term, the multiple-set group demonstrated greater increases in upper and lower body strength, power, speed, and high-intensity local muscle endurance as compared with the single-set group training group at 24 weeks. Similar findings have been reported in men (36,37), which challenge the notion that single and multiple set programs yield comparable benefits, at least over the long term.

Sarcopenia (i.e., loss of skeletal muscle mass that normally accompanies aging) is one of the major reasons for impaired muscle performance and the loss of functional independence in elderly people. This is especially noteworthy since the Framingham Heart Study found that about half of women over age 65 could not lift 10 pounds! To what extent these age-related changes can be counteracted by lifestyle interventions, such as increasing the level of physical activity has, until recently, remained unclear.

Resistance training can augment muscular strength and endurance in both men and women of all ages by 25% to 100%, depending on the training stimulus and initial level of strength (38). Moreover, some of the greatest improvements have been reported in elderly people. One study of 10 elderly men and women who ranged in age from 87 to 96 years, in a noncardiac rehabilitation setting, showed that high-intensity strength training improved average muscle strength, walking speed, and mid-thigh muscle girth by 174%, 48%, and 9%, respectively (39). Other contemporary studies have reported significant increases in type II fiber area and skeletal muscle hypertrophy in healthy, elderly women following resistance training programs (40,41).

To evaluate the cardiovascular tolerance of healthy elderly subjects to weight-lifting exercises, Bermon et al. (42) studied 32 men and 33 women between the ages of 65 and 80 who performed two sets of 12 repetitions and four sets of five repetitions on three resistance training devices (horizontal leg press, seated chest press, and bilateral leg extension). Hemodynamic strain and myocardial tolerance were assessed by measuring heart rate and blood pressure responses continuously during exercise, and cardiac troponin I blood concentrations before and 6 hours postexercise. Although there were significant increases in the exercise systolic and diastolic blood pressures, as well as heart rate, especially during the horizontal leg press, serum enzymes heralding myocardial damage or necrosis remained unchanged. The investigators concluded that older men and women could perform resistance training without clinical, electrocardiographic, or biological signs or symptoms of myocardial ischemia, if appropriate selection criteria and proper respiratory techniques during exercise were employed.

Recently, investigators reported on the effects of a 6-month program of home-based resistance training, complemented by selected aerobic components (e.g. stairclimbing) in an 85-year-old woman with a history of severe CAD and chronic heart failure (43). Training loads were initiated in the range of 30% to 40% of 1-RM, using fabricated weights (i.e., canned foods loaded in a handled canvas bag). Five different exercises were performed (biceps curls, upright rowing, lower leg extension, shoulder presses, and squats) for one set of 10 to 15 repetitions; this regime was progressed to 2 sets after 1 month of exercise, and weight loads were increased as tolerated. The subject experienced a 5% increase in lean body mass, whereas isokinetic leg extension, handgrip strength, and measured $\dot{V}O_2$max increased 58%, 15%, and 36%, respectively. Improvements were also noted in the subject's capacity to perform ac-

tivities of daily living and general well-being (i.e., four of eight components on the Medical Outcomes Study Short Form-36) (44), along with a decreased geriatric depression score (7/15 to 3/15 [clinical depression suggested by 5/15]) (45). The investigators concluded that these favorable results, in a single subject, may warrant expansion of the intervention to a controlled clinical trial.

## Post-MI and Coronary Revascularization Patients

Exercise-based cardiac rehabilitation programs are designed to return patients to daily occupational and leisure-time activities to the greatest extent possible. Although aerobic exercise has traditionally served as the predominant mode of training, many activities of daily living require significant amounts of muscular strength and endurance. Until recently, however, few data were available regarding the safety and effectiveness of adjunctive weight training soon after acute coronary events or interventions.

Stretching or flexibility exercises can begin as early as 1 and 2 days after coronary bypass surgery or uncomplicated acute MI, respectively (19). Low-intensity resistance training (e.g., elastic resistance bands, light [2 to 5 pound] hand weights) should probably not begin sooner than 2 to 3 weeks post-MI (20). Nevertheless, many clinically stable patients can safely perform static-dynamic activity equivalent to carrying up to 30 pounds at this time (46). After the convalescence stage of recovery, usually 4 to 6 weeks post-MI, regular barbells, weight machines, or both, may be initiated. On the other hand, surgical patients should probably avoid traditional resistance training exercises (with moderate-to-heavy weights), which may cause pulling on the sternum within 3 months of coronary artery bypass surgery or sternotomy (19).

Adding a low-to-moderate intensity (20% to 60% of 1-RM) resistance training program to aerobic exercise in low-risk men as soon as 4 to 6 weeks post-MI has been shown to improve aerobic fitness and muscle strength more than endurance exercise alone, without eliciting signs or symptoms of myocardial ischemia, abnormal hemodynamics, adverse changes in left ventricular function and structure, and cardiovascular complications (47,48). Average improvements in muscular strength were similar for patients performing 20 reps at 20% of 1-RM versus those performing 7 reps at 60% of 1-RM, 10.5% and 13.5%, respectively (48). Collectively, these randomized, controlled trials suggest that the timeline between acute MI and the restoration and enhancement of aerobic fitness and strength may be dramatically shortened by complementing endurance exercise with resistance training, even at very low intensities (i.e. 20% of 1-RM). Such findings have important clinical significance when higher risk patient populations are referred for rehabilitation therapy.

## Patients With Congestive Heart Failure

Numerous studies have now shown that aerobic exercise training improves endurance capacity in patients with congestive heart failure (CHF) (49). Nevertheless, such exercise would be expected to have only minimal effects on the skeletal muscle wasting that commonly occurs with CHF, accounting for a high percentage of the individual variation in aerobic fitness. Until recently, there has been reluctance in applying resistance training to this population. This reluctance, no doubt, stems from the increase in systemic vascular resistance and the concomitant decrease in left ventricular ejection fraction and stroke work index that occurs during sustained isometric exercise, indicating acute overload of the left ventricle (50,51). In contrast, a recent comparison of the cardiovascular responses to resistance exercise with steady-state submaximal cycle ergometry at the same relative intensity (70% of 1-RM versus 70% of peak $\dot{V}O_2$) in patients with CHF demonstrated a lower rate-pressure product and a higher diastolic blood pressure during the former, suggesting a more favorable myocardial oxygen supply/demand relationship (52). Other studies of resistance exercise in well-compensated CHF patients (i.e. on optimal drug therapy) have shown an increased left ventricular stroke work index and decreased systemic vascular resistance, suggesting enhanced left ventricular function (53). Although muscular hypertrophy may not necessarily occur in these patients, increases in muscle motor unit recruitment and/or the frequency of impulses within a single motor unit may play an important role in improving the patient's physical work capacity for occupational and leisure-time activities (54).

Recently, investigators examined the effects of combined aerobic and resistance training in 14 outpatients (mean age = 57 years) with advanced CHF (mean ± SD ejection fraction = 29 ± 10%) over a 6-month duration (80 sessions) (55). The physical training program involved 3 sessions/week, including 30 minutes of aerobic exercise at 60% $\dot{V}O_2$ max.

Resistance training included 3 sets of 15 repetitions at 60% to 80% of 1-RM on 6 different upper and lower extremity devices. Both endurance and strength were periodically re-evaluated and progressively increased. Strength improved by 25% for knee extensors and 18% for knee flexors, whereas $\dot{V}O_2$ max increased 10%. There were no untoward events or medical complications as a result of the training regimen, and compliance was 89%.

Aside from the physical benefits of resistance training in clinically stable patients with CHF, the potential psychological benefits should also be considered. Activity restrictions from symptomatic CHF often lead to a decreased quality of life and depression, further diminishing the patient's rehabilitative potential and motivation to exercise. Patients with CHF undergoing an innovative home-based walking and resistance training program demonstrated significant improvements in symptoms of fatigue, dyspnea and quality of life parameters (e.g. emotional function and mastery) and an excellent exercise adherence (90%), with no adverse cardiovascular events (56). These benefits occurred in the absence of appreciable fitness improvements, suggesting that other factors may contribute to the patient's perception of symptoms and well-being.

In summary, incorporating resistance training into a traditional regimen of aerobic exercise in stable patients with CHF may provide important physiological and/or psychological benefits, including reduced symptoms and improved muscular strength, peak $\dot{V}O_2$, and quality of life. Resistance training programs for CHF patients should be individually prescribed, medically supervised, and carefully monitored for signs or symptoms of myocardial ischemia and malignant ventricular arrhythmias. Intensity and muscle group specificity should be the primary considerations, utilizing segmental exercises involving single or small peripheral muscle groups to avoid the high cardiovascular stress that can occur during multiple muscle-group training. The prescribed regimen should include short exercise bouts of 10 to 12 repetitions/set at intensities up to 60% to 80% of 1-RM (52,53), allowing for a rest period approximating twice that of the work period (54).

## Exercise Prescription for Resistance Training

Although the traditional prescription involved performing 3 sets of each exercise at 10 repetitions per set, a recent review suggested that one set provides nearly the same improvement in muscular strength and endurance, at least over the short term (57). Consequently, for unfit individuals beginning a resistance training regimen, single set programs to volitional fatigue, using weight loads that approximate 50 ± 10% of 1-RM, are recommended over multiple set because they are highly effective and less time consuming. Because ~ 75% of the improvement that occurs with a 3-days-per-week resistance training program can be attained with a 2-day-per week schedule, novice lifters are advised to start with the latter and, if time permits, progress to the former (57). Such regimens should include 8 to 10 different exercises (e.g., chest press, should press, triceps extension, biceps curl, pull-down [upper back], lower back extension, abdominal crunch/curl-up, quadriceps extension or leg press, leg curls [hamstrings], calf raise) at a load that permits 8 to 12 repetitions for healthy participants younger than 50 to 60 years of age and 10 to 15 repetitions at a lower relative resistance for cardiac patients and healthy older participants (figure 28.2). The increased repetition range at a lower relative effort for more fragile patients is designed for injury prevention.

Although contemporary resistance exercise guidelines continue to focus on the value of single set, low-to-moderate intensity training, especially during the initial weeks of a weight lifting regimen, high-intensity strength training (60% to 80% of 1-RM), especially when combined with aerobic exercise, has been shown to be safe and effective in varied patient populations, including subsets of high-risk cardiac patients (58-60). Such programs facilitate significant improvements in muscular strength, local muscle endurance, treadmill time and body composition, enabling participants to complete activities of daily living at lower levels of perceived exertion. In one study, coronary patients enrolled in a high-intensity strength training regimen demonstrated significant improvements in self efficacy, mood states, and overall perceptions of physical and emotional well being when compared with their flexibility-trained control counterparts (60).

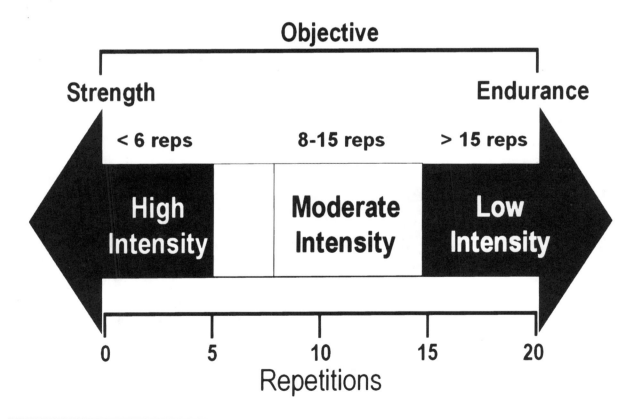

**Figure 28.2**  Classification of weight training intensity (resistance). A moderate training intensity will generally facilitate improvements in muscular strength and endurance, considering age and health status.

## Patient Eligibility/Contraindications

Eligibility criteria for resistance training are similar to those used for the endurance component of adult fitness or exercise-based cardiac rehabilitation programs (19). Most previous strength-training studies involved small numbers of low-risk male patients with CAD who had normal or near-normal aerobic fitness and left ventricular function. Moreover, circuit weight training was generally added to the physical conditioning programs of coronary patients who had already undergone 3 or more months of aerobic exercise training (1). The extent to which these data can be generalized to other populations of coronary patients (e.g. low-level angina, patients with permanent pacemakers or an implantable cardioverter defibrillator, cardiac transplant recipients) remains unclear. Accordingly, these patient subsets may require more careful evaluation, progression, and initial and serial surveillance.

Absolute contraindications to traditional resistance training (i.e. using weight loads corresponding to >50% of 1-RM) include unstable angina, stage 2 or 3 hypertension (systolic blood pressure >160 mmHg and/or diastolic blood pressure >100 mmHg), uncontrolled atrial and/or threatening ventricular dysrhythmias, a recent history of CHF that has not been evaluated and effectively treated, severe stenotic or regurgitant valvular disease, and hypertrophic cardiomyopathy (19). It should be emphasized that these contraindications have been developed as guidelines, and that a patient's participation in moderate-to-high intensity weight training should be contingent on approval of the medical director or his or her internist or cardiologist. Many programs, however, have adopted a more flexible approach for high risk patients or those with absolute contraindications to traditional resistance training. Oftentimes, body weight (calisthenics), rubber band or spring devices, pulley weights, light dumbbells or wrist weights, or fabricated weights (e.g. canned foods loaded in a handled canvas bag) can be safely adapted for such program participants.

## Summary and Conclusions

Patients with and without CAD require a minimum level of strength for daily living and functional independence. Unfortunately, many individuals lack the physical strength to perform common tasks like rising from a chair, carrying groceries, or opening windows. Resistance training, even at low-to-moderate intensities (i.e., 20-40% of 1-RM), can provide a safe and effective method for improving muscular strength and endurance, favorably modifying body composition and coronary risk factors, and enhancing self-efficacy and psychosocial well-being. Following a resistance training program, the rate-pressure product is reduced when lifting any given load (31). Thus, strength training can decrease cardiac demands during daily activities requiring upper extremity efforts (e.g. lifting or carrying objects). Because long-term compliance remains a problem for exercise-based preventive and rehabilitative programs, resistance training can provide a means for maintaining interest and diversity. Nevertheless, it should serve as a complement to, rather than a replacement for, the patient's aerobic exercise prescription.

## References

1. Wenger NK, Froelicher ES, Smith LK, et al: Cardiac Rehabilitation. Clinical Practice Guideline No. 17. Rockville, MD: U.S. Department of Health and Human Services, Public Health Service, Agency for Health Care Policy and Research and the National Heart, Lung, and Blood Institute. AHCPR Publication No. 96-0672. October 1995.

2. Kelemen MH: Resistance training safety and essential guidelines for cardiac and coronary prone patients. *Med Sci Sports Exerc* 1989;21:675-677.

3. Wilke NA, Sheldahl LM, Levandoski SG, Hoffman MD, Dougherty SM, Tristani FE: Transfer effect of upper extremity training to weight carrying in men with ischemic heart disease. *J Cardiopulmonary Rehabil* 1991;11:365-372.

4. Butler RM, Palmer G, Rogers FJ: Circuit weight training in early cardiac rehabilitation. *J Am Osteopath Assoc* 1992;92:77-89.

5. McCartney N, McKelvie RS, Haslam DR, Jones NL: Usefulness of weightlifting training in improving strength and maximal power output in coronary artery disease. *Am J Cardiol* 1991;67:939-945.

6. Sparling PB, Cantwell JD, Dolan CM Niederman RK: Strength training in a cardiac rehabilitation program: a six-month follow-up. *Arch Phys Med Rehabil* 1990;71:148-152.

7. Stewart KJ, Mason M, Kelemen MH: Three-year participation in circuit weight training improves muscular strength and self-efficacy in cardiac patients. *J Cardiopulmonary Rehabil* 1988;8:292-296.

8. Crozier Ghilarducci LE, Holly RG, Amsterdam EA: Effects of high resistance training in coronary artery disease. *Am J Cardiol* 1989;64:866-870.

9. Amos KR, Porcari JP, Bauer SR, Wilson PK: The safety and effectiveness of walking with ankle weights and wrist weights for patients with cardiac disease. *J Cardiopulmonary Rehabil* 1992; 12:254-260.

10. Faigenbaum AD, Skrinar GS, Cesare WF, Kraemer WJ, Thomas HE: Physiologic and symptomatic responses of cardiac patients to resistance exercise. *Arch Phys Med Rehabil* 1990;71:395-398.

11. Featherstone JF, Holly RG, Amsterdam EA: Physiologic response to weight lifting in coronary artery disease. *Am J Cardiol* 1993;71:287-292.

12. Schram V, Hanson P: Cardiovascular and metabolic responses to weight-loaded walking in cardiac rehabilitation patients. *J Cardiopulmonary Rehabil* 1988;8:28-32.

13. Sheldahl M, Wilke NA, Tristani FE, Kalbfleisch JH: Response of patients after myocardial infarction to carrying a graded series of weight loads. *Am J Cardiol* 1983;52:698-703.

14. De Busk RF, Valdez R, Houston N, Haskell W: Cardiovascular responses to dynamic and static effort soon after myocardial infarction: Application to occupational work assessment. *Circulation* 1978;58:368-375.

15. Kerber RE, Miller RA, Najjar SM: Myocardial ischemic effects of isometric, dynamic and combined exercise in coronary artery disease. *Chest* 1975;67:388-394.

16. De Busk R, Pitts W, Haskell W, Houston N: Comparison of cardiovascular responses to static-dynamic effort and dynamic effort alone in patients with chronic ischemic heart disease. *Circulation* 1979;59:977-984.

17. Bertagnoli K, Hanson P, Ward A: Attenuation of exercise-induced ST depression during combined isometric and dynamic exercise in coronary artery disease. *Am J Cardiol* 1990;65:314-317.

18. American College of Sports Medicine position stand: the recommended quantity and quality of exercise for developing and maintaining cardiorespiratory and muscular fitness and flexibility in healthy adults. *Med Sci Sports Exerc* 1998;30:975-991.

19. Pollock ML, Franklin BA, Balady GJ, et al: Resistance exercise in individuals with and without cardiovascular disease: benefits, rationale, safety, and prescription. *Circulation* 2000;101: 828-833.

20. American Association of Cardiovascular and Pulmonary Rehabilitation. Guidelines for Cardiac Rehabilitation and Secondary Prevention Programs. Ed. 3. Champaign, IL: Human Kinetics; 1999.

21. US Department of Health and Human Services: Physical Activity and Health: A Report of the Surgeon General. Atlanta, GA: US Department of Health and Human Services, Centers for Disease Control and Prevention, National Center for Chronic Disease Prevention and Health Promotion; 1996.

22. Fiatarone MA, Evans WJ: The etiology and reversibility of muscle dysfunction in the aged. *J Gerontol* 1993;48:77-83.

23. Pollock ML, Vincent KR: Resistance training for health. The President's Council on Physical Fitness and Sports Research Digest. December 1996; Series 2, No. 8.

24. Goldberg L, Elliot LD, Schutz RW, Kloster FE: Changes in lipid and lipoprotein levels after weight training. *JAMA* 1984;252:504-506.

25. Hurley BF, Hagberg JM, Goldberg AP, et al: Resistive training can reduce coronary risk factors without altering $VO_2$ max or percent body fat. *Med Sci Sports Exerc* 1988;20:150-154.

26. Harris KA, Holly RG: Physiologic response to circuit weight training in borderline hypertensive subjects. *Med Sci Sports Exerc* 1987;19:246-252.

27. Lind AR, Taylor SH, Humphreys PW, Kennelly BM, Donald KW: Circulatory effects of sustained voluntary muscle contraction. *Clin Sci* 1964;27:229-244.

28. Mitchell JH, Payne FC, Saltin B, Schibye B: The role of muscle mass in the cardiovascular response to static contractions. *J Physiol* 1980;309: 45-54.

29. Buck JA, Amundsen LR, Nielsen DH: Systolic blood pressure responses during isometric contractions of large and small muscle groups. *Med Sci Sports Exerc* 1980;12:145-147.

30. Seals DR, Washburn RA, Hanson PG, Painter PL, Nagle FJ: Increased cardiovascular response to static contraction of larger muscle groups. *J Appl Physiol* 1983;54:434-437.

31. McCartney N, McKelvie RS, Martin J, Sale DG, MacDougall JD: Weight-training-induced attenuation of the circulatory response of older males to weight lifting. *J Appl Physiol* 1993;74:1056-1060.

32. Hickson RC, Rosenkoetter MA, Brown MM: Strength training effects on aerobic power and short-term endurance. *Med Sci Sports Exerc* 1980;12:336-339.

33. Ades PA, Ballor DL, Ashikaga T, Utton JL, Nair KS: Weight training improves walking endurance in healthy elderly persons. *Ann Intern Med* 1996;124:568-572.

34. Resistance Training for Health and Rehabilitation. Graves JE, Franklin BA, eds. Champaign, IL: Human Kinetics, 2001.

35. Marx JO, Ratamess NA, Nindl BC, et al: Low-volume circuit versus high-volume periodized resistance training in women. *Med Sci Sports Exerc* 2001;33:635-643.

36. Kramer JB, Stone MH, O'Bryant HS, et al: Effects of single vs. multiple sets of weight training: impact of volume, intensity, and variation. *J Strength Cond Res* 1997;11:143-147.

37. Fleck SJ: Periodized strength training: a critical review. *J Strength Cond Res* 1999;13:82-89.

38. Fleck SJ, Kraemer WJ: Designing Resistance Training Programs. Ed. 2. Champaign, IL: Human Kinetics; 1997.

39. Fiatarone MA, Marks EC, Ryan ND, Meredith CN, Lipsitz LA, Evans WJ: High-intensity strength training in nonagenarians: effects on skeletal muscle. *JAMA* 1990;263:3029-3034.

40. Charette SL, McEvoy L, Pyka G, et al: Muscle hypertrophy to resistance training in older women. *J Appl Physiol* 1991;70:1912-1916.

41. Sipilä S, Suominen H: Effects of strength and endurance training on thigh and leg muscle mass and composition in elderly women. *J Appl Physiol* 1995;78:334-340.

42. Bermon S, Rama D, Dolisi C: Cardiovascular tolerance of healthy elderly subjects to weight-lifting exercises. *Med Sci Sports Exerc* 2000;32:1845-1848.

43. King PA, Savage P, Ades PA: Home resistance training in an elderly woman with coronary heart disease. *J Cardiopulmonary Rehabil* 2000;20:126-129.

44. Stewart AL, Hays RD, Ware JE: The MOS short-form general health survey: reliability and validity in a patient population. *Med Care* 1988;26:724-735.

45. Yesavage JA, Brink TL, Rose TL: Development and validation of a geriatric depression screening scale: a preliminary report. *J Psychiatr Res* 1983:17;37-49.

46. Wilke NA, Sheldahl LM, Tristani FE, et al: The safety of static-dynamic effort soon after myocardial infarction. *Am Heart J* 1985;110:542-545.

47. Stewart KJ, McFarland LD, Weinhofer JJ, Cottrell E, Brown CS, Shapiro EP: Safety and efficacy of weight training soon after acute myocardial infarction. *J Cardiopulmonary Rehabil* 1998;18:37-44.

48. Daub WD, Knapik GP, Black WR: Strength training early after myocardial infarction. *J Cardiopulmonary Rehabil* 1996;16:100-108.

49. American College of Sports Medicine: ACSM's Guidelines for Exercise Testing and Prescription. Ed. 6. Franklin BA, Howley E, Whaley M, eds. Baltimore, MD: Lippincott Williams and Wilkins, 2000.

50. Elkayam U, Roth A, Weber L, et al: Isometric exercise in patients with chronic advanced heart failure: hemodynamic and neurohumoral evaluation. *Circulation* 1985;72:975-981.

51. Reddy HK, Weber KT, Janicki JS, McElroy PA: Hemodynamic, ventilatory and metabolic effects of light isometric exercise in patients with chronic heart failure. *J Am Coll Cardiol* 1988;12:353-358.

52. McKelvie RS, McCartney N, Tomlinson C, Bauer R, MacDougall JD: Comparison of hemodynamic responses to cycling and resistance exercise in congestive heart failure secondary to ischemic cardiomyopathy. *Am J Cardiol* 1995;76:977-979.

53. Meyer K, Hajric R, Westbrook S, et al: Hemodynamic responses during leg press exercise in patients with chronic congestive heart failure. *Am J Cardiol* 1999;83:1537-1543.

54. Meyer K: Exercise training in heart failure: recommendations based on current research. *Med Sci Sports Exerc* 2001;33:525-531.

55. Delagardelle C, Feiereisen P, Krecké R, Essamri B, Beissel J: Objective effects of a 6 months' endurance and strength training program in outpatients with congestive heart failure. *Med Sci Sports Exerc* 1999;31:1102-1107.

56. Oka RK, DeMarco T, Haskell WL, et al: Impact of a home-based walking and resistance training program on quality of life in patients with heart failure. *Am J Cardiol* 2000;85:365-369.

57. Feigenbaum MS, Pollock ML: Strength training: rationale for current guidelines for adult fitness programs. *The Physician and Sportsmedicine* 1997;25(2):44-64.

58. Beniamini Y, Rubenstein JJ, Faigenbaum AD, Lichtenstein AH, Crim MC: High-intensity strength training of patients enrolled in an outpatient cardiac rehabilitation program. *J Cardiopulmonary Rehabil* 1999;19:8-17.

59. Adams KJ, Barnard KL, Swank AM, Mann E, Kushnick MR, Denny DM: Combined high-intensity strength and aerobic training in diverse phase II cardiac rehabilitation patients. *J Cardiopulmonary Rehabil* 1999;19:209-215.

60. Beniamini Y, Rubenstein JJ, Zaichkowsky LD, Crim MC: Effects of high-intensity strength training on quality-of-life parameters in cardiac rehabilitation patients. *Am J Cardiol* 1997;80:841-846.

Chapter 29

# Beneficial Impact of Exercise In Subjects With Diabetes and Heart Disease

Paul Poirier, MD, Carmen Paquette, BSc, Bruno Pilote, RN, Peter Bogaty, MD, Canada

## Introduction

Diabetes mellitus is among the top 5 causes of mortality in industrialized countries and there is increasing evidence that diabetes mellitus is attaining epidemic proportions in the third world (1). Diabetes mellitus is found in most countries and epidemiological studies suggest that without appropriate prevention, the incidence and prevalence will grow tremendously worldwide (1). Complications associated with diabetes, which are mainly coronary artery disease, peripheral arterial disease, stroke, neuropathy, renal disease and retinopathy, result in increased morbidity, reduced life expectancy and implicate enormous costs to the health system (2). Therefore, diabetes mellitus may well become the major health problem of the 21$^{st}$ century. Diabetes mellitus is characterized by abnormal glucose metabolism with hyperglycemia resulting from blunted insulin secretion/action. Chronic hyperglycemia results in long-term organ damage (kidney, eye, nerve, heart and arteries).

Diabetes mellitus is frequent and meets the criteria of a major public health problem which are: 1) a very high morbidity, 2) a chronic progressive condition, and 3) an uncontrolled situation of an underestimated gravity (2,3). Subjects are often asymptomatic during the decade prior to diagnosis and discovery is often associated with complications characteristic of the disease (2). During this long insidious undiagnosed period, diabetes mellitus is literally ravaging the organism. Indeed at the time of diagnosis, 15-20% of subjects already have significant retinopathy whereas 5 to 10% have proteinuria (2). Diabetes mellitus is associated with obesity and there is a strong familial aggregation but the exact genes involved are yet to be well defined (4). In 1997, type 2 diabetes mellitus represented the vast majority of cases of diabetes (97%) (1). Diabetes is destined to become an increasing problem in most countries because of the worldwide tendency to adopt deleterious lifestyles (decreased physical activity with increasing obesity, unhealthy choices of food). Most patients with type 2 diabetes will die of cardiovascular disease (5). In terms of public health, the cost associated with diabetes mellitus may be alleviated with appropriate and judicious screening and aggressive management (2,6-12) since the prognosis of subjects with diabetes is influenced by the duration of the condition and the adequacy of metabolic control (7,8,10,13). Life expectancy is reduced by 5 to 10 years and the mortality rate is approximately twice that of populations without diabetes (1,2,14). Importantly, increased mortality is found similarly in both men and women (14).

## Prevention of Type 2 Diabetes

Prospective studies have reported factors associated with increased risk of developing type 2 diabetes (15-18). These include age, ethnicity, obesity (particularly abdominal obesity), sedentarity, gestational diabetes, coronary artery disease, elevated fasting insulin levels and glucose intolerance (19,20). Two non-randomized studies have shown that dietary guidance with aerobic exercise may reduce the incidence of diabetes by 25 to 50% over a 6-year period (21,22). These findings from Sweden (22) and China (21) have been recently confirmed. The Finnish Diabetes Prevention Study Group has nicely shown with a randomized prospective protocol and a mean duration of three years that weight loss of ~5% combined with increased physical activity decreased the cumulative incidence of diabetes by 58% (23). Of interest is that in subjects who did not lose weight, 4 hrs of weekly exercise was associated with a significant reduction in the risk of diabetes (23). Consequently, weight control, healthy alimentation and daily physical activity should be strongly recommended in individuals with glucose intolerance or type 2 diabetes. In general terms, prevention aims at maintaining good health while avoiding acute and chronic complications. There is good evidence that near normal glycemia and improvement of lipid profile reduces microvascular complications and coronary artery disease manifestations (7,10,13,24). Nevertheless, silent ischemia and myocardial infarction are frequent and are associated with increased morbidity and mortality in patients with type 2 diabetes compared to patients without diabetes (25,26). Indeed, following an acute myocardial infarction, patients with diabetes demonstrate increased predisposition to heart failure and recurrent myocardial infarction with decreased survival (25,26).

## Physical Activity, Exercise and Type 2 Diabetes

Active lifestyle favors good cardiovascular health and well-being, increases insulin sensitivity, reduces arterial blood pressure and improves lipid profile in subjects with and without diabetes (27-29). Gradual and regular practice of physical activity may help to better control blood glucose and reduce the need for hypoglycemic drugs in patients with type 2 diabetes. There is, however, an equilibrium between the advantages and risks of physical activity in this particular population. For example, patients with type 2 diabetes with macroangiopathy are vulnerable to ischemic events (cardiac and non cardiac) and arrhythmias. Patients with proliferative retinopathy may be at risk of bleeding whereas patients with peripheral neuropathy are vulnerable to foot lesions. Some of these aspects will be discussed further.

Aerobic exercise training has long been considered an important part of the treatment of subjects with type 2 diabetes (30,31). Lawrence et al. were among the first to report the impact of exercise on blood glucose in subjects with diabetes treated with insulin (30). Even if the beneficial effects of regular physical activity are well established in non-diabetic populations, the literature is less abundant and conclusive in patients with type 2 diabetes (32,33). Moreover, even if walking seems to be the activity of choice, it has been reported that individuals with

type 2 diabetes are less prone to be regularly active in comparison to their non-diabetic counterparts (34% vs. 41% respectively) (34). As stated before, regular physical exercise in subjects with type 2 diabetes is associated with improvement in co-morbidities associated with diabetes (arterial blood pressure, lipid profile and insulin sensitivity) and contributes to generate weight loss and weight maintenance (29). The following sections will specifically review the available literature.

## Impact of Regular Physical Activity on Diabetes Prevention

The goal of primary prevention is to eliminate or lessen the incidence of a disease i.e. apparition of new cases in the population. Numerous prospective epidemiological studies have demonstrated that regular physical activity prevents the occurrence of diabetes (16,17,35-40).

After adjustment for age, baseline glycemia, body mass index (BMI), triglyceride levels, family history and alcohol consumption, physical activity at $\geq 5.5$ METs over a 40 minute period per week was associated with a reduced risk (56%) of the development of diabetes (41). Less intense activity (< 5.5 METs), whatever the duration, was not protective. More precisely, $\dot{V}O_2 max \geq 31$ ml/kg/min was protective. Moreover, a subgroup of high risk obese and hypertensive men, with a positive family history, had a more reduced risk (64%) with the practice of physical activity at moderate intensity ($\geq 5.5$ METs, 40 minutes/week) (41).

The association between regular vigorous exercise and incidence of type 2 diabetes was also evaluated prospectively in a cohort of 87,253 women aged 34-59 years (40). After an 8-year follow-up, women who were involved in vigorous activity at least once a week demonstrated a reduction in the relative risk (RR: 0.67) of developing diabetes compared to sedentary women. After adjusting for BMI, physical activity was still beneficial in protecting from the development of diabetes (RR: 0.84). In this study, there was no dose-response physical activity effect (40). Inexplicably, risk of developing diabetes appeared similar between obese and non-obese women. Furthermore, age and positive family history did not significantly influence the protective effect of physical activity on the onset of diabetes. Another study from a cohort composed of 21,271 men reported that men who practice one hour of physical activity per week diminish their risk of developing diabetes by 29%, independently of age and BMI (17).

The study of Helmrich et al. (Alumni Health Study) showed that an energy expenditure of 2000 Kcal/week was associated with a 24% decrease in the risk of developing diabetes over a 14-year period (39). An energy expenditure of 2000 Kcal corresponds to a 1-hour daily walk. In the same study, the incidence of diabetes was almost halved (26.3 to 13.7 case/1000 patients-years) when the physical activity index increased from < 500 Kcal/week to > 3500 Kcal/week (39). Finally, the Cooper clinic study (8633 men) confirmed the same findings (42). After a 6-year follow-up, men within the group with lower cardiorespiratory fitness ($\dot{V}O_2$max) presented 3.7 times the risk of developing diabetes compared to the better-trained group. This relation was adjusted for age, BMI, blood pressure, triglyceride levels and positive family history of diabetes (42).

Taken together with the recent findings from the Finnish group that has been previously discussed (23), these results in different groups reinforce the notion that individuals at high risk of developing diabetes should be highly encouraged to maintain a minimum of regular physical exercise in their daily lives (43).

## Impact of Acute Aerobic Exercise on Glycemic Control

In subjects with type 2 diabetes, exercise may help lower blood glucose levels. Indeed, regular exercise is considered to be one of the cornerstones in the management of blood glucose in patients with type 2 diabetes. Nonetheless, this well-established notion is not that clearly defined in the literature. It has been demonstrated in subjects with type 2 diabetes that hepatic glucose production is decreased during exercise (44,45). The decrease in hepatic glucose production is not related to lower glucagon, cortisol or growth hormone levels (44,45). Besides, glucose uptake in lower limbs as evaluated by vein and femoral artery catheterization, is higher in subjects with type 2 diabetes compared to controls (46). At rest, a higher proportion of splanchnic glucose production is derived from neoglucogenesis in subjects with type 2 diabetes whereas during exercise, glucose production is mainly via glycogenolysis at a rate similar to that in subjects without diabetes (46). Therefore, hepatic glucose production is derived from glycogenolysis but peripheral uptake, which is higher than production, generates a net

decrement in blood glucose (46). However, this adaptation in glucose metabolism during exercise does not operate equally in every individual with type 2 diabetes and may be heterogeneous (44,45). In the study by Jenkins et al., fasting subjects with type 2 diabetes experienced a decrease, an increase or no change in blood glucose levels. The authors suggested that hepatic feedback from blood glucose levels is altered in subjects with type 2 diabetes resulting in an erratic blood glucose response to exercise and hepatic insulin resistance results in an abnormal balance between glucose production and peripheral glucose utilization in subjects with type 2 diabetes (45). Of note, however, there are some technical problems associated with isotopic glucose tracers in subjects with type 2 diabetes i.e. distribution volume being increased in these subjects (47).

Numerous studies have investigated the impact of one aerobic exercise session on blood glucose in subjects with type 2 diabetes (44-46,48-54). In contrast to the belief of most health care professionals, the blood lowering influence of a single exercise session is modest in subjects with type 2 diabetes (~1.5 mmol/l) (46,49,50,53-55), or even inexistent when exercise is performed in the fasting state (45,52). However, the higher the blood glucose levels at the beginning of exercise, the higher the blood glucose lowering effect of exercise (49). Since exercise may potentially induce hypoglycemia in subjects with type 2 diabetes treated with sulphonylureas, health care professionals are generally reluctant to encourage the patient to exercise in the fasting state. In contrast, a study has reported that hypoglycemia defined as blood glucose < 3.3 mmol/l, occurred in 5 subjects out of 98 who exercised in the postprandial state with medication taken the morning of the exercise session (54). Several reports have evaluated the impact of exercise with type 2 diabetes in the fasting state (44-46,49,50,52) with hypoglycemic drug interruption for a significative period before the exercise study (45,46,49). However, this is not representative of the real life situation for subjects with type 2 diabetes who exercise regularly. Only two studies have investigated the impact of exercise in subjects with type 2 diabetes in the postprandial state (48,54). Larsen et al. studied blood glucose responses after a meal (breakfast) with and without exercise in subjects with type 2 diabetes (48). They found that exercise enhances the blood glucose response compared to control (without exercise). Of interest, all subjects were controlled with diet alone and blood glucose returned to baseline before the next meal (lunch) in both situations (48). Consequently, these findings may not be representative of subjects with type 2 diabetes with more important insulin resistance necessitating treatment with oral hypoglycemic agents. From a clinical viewpoint, the latter population is rather worrisome for the health care professional when the time comes to prescribe exercise.

Therefore, the nutritional status of the subject (fasting vs. postprandial state) is primordial for the health care professional. This is important since the vast majority of subjects with type 2 diabetes exercise in the postprandial state because of the fear of exercise-induced hypoglycemia in the fasting state (29,56,57). Surprisingly, in the literature (44,46,49,50, 52,53,55), there is no report of exercise-induced hypoglycemia when subjects with type 2 diabetes were exercising in the fasting state (45). Surprisingly, little information is available regarding the glucose level changes that occur in subjects with type 2 diabetes after an acute bout of exercise in relation to the time interval from the last meal. Exercise-induced hypoglycemia in subjects with type 2 diabetes treated with sulphonylureas is a practical concern since there is a potentially increased risk of hypoglycemia with exercise in patients with type 2 diabetes on sulphonylurea therapy. Again, the risk is generally perceived by clinicians to be greater when ex-

ercise is performed in the fasted state (45,49,53). In addition, in daily life, physical exercise is usually performed in the postprandial rather than in the fasted state. Because hypoglycemia can precipitate myocardial ischemia (58), knowledge about the expected decline in blood glucose following exercise is important.

We evaluated the influence of the time interval from the last meal on the blood glucose response to exercise in men with type 2 diabetes (n = 1045 exercise sessions) (59). There was no change in blood glucose levels when individuals were in the fasted state (8.1 ± 0.2 vs. 8.1 ± 0.1 mmol/l, mean ± SE, before vs. after exercise, respectively). However, blood glucose decreased by 28 ± 1% at 0-1 hr, 33 ± 1% at 1-2 hr, 35 ± 1% at 2-3 hr, 38 ± 2% at 3-4 hr, 43 ± 2% at 4-5 hr, and 23 ± 3% at 5-8 hr (all p<0.001). Thus 1 hour of ergocycle exercise has no significant clinical impact on blood glucose when performed in the fasted state in men with type 2 diabetes whereas a significant decrease in blood glucose should be expected when the same exercise is performed postprandially (figure 29.1). Of particular interest is that even if preexercise blood glucose levels were comparable in the fasted state and 5-8 hr postprandially, blood glucose levels decreased significantly

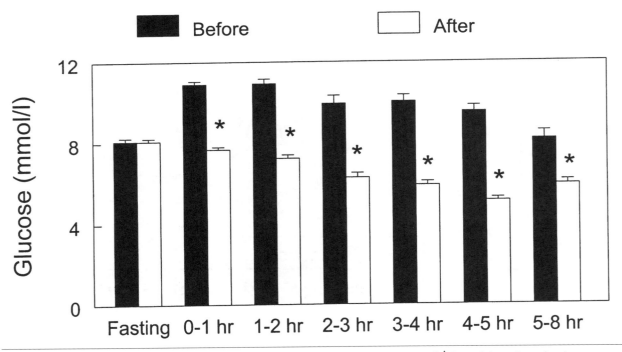

**Figure 29.1**    Glucose levels before and after one hour of aerobic exercise at 60% of $\dot{V}O_2$peak based on the time interval from the last meal (fasted overnight, n=80 sessions; 0-1 hr, n=351 sessions; 1-2 hr, n=254 sessions; 2-3 hr, n=88 sessions; 3-4 hr, n=126 sessions; 4-5 hr, n=102 sessions; and 5-8 hr, n=44 sessions). * = P < 0.001 before versus after. (From Poirier et al, *Journal Clinical Endocrinology Metabolism* 85:2860-2864, 2000)

only in subjects who were in the postprandial state (8.2 ± 0.4 decreasing to 6.0 ± 0.2 mmol/l, p<0.001). No subject suffered from clinical hypoglycemia during the exercise session. Of note, few exercise sessions (n = 14) ended with blood glucose ≤ 3.3 mmol/l (range: 2.8-3.3 mmol/l) and all of them were carried out in the postprandial state. Thus, importantly and contrary to a frequently held belief, the risk of a hypoglycemic event may be greater when subjects with type 2 diabetes performed exercise after a meal than in the fasted state (59). Blood glucose surveillance after exercise may have both safety and motivational features in subjects with type 2 diabetes. Long-term compliance to an exercise program tends to become low (28,60) and motivation needs to be reinforced. Lowering of blood glucose may be used as part of the motivation and knowledge about the degree of lowering that can be expected postprandially with exercise will help both in encouraging subjects to exercise regularly and in prescribing a safe exercise program. However, in addition to nutritional status, many other

factors such as the intensity and duration of the exercise session, type of treatment and metabolic control, may also influence the blood glucose response to exercise in subjects with type 2 diabetes.

To isolate the influence of dietary status on changes in blood glucose levels in subjects with type 2 diabetes, we evaluated the glucoregulatory response to 1 hr of exercise at 60% $\dot{V}O_2$ peak performed either in the fasted state or 2 hrs after a standardized breakfast in the same individuals in a random order (61). In accordance with previous results (59), we found that 1 hr of exercise in the fasting state has a minimal impact on blood glucose levels whereas prior breakfast enhances the glucose lowering effect of exercise (figure 29.2) (61). The higher insulin levels during exercise in the fed state have probably blunted hepatic glucose production, resulting in a glucose production/utilization imbalance and in a greater decrease in glucose blood levels (figure 29.3).

Published studies have evaluated the impact of exercise in subjects with type 2 diabetes using different exercise durations [20 minutes to 3 hours,

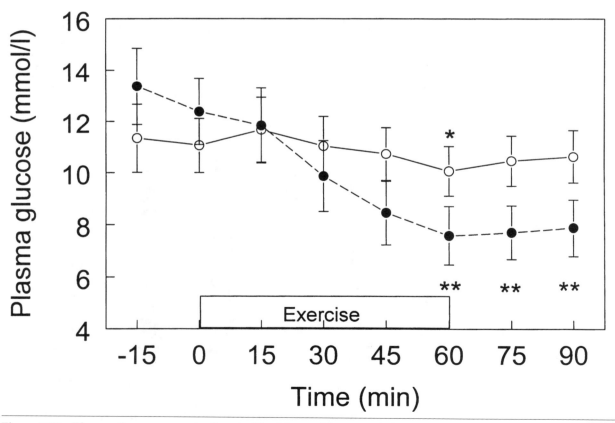

**Figure 29.2**   Plasma glucose concentrations in 10 subjects with type 2 diabetes in the fasted state (open symbols) and in the fed state (closed symbols) measured at 15-min intervals starting 15 minutes prior to exercise and up to 30 minutes after a 60-min exercise period. * = P < 0.01 baseline vs. after 60 minutes of exercise. ** = P < 0.001 vs baseline. (From Poirier et al, *Medicine Science Sports Exercise* 33:1259-1264,2001)

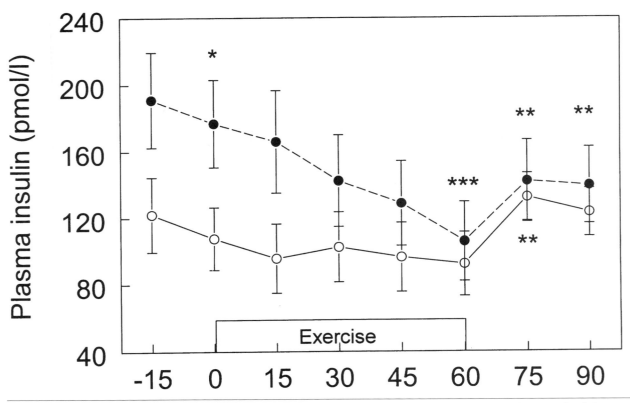

**Figure 29.3**   Plasma insulin in 10 subjects with type 2 diabetes in the fasted state (open symbols) and in the fed state (closed symbols) measured at 15-min intervals starting 15 minutes prior to exercise and up to 30 minutes after a 60-min exercise period. * = P < 0.05 fasted vs. fed state. ** = P < 0.01 baseline vs. recovery period (75 and 90 minutes). *** = P < 0.001 baseline vs. after 60 minutes of exercise. (From Poirier et al, *Medicine Science Sports Exercise*, 33:1259-1264,2001)

(51,55)] and intensities [40 to 70% of V̇O₂max (50-52)]. Heterogeneous diabetic populations were studied in terms of treatment [diet only (45,48,51)] and use of oral hypoglycemic agents (49,50). Interestingly, when sub-maximal exercise intensity is matched for exercise duration, the blood glucose response is comparable. Thus, it has been shown that changes in plasma glucose levels are similar following 70 min of exercise at 50% V̇O₂peak compared to 50 minutes at 70% of V̇O₂peak, which induced a similar negative caloric deficit (50).

## Effect of Exercise Training on Insulin Sensitivity

Numerous studies have reported beneficial results in term of glucose tolerance following aerobic exercise training (28,62-71), interval training (72,73), or weight resistance training in subjects with type 2 diabetes (74,75). On the other hand, other studies have not shown a beneficial impact of aerobic exer-

cise training on insulin sensitivity in older populations of subjects with type 2 diabetes (> 60 yr.) (57,60). In numerous studies (28,63-65,67,69-71,76,77), the specific impact of exercise training *per se* is difficult to appreciate since the concomitant weight loss by itself may favorably influence insulin sensitivity. Nevertheless, there is evidence that exercise training enhances insulin sensitivity in the absence of significative weight loss (62,64,66,68,71,72,74,78). However, insulin sensitivity was assessed using different techniques, which complicates interpretation of the results. Insulin sensitivity was evaluated with; 1) fasting glucose (28,60,63,65,70,73,75,77,79), 2) 50 to 100 g oral glucose tolerance test (60,62,64-66,68,72,73,75,76,78-82), 3) intra-venous glucose tolerance test (62,68,78), 4) glycated hemoglobin (28,57,63,65,67,68,74,75,77,78,80,83,84), 5) euglycemic hyperinsulinemic clamp study (69,72-74) and, 6) insulin tolerance test (57,63). Another important issue is the time interval separating the last exercise session from the time of evaluation of insulin sensitivity, enable one to dissociate the acute effect from the chronic effect of exercise (85).

Furthermore, individuals with type 2 diabetes are heterogeneous in terms of weight, diabetes duration and diabetes treatment. Numerous cohorts of lean subjects with type 2 diabetes were constituted (60,64,74,76,78), subjects treated with diet only (62,65,66,68,78) or with oral hypoglycemic agents (57,63,65,66,72,74). Moreover, it is well known that the medication used to treat concomitant pathologies associated with diabetes (hypertension and angina pectoris) may influence insulin sensitivity (57,65). Finally, only few studies have evaluated the effect of exercise in obese subjects with type 2 diabetes (57,63,69,70,72,73). Several studies have evaluated the impact of aerobic exercise training on insulin sensitivity in subjects treated with oral hypoglycemic agents (57,63,65,66,70,72,79). However, of these, only the study of Krotkiewski et al. used euglycemic hyperinsulinemic clamps (72). The exercise program was based on interval training and only 10/33 subjects were evaluated with the clamp. The characteristics of these 10 subjects were not reported. On the other hand, studies investigating in obese subjects with type 2 diabetes the impact of aerobic physical exercise without fat mass loss on insulin sensitivity are sparse and have reported no beneficial effect of exercise training on insulin sensitivity in obese subjects with type 2 diabetes (57,73). In contrast, using the glucose clamp technique, Trovati et al. reported increased insulin sensitivity in lean subjects with type 2 diabetes (73). Accordingly, some evidence suggests that in order to enhance insulin sensitivity in obese subjects with type 2 diabetes, exercise training must be associated with a substantial visceral fat loss (63,86). The additive effect of diabetes and obesity on insulin resistance may be too important to allow a beneficial response to an exercise training stimulus alone (73), in contrast to nonobese subjects with type 2 diabetes (51,68). Consistent with this concept, Kelley et al. (87) showed that, together with the impaired glucose transport associated with obesity, subjects with type 2 diabetes have additional impairment in glucose phosphorylation. This is supported by a study showing that 7 consecutive days of 50 minutes cycling at 70% $\dot{V}O_2$max improved insulin sensitivity in obese individuals without diabetes whereas no change was demonstrated in obese subjects with type 2 diabetes (79). The increase in skeletal muscle insulin sensitivity following aerobic physical training is largely attributable to the last exercise session and is short-lived (24-48 hrs) (85) and one exercise session increases hepatic insulin sensitivity for 12 to 16 hrs duration to reconstitute the glycogen reserve (85). Thus, it is essential to emphasize from an insulin sensitivity viewpoint that total energy expenditure is probably more important than exercise intensity or duration (79,84). Finally, the available evidence suggests that without weight loss or fat loss, the impact of exercise on insulin sensitivity is due to the residual effect of the last exercise session.

## Effect of Aerobic Exercise Training on Lipid Profile

Aerobic physical training may be beneficial in subjects without diabetes by increasing high-density lipoprotein (HDL) and decreasing low-density lipoprotein (LDL) and triglyceride (88). Of interest, Wood et al. compared the influence of diet-induced weight loss to exercise-induced weight loss in obese subjects. Fat mass loss was the better predictor of the increment in HDL-cholesterol and triglycerides following both experimental conditions (89). Thus, fat mass loss induced with exercise is important when evaluating the real influence of exercise on lipid profile in subjects with diabetes. There are numerous studies that have evaluated the impact of aerobic exercise training on lipid profile in subjects with type 2 diabetes (28,57,60,62,67,70-72,77,80,81,83,90-92). It is interesting to note that there was no beneficial impact of exercise training on total cholesterol and triglyceride levels in the absence of exercise training-induced weight loss (28,57,60,62,72,80,81,83,90), even after a strenuous training regimen (90). On the other hand all the studies inducing fat mass loss following the exercise training program regimen have demonstrated an improvement in lipid profile especially a fall in triglyceride levels (28,67,70,71,77,92). Weight loss in these studies is approximately 2 kg (28,92). Generally, the total cholesterol decrease is modest (4 to 13%) (67,91,92) and triglycerides decrement may reach 12 to 20% (28,70,83,92), but all these studies were associated with concomitant weight loss. Thus in subjects with type 2 diabetes, the beneficial impact of exercise training on lipid profile is also largely attributed to concomitant weight loss. Although body fat mass has been measured (80,91,93) or estimated (77,81) in some of these studies, the relationship between the training-induced changes in body fat mass and changes in the plasma lipid sub fractions in subjects with type 2 diabetes have been reported by our group. We examined the impact of a 6-month training program on the plasma lipid profile in men with type 2 diabetes treated with diet and oral hypoglycemic agents (94). In accordance with previous literature (28,67,70,71,77,92), our data indicate that fat loss, and not training *per se*, favorably alters the lipid profile of subjects with type 2 diabetes who participate in an aerobic physical conditioning program (94).

## Influence of Diabetes on the Cardiovascular System

In subjects with type 2 diabetes, regular exercise is associated with a decrease in both resting (28,67,70, 82,83) and exercise blood pressure (28,72) as well as a decrease in resting heart rate (70,83). In previous exercise training studies involving subjects with type 2 diabetes, it has been observed that these individuals exhibit lower maximal oxygen uptake ($\dot{V}O_2$max) than matched nondiabetic subjects (28,62, 64,78,95). This decrease in maximal exercise capacity does not appear to be associated with autonomic cardiac neuropathy or different lifestyle habits in subjects with and without diabetes (28). Even following a 3-month training program (3-4 sessions per week with a 40-60 minute duration per session), maximal capacity remains lower in subjects with type 2 diabetes (28). Although dysfunctional autonomic system regulation may alter the response to exercise (96,97), the decreased performance was demonstrated in subjects with type 2 diabetes both with

and without autonomic neuropathy (15,84,98,99) and exercise performance is altered both on ergocycle (96,99,100) and on treadmill (97,98). In subjects with diabetes, left ventricular (LV) diastolic dysfunction may be the first manifestation of diabetic cardiomyopathy (101-104). LV diastolic dysfunction has been shown to limit exercise performance in nondiabetic subjects. It has been shown that although age, gender and LV diastolic dysfunction influence exercise performance, in a step-wise multiple regression analysis, LV diastolic dysfunction was the most powerful predictor of $\dot{V}O_2$max (105).

We have investigated the role of LV diastolic dysfunction on exercise capacity using well-standardized echocardiographic technique in normotensive subjects with well-controlled type 2 diabetes mellitus (104,106,107). Although there were no differences in maximal heart rate, maximal systolic and diastolic blood pressures and maximal rate-pressure product at the end of exercise, exercise duration was decreased by 18% in subjects with type 2 diabetes with LV diastolic dysfunction compared to subjects with type 2 diabetes with normal LV diastolic function (108). As well, exercise performance expressed in METs was decreased by 17% in subjects with LV diastolic dysfunction compared to subjects with normal LV diastolic function (108) (Figure 29.4). As

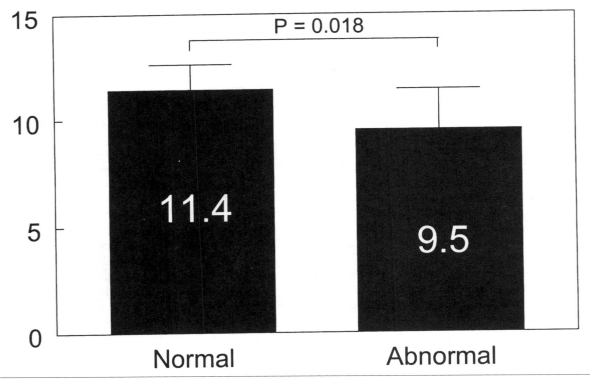

**Figure 29.4** Performance (METs) between subjects with well-controlled type 2 diabetes with normal and abnormal left ventricular diastolic function. (From Poirier et al, *American Journal Cardiology* 85:473-477, 2000).

postulated by other investigators (96,100,109), the observed differences were probably the result of a reduction in preload due to a decreased LV compliance. Finally, supporting the findings of a more invasive study (110), it has been observed that subjects with type 2 diabetes have an impaired cardiac output response to increasing workload compared to subjects without diabetes (111). Mechanistically, impaired LV diastolic function may increase pulmonary artery wedge pressure. This in turn could alter total lung perfusion as well as the distribution of pulmonary blood flow, and could induce relative pulmonary congestion. It may also be that a relatively fixed systolic volume induced by LV diastolic dysfunction limited cardiac output during maximal performance thus limiting $\dot{V}O_2$max. This mechanical constraint, which does not limit daily life activities, may become a limiting factor when a greater exercise performance is required.

## Discussion

Exercise is an essential part of the proper management of subjects with type 2 diabetes. Guidelines of the American Diabetes Association and the American College of Sports Medicine have been published recently (29,112). Since the vast majority of subjects with and without type 2 diabetes did not meet national standards for the practice of leisure physical activity (34), it is of major importance to reinforce the value of aerobic physical activity in the management of diabetes. The participation of the spouse is primordial for better long-term compliance (28). If our sedentary society is to change and become more active physically, health care institutions must educate the public about the guidelines regarding the quantity and type of exercise conductive to healthier life style. Epidemiological and observational studies have demonstrated the prophylactic value of aerobic exercise (27). Adults should practice 30 minutes or more daily of moderate physical activity (27). Moderate physical activity represents an activity corresponding to 3 to 6 METs i.e., equivalent to a brisk walk at 3-4 mph (4.8-6.4 km/hr) (27). In the particular context of diabetes, it is clear that the worldwide epidemic is, in part, secondary to a decrease in physical activity and to the increased prevalence of obesity. Therefore, promotion of exercise is a vital component of prevention and treatment of subjects with type 2 diabetes that should be considered a high priority.

Cardiovascular disease is the principal cause of mortality in subjects with type 2 diabetes (25). It is clear that diabetes is not a benign state and is associated with significant morbidity and mortality (113,114). This pathology is associated with several other risks factor for coronary heart disease (6). Blood pressure and lipid profile are very often abnormal in these individuals. Approximately 74% of subjects with diabetes show high blood pressure (> 140/90 mmHg) and 71% have total cholesterol >200 mg/dl (> 5.2 mmol/l) (2). These are reasons why changes in lifestyle should always be advocated as a nonpharmacological approach to prevent the onset, or assist in the management, type 2 diabetes (23). Nevertheless, the utilization of exercise in clinical practice is limited and several health care professionals are preoccupied by the risk-benefit ratio of exercise in this high-risk population (56,60). Indeed, when the patient presents with complications associated with diabetes, the role of exercise is generally neglected (33). The options and precautions in regard to exercise in individuals with type 2 diabetes suffering from complications are available (28,60). Thus, health care professionals should evaluate the advantages and limitations of exercise when it is time to prescribe an exercise regimen. Gradual increase in physical activity adapted to lifestyle must be an important aspect of treatment of every individual with type 2 diabetes. This approach must include an adapted exercise-training regimen in subjects with macrovascular disease, diabetic neuropathy or microvascular complications. The introduction of a program of vigorous physical exercise into the treatment regimen of subjects with type 2 diabetes requires health care professional interventions with specific evaluations. Subjects with type 2 diabetes who wish to exercise should wear appropriate shoes; examine their feet regularly and after each exercise session. Health care professionals should recommend avoiding exercise when metabolic control is unsatisfactory. Sugar should be absorbed before exercise if blood glucose is below 5 mmol/l and exercise should be avoided in extremely cold or hot temperatures (57,78). In subjects with type 2 diabetes, there are also psychological benefits to exercise (115). These benefits disappear 8 weeks after exercise training cessation (115). Individualized exercise programs with realistic goals will generally result in good compliance with better management of risk factors (70,115).

It is recommended that individuals with type 2 diabetes be evaluated by a health care professional before engaging in an exercise program. Thus, any individuals with type 2 diabetes older than 35 years or with diabetes duration longer than 10 years should have a complete medical examination with an exercise stress test (1,116). These precautions may unmask silent ischemia or manifestations of diabetes complications (28,33,60). Stress testing will provide information about maximal functional capacity and heart rate and blood pressure response to exercise (96,117-120). In individuals with non-specific ECG anomalies during the stress test, more specialized evaluation modalities should be considered like nuclear imaging or echocardiographic techniques (121-123).

In conclusion, exercise is associated with several benefits both from a metabolic and a cardiovascular viewpoint. Physical activity should be strongly advocated both in patients at high-risk of developing diabetes and in patients with overt diabetes. This is primordial since exercise has been shown to increase survival in men and women with diabetes (124,125).

# References

1. Amos, A. F., McCarty, D. J., and Zimmet, P. 1997. The rising global burden of diabetes and its complications: estimates and projections to the year. *Diabet Med* 2010;14:S1-S85.
2. Roman, S. H. and Harris, M. I. Management of diabetes mellitus from a public health perspective. *Endocrinol Metab Clin North Am* 1997;26:443-474.
3. Meltzer, S., Leiter, L., Daneman, D., Gerstein, H. C., Lau, D., Ludwig, S., Yale, J. F., Zinman, B., and Lillie, D. 1998 clinical practice guidelines for the management of diabetes in Canada. Canadian Diabetes Association. *CMAJ.1998* 159:S1-S29.
4. Newman, B., Selby, J. V., King, M. C., Slemenda, C., Fabsitz, R., and Friedman, G. D. Concordance for type 2 (non-insulin-dependent) diabetes mellitus in male twins. *Diabetologia* 1987;30:763-768.
5. Wingard, D. L. and Barrett-Connor, E. Heart disease and diabetes. In National Diabetes Data Group, ed., *Diabetes in America*, pp. 429-448. NIH Publication 95-1468, National Institutes of Health, 1995.
6. Stamler, J., Vaccaro, O., Neaton, J. D., and Wentworth, D. Diabetes, other risk factors, and 12-yr cardiovascular mortality for men screened in the Multiple Risk Factor Intervention Trial. *Diabetes Care* 1993;16:434-444.
7. Intensive blood-glucose control with sulphonylureas or insulin compared with conventional treatment and risk of complications in patients with type 2 diabetes (UKPDS 33). UK Prospective Diabetes Study (UKPDS) Group. *Lancet* 1998;352:837-853.
8. Tight blood pressure control and risk of macrovascular and microvascular complications in type 2 diabetes: UKPDS 38. UK Prospective Diabetes Study Group [see comments]. *BMJ* 1998;317:703-713.
9. Efficacy of atenolol and captopril in reducing risk of macrovascular and microvascular complications in type 2 diabetes: UKPDS 39. UK Prospective Diabetes Study Group. *BMJ* 1998;317:713-720.
10. Effect of intensive blood-glucose control with metformin on complications in overweight patients with type 2 diabetes (UKPDS 34). UK Prospective Diabetes Study (UKPDS) Group. *Lancet* 1998;352:854-865.
11. The effect of intensive treatment of diabetes on the development and progression of long-term complications in insulin-dependent diabetes mellitus. The Diabetes Control and Complications Trial Research Group. *N Engl J Med* 1993;329:977-986.
12. Cost effectiveness analysis of improved blood pressure control in hypertensive patients with type 2 diabetes: UKPDS 40. UK Prospective Diabetes Study Group. *BMJ* 1998;317:720-726.
13. Ohkubo, Y., Kishikawa, H., Araki, E., Miyata, T., Isami, S., Motoyoshi, S., Kojima, Y., Furuyoshi, N., and Shichiri, M. Intensive insulin therapy prevents the progression of diabetic microvascular complications in Japanese patients with non-insulin-dependent diabetes mellitus: a randomized prospective 6-year study. *Diabetes Res Clin Pract* 1995;28:103-117.
14. Panzram, G. Mortality and survival in type 2 (non-insulin-dependent) diabetes mellitus. *Diabetologia* 1987;30:123-131.
15. Perry, I. J., Wannamethee, S. G., Walker, M. K., Thomson, A. G., Whincup, P. H., and Shaper, A. G. Prospective study of risk factors for development of non-insulin dependent diabetes in middle aged British men. *BMJ* 1995;310:560-564.
16. Helmrich, S. P., Ragland, D. R., and Paffenbarger, R. S. J. Prevention of non-insulin-dependent diabetes mellitus with physical activity. *Med Sci Sports Exerc* 1994;26:824-830.
17. Manson, J. E., Nathan, D. M., Krolewski, A. S., Stampfer, M. J., Willett, W. C., and Hennekens, C. H. A prospective study of exercise and incidence of diabetes among US male physicians. *JAMA* 1992;268:63-67.

18. Monterrosa, A. E., Haffner, S. M., Stern, M. P., and Hazuda, H. P. Sex difference in lifestyle factors predictive of diabetes in Mexican-Americans. *Diabetes Care* 1995;18:448-456.

19. Keen, H., Jarrett, R. J., and McCartney, P. The ten-year follow-up of the Bedford survey (1962-1972): glucose tolerance and diabetes. *Diabetologia* 1982;22:73-78.

20. Jarrett, R. J., Keen, H., Fuller, J. H., and McCartney, M. Worsening to diabetes in men with impaired glucose tolerance ("borderline diabetes"). *Diabetologia* 1979;16:25-30.

21. Pan, X. R., Li, G. W., Hu, Y. H., Wang, J. X., Yang, W. Y., An, Z. X., Hu, Z. X., Lin, J., Xiao, J. Z., Cao, H. B., Liu, P. A., Jiang, X. G., Jiang, Y. Y., Wang, J. P., Zheng, H., Zhang, H., Bennett, P. H., and Howard, B. V. Effects of diet and exercise in preventing NIDDM in people with impaired glucose tolerance. The Da Qing IGT and Diabetes Study. *Diabetes Care* 1997;20:537-544.

22. Eriksson, K. F. and Lindgarde, F. Prevention of type 2 (non-insulin-dependent) diabetes mellitus by diet and physical exercise. The 6-year Malmo feasibility study. *Diabetologia* 1991;34:891-898.

23. Tuomilehto, J., Lindstrom, J., Eriksson, J. G., Valle, T. T., Hamalainen, H., Ilanne-Parikka, P., Keinanen-Kiukaanniemi, S., Laakso, M., Louheranta, A., Rastas, M., Salminen, V., and Uusitupa, M. Prevention of type 2 diabetes mellitus by changes in lifestyle among subjects with impaired glucose tolerance. *N Engl J Med* 2001;344:1343-1350.

24. Pyorala, K., Pedersen, T. R., Kjekshus, J., Faergeman, O., Olsson, A. G., and Thorgeirsson, G. Cholesterol lowering with simvastatin improves prognosis of diabetic patients with coronary heart disease. A subgroup analysis of the Scandinavian Simvastatin Survival Study (4S). *Diabetes Care* 1997;20:614-620.

25. Aronson, D., Rayfield, E. J., and Chesebro, J. H. Mechanisms determining course and outcome of diabetic patients who have had acute myocardial infarction. *Ann Intern Med* 1997;126:296-306.

26. Mak, K. H., Moliterno, D. J., Granger, C. B., Miller, D. P., White, H. D., Wilcox, R. G., Califf, R. M., and Topol, E. J. Influence of diabetes mellitus on clinical outcome in the thrombolytic era of acute myocardial infarction. GUSTO-I Investigators. Global Utilization of Streptokinase and Tissue Plasminogen Activator for Occluded Coronary Arteries. *J Am Coll Cardiol* 1997;30:171-179.

27. Pate, R. R., Pratt, M., Blair, S. N., Haskell, W. L., Macera, C. A., Bouchard, C., Buchner, D., Ettinger, W., Heath, G. W., and King, A. C. Physical activity and public health. A recommendation from the Centers for Disease Control and Prevention and the American College of Sports Medicine. *JAMA* 1995;273:402-407.

28. Schneider, S. H., Khachadurian, A. K., Amorosa, L. F., Clemow, L., and Ruderman, N. B. Ten-year experience with an exercise-based outpatient life-style modification program in the treatment of diabetes mellitus. *Diabetes Care* 1992;15:1800-1810.

29. American College of Sports Medicine and American Diabetes Association joint position statement. Diabetes mellitus and exercise. *Med Sci Sports Exerc* 1997;29:i-vi.

30. Lawrence, R. H. The effects of exercise on insulin action in diabetes. *Br Med J* 1926;1:648-650.

31. Joslin, E. P., Root, H. F., White, P., and Marble, A. *The treatment of diabetes mellitus*, 5th ed. Lea & Febiger, Philadelphia 1935.

32. Gautier, J. F., Scheen, A., and Lefebvre, P. J. Exercise in the management of non-insulin-dependent (type 2) diabetes mellitus. *Int J Obes Relat Metab Disord* 1995;19 Suppl 4:S58-61:S58-S61.

33. Samaras, K., Ashwell, S., Mackintosh, A. M., Campbell, L. V., and Chisholm, D. J. Exercise in NIDDM: are we missing the point? *Diabet Med* 1996;13:780-781.

34. Ford, E. S. and Herman, W. H. Leisure-time physical activity patterns in the U.S. diabetic population. Findings from the 1990 National Health Interview Survey—Health Promotion and Disease Prevention Supplement. *Diabetes Care* 1995;1:27-33.

35. Frisch, R. E., Wyshak, G., Albright, T. E., Albright, N. L., and Schiff, I. Lower prevalence of diabetes in female former college athletes compared with nonathletes. *Diabetes* 1986;35:1101-1105.

36. Lipton, R. B., Liao, Y., Cao, G., Cooper, R. S., and McGee, D. Determinants of incident non-insulin-dependent diabetes mellitus among blacks and whites in a national sample. The NHANES I Epidemiologic Follow-up Study. *Am J Epidemiol* 1993;138:826-839.

37. Schranz, A., Tuomilehto, J., Marti, B., Jarrett, R. J., Grabauskas, V., and Vassallo, A. Low physical activity and worsening of glucose tol-

erance: results from a 2-year follow-up of a population sample in Malta. *Diabetes Res Clin Pract* 1991;11:127-136.

38. Burchfiel, C. M., Sharp, D. S., Curb, J. D., Rodriguez, B. L., Hwang, L. J., Marcus, E. B., and Yano, K. Physical activity and incidence of diabetes: the Honolulu Heart Program. *Am J Epidemiol* 1995;141:360-368.

39. Helmrich, S. P., Ragland, D. R., Leung, R. W., and Paffenbarger, R. S. J. Physical activity and reduced occurrence of non-insulin-dependent diabetes mellitus. *N Engl J Med* 1991;325:147-152.

40. Manson, J. E., Rimm, E. B., Stampfer, M. J., Colditz, G. A., Willett, W. C., Krolewski, A. S., Rosner, B., Hennekens, C. H., and Speizer, F. E. Physical activity and incidence of non-insulin-dependent diabetes mellitus in women. *Lancet* 1991;338:774-778.

41. Lynch, J., Helmrich, S. P., Lakka, T. A., Kaplan, G. A., Cohen, R. D., Salonen, R., and Salonen, J. T. Moderately intense physical activities and high levels of cardiorespiratory fitness reduce the risk of non-insulin-dependent diabetes mellitus in middle-aged men. *Arch Intern Med* 1996;156:1307-1314.

42. Wei, M., Gibbons, L. W., Mitchell, T. L., Kampert, J. B., Lee, C. D., and Blair, S. N. The association between cardiorespiratory fitness and impaired fasting glucose and type 2 diabetes mellitus in men. *Ann Intern Med* 1999;130:89-96.

43. Tuomilehto, J., Knowler, W. C., and Zimmet, P. Primary prevention of non-insulin-dependent diabetes mellitus. *Diabetes Metab Rev* 1992;8:339-353.

44. Minuk, H. L., Vranic, M., Marliss, E. B., Hanna, A. K., Albisser, A. M., and Zinman, B. Glucoregulatory and metabolic response to exercise in obese noninsulin-dependent diabetes. *Am J Physiol* 1981;240:E458-E464.

45. Jenkins, A. B., Furler, S. M., Bruce, D. G., and Chisholm, D. J. Regulation of hepatic glucose output during moderate exercise in non-insulin-dependent diabetes. *Metabolism* 1988; 37:966-972.

46. Martin, I. K., Katz, A., and Wahren, J. Splanchnic and muscle metabolism during exercise in NIDDM patients. *Am J Physiol* 1995;269:E583-E590.

47. Hother-Nielsen, O. and Beck-Nielsen, H. On the determination of basal glucose production rate in patients with type 2 (non-insulin-dependent) diabetes mellitus using primed-continuous 3-3H-glucose infusion. *Diabetologia* 1990;33:603-610.

48. Larsen, J. J., Dela, F., Kjaer, M., and Galbo, H. The effect of moderate exercise on postprandial glucose homeostasis in NIDDM patients. *Diabetologia* 1997;40:447-453.

49. Riddle, M. C., McDaniel, P. A., and Tive, L. A. Glipizide-GITS does not increase the hypoglycemic effect of mild exercise during fasting in NIDDM. *Diabetes Care* 1997;20:992-994.

50. Kang, J., Kelley, D. E., Robertson, R. J., Goss, F. L., Suminski, R. R., Utter, A. C., and DaSilva, S. G. Substrate utilization and glucose turnover during exercise of varying intensities in individuals with NIDDM. *Med Sci Sports Exerc* 1999;31:82-89.

51. Koivisto, V. A. and DeFronzo, R. A. Exercise in the treatment of type II diabetes. *Acta Endocrinol (Copenh.)* 1984;Suppl 262:107-111.

52. Colberg, S. R., Hagberg, J. M., McCole, S. D., Zmuda, J. M., Thompson, P. D., and Kelley, D. E. Utilization of glycogen but not plasma glucose is reduced in individuals with NIDDM during mild-intensity exercise. *J Appl Physiol* 1996;81:2027-2033.

53. Gudat, U., Bungert, S., Kemmer, F., and Heinemann, L. The blood glucose lowering effects of exercise and glibenclamide in patients with type 2 diabetes mellitus. *Diabet Med* 1998;15:194-198.

54. Massi-Benedetti, M., Herz, M., and Pfeiffer, C. The effects of acute exercise on metabolic control in type II diabetic patients treated with glimepiride or glibenclamide. *Horm Metab Res* 1996;28:451-455.

55. Paternostro-Bayles, M., Wing, R. R., and Robertson, R. J. Effect of life-style activity of varying duration on glycemic control in type II diabetic women. *Diabetes Care* 1989;12:34-37.

56. Zierath, J. R. and Wallberg-Henriksson, H. Exercise training in obese diabetic patients. Special considerations. *Sports Med* 1992;14:171-189.

57. Ligtenberg, P. C., Hoekstra, J. B., Bol, E., Zonderland, M. L., and Erkelens, D. W. Effects of physical training on metabolic control in elderly type 2 diabetes mellitus patients. *Clin Sci* 1997;93:127-135.

58. Duh, E. and Feinglos, M. Hypoglycemia-induced angina pectoris in a patient with diabetes mellitus. *Ann Intern Med* 1994;121:945-946.

59. Poirier, P., Tremblay, A., Catellier, C., Tancrede, G., Garneau, C., and Nadeau, A. Impact of time interval from the last meal on glucose response to exercise in subjects with type 2 diabetes. *J Clin Endocrinol Metab* 2000;85:2860-2864.

60. Skarfors, E. T., Wegener, T. A., Lithell, H., and Selinus, I. Physical training as treatment for type 2 (non-insulin-dependent) diabetes in elderly men. A feasibility study over 2 years. *Diabetologia* 1987;12:930-933.

61. Poirier, P., MaWhinney, S., Grondin, L., Tremblay, A., Broderick, T. L., Cleroux, J., Catellier, C., Tancrede, G., and Nadeau, A. Prior meal enhances the plasma glucose lowering effect of exercise in type 2 diabetes. *Med Sci Sports Exerc* 2001;33:1259-1264.

62. Ruderman, N. B., Ganda, O. P., and Johansen, K. The effect of physical training on glucose tolerance and plasma lipids in maturity-onset diabetes. *Diabetes* 1979;28 Suppl 1:89-92.

63. Mourier, A., Gautier, J. F., De Kerviler, E., Bigard, A. X., Villette, J. M., Garnier, J. P., Duvallet, A., Guezennec, C. Y., and Cathelineau, G. Mobilization of visceral adipose tissue related to the improvement in insulin sensitivity in response to physical training in NIDDM. Effects of branched-chain amino acid supplements. *Diabetes Care* 1997;20:385-391.

64. Saltin, B., Lindgarde, F., Houston, M., Horlin, R., Nygaard, E., and Gad, P. Physical training and glucose tolerance in middle-aged men with chemical diabetes. *Diabetes* 1979;28 Suppl 1:30-32.

65. Ronnemaa, T., Mattila, K., Lehtonen, A., and Kallio, V. A controlled randomized study on the effect of long-term physical exercise on the metabolic control in type 2 diabetic patients. *Acta Med Scand* 1986;220:219-224.

66. Lindgarde, F., Malmquist, J., and Balke, B. Physical fitness, insulin secretion, and glucose tolerance in healthy males and mild type-2 diabetes. *Acta Diabetol Lat* 1983;20:33-40.

67. Wing, R. R., Epstein, L. H., Paternostro-Bayles, M., Kriska, A., Nowalk, M. P., and Gooding, W. Exercise in a behavioural weight control programme for obese patients with Type 2 (non-insulin-dependent) diabetes. *Diabetologia* 1988;31:902-909.

68. Trovati, M., Carta, Q., Cavalot, F., Vitali, S., Banaudi, C., Lucchina, P. G., Fiocchi, F., Emanuelli, G., and Lenti, G. Influence of physical training on blood glucose control, glucose tolerance, insulin secretion, and insulin action in non-insulin-dependent diabetic patients. *Diabetes Care* 1984;7:416-420.

69. Yamanouchi, K., Shinozaki, T., Chikada, K., Nishikawa, T., Ito, K., Shimizu, S., Ozawa, N., Suzuki, Y., Maeno, H., and Kato, K. Daily walking combined with diet therapy is a useful means for obese NIDDM patients not only to reduce body weight but also to improve insulin sensitivity. *Diabetes Care* 1995;18:775-778.

70. Lehmann, R., Vokac, A., Niedermann, K., Agosti, K., and Spinas, G. A. Loss of abdominal fat and improvement of the cardiovascular risk profile by regular moderate exercise training in patients with NIDDM. *Diabetologia* 1995;38:1313-1319.

71. Barnard, R. J., Lattimore, L., Holly, R. G., Cherny, S., and Pritikin, N. Response of non-insulin-dependent diabetic patients to an intensive program of diet and exercise. *Diabetes Care* 1982;5:370-374.

72. Krotkiewski, M., Lonnroth, P., Mandroukas, K., Wroblewski, Z., Rebuffe, S., Holm, G., Smith, U., and Bjorntorp, P. The effects of physical training on insulin secretion and effectiveness and on glucose metabolism in obesity and type 2 (non-insulin-dependent) diabetes mellitus. *Diabetologia* 1985;28:881-890.

73. Reitman, J. S., Vasquez, B., Klimes, I., and Nagulesparan, M. Improvement of glucose homeostasis after exercise training in non-insulin-dependent diabetes. *Diabetes Care* 1984;7:434-441.

74. Ishii, T., Yamakita, T., Sato, T., Tanaka, S., and Fujii, S. Resistance training improves insulin sensitivity in NIDDM subjects without altering maximal oxygen uptake. *Diabetes Care* 1998;21:1353-1355.

75. Dunstan, D. W., Puddey, I. B., Beilin, L. J., Burke, V., Morton, A. R., and Stanton, K. G. Effects of a short-term circuit weight training program on glycaemic control in NIDDM. *Diabetes Res Clin Pract* 1998;40:53-61.

76. Fujii, S., Okuno, Y., Okada, K., Tanaka, S., Seki, J., Wada, M., and Iseki, T. Effects of physical training on glucose tolerance and insulin response in diabetics. *Osaka City Med J* 1982;28:1-8.

77. Vanninen, E., Uusitupa, M., Siitonen, O., Laitinen, J., and Lansimies, E. Habitual physical activity, aerobic capacity and metabolic control in patients with newly-diagnosed type 2 (non-insulin-dependent) diabetes mellitus: effect of 1-year diet and exercise intervention. *Diabetologia* 1992;35:340-346.

78. Schneider, S. H., Amorosa, L. F., Khachadurian, A. K., and Ruderman, N. B. Studies on the mechanism of improved glucose control during regular exercise in type 2 (non-insulin-dependent) diabetes. *Diabetologia* 1984;26:355-360.

79. Kang, J., Robertson, R. J., Hagberg, J. M., Kelley, D. E., Goss, F. L., DaSilva, S. G., Suminski, R. R., and Utter, A. C. Effect of exercise intensity on glucose and insulin metabolism in obese individuals and obese NIDDM patients. *Diabetes Care* 1996;19:341-349.

80. Allenberg, K., Johansen, K., and Saltin, B. Skeletal muscle adaptations to physical training in type II (non-insulin-dependent) diabetes mellitus. *Acta Med Scand* 1988;223:365-373.

81. Leon, A. S., Conrad, J. C., Casal, D. C., Serfass, R., Bonnard, R. A., Goetz, F. C., and Blackburn, T. Exercise for diabetics: Effects of conditioning at constant body weight. *J Cardiac Rehabil* 1984;4:278-286.

82. Rogers, M. A., Yamamoto, C., King, D. S., Hagberg, J. M., Ehsani, A. A., and Holloszy, J. O. Improvement in glucose tolerance after 1 wk of exercise in patients with mild NIDDM. *Diabetes Care* 1988;11:613-618.

83. Yeater, R. A., Ullrich, I. H., Maxwell, L. P., and Goetsch, V. L. Coronary risk factors in type II diabetes: response to low-intensity aerobic exercise. *W V Med J* 1990;86:287-290.

84. Knowler, W. C., Narayan, K. M., Hanson, R. L., Nelson, R. G., Bennett, P. H., Tuomilehto, J., Schersten, B., and Pettitt, D. J. Preventing non-insulin-dependent diabetes. *Diabetes* 1995;44:483-488.

85. Devlin, J. T., Hirshman, M., Horton, E. D., and Horton, E. S. Enhanced peripheral and splanchnic insulin sensitivity in NIDDM men after single bout of exercise. *Diabetes* 1987; 36:434-439.

86. Walker, K. Z., Piers, L. S., Putt, R. S., Jones, J. A., and O'Dea, K. Effects of regular walking on cardiovascular risk factors and body composition in normoglycemic women and women with type 2 diabetes. *Diabetes Care* 1999;22:555-561.

87. Kelley, D. E., Mintun, M. A., Watkins, S. C., Simoneau, J. A., Jadali, F., Fredrickson, Beattie, J., and Theriault, R. The effect of non-insulin-dependent diabetes mellitus and obesity on glucose transport and phosphorylation in skeletal muscle. *J Clin Invest* 1996;97:2705-2713.

88. Després, J. P. and Lamarche, B. Low-intensity endurance exercise training, plasma lipoproteins and the risk of coronary heart disease. *J Intern Med* 1994;236:7-22.

89. Wood, P. D., Stefanick, M. L., Dreon, D. M., Frey-Hewitt, B., Garay, S. C., Williams, P. T., Superko, H. R., Fortmann, S. P., Albers, J. J., and Vranizan, K. M. Changes in plasma lipids and lipoproteins in overweight men during weight loss through dieting as compared with exercise. *N Engl J Med* 1988;319:1173-1179.

90. Trovati, M. Physical training and plasma lipids in type 2 (non-insulin-dependent) diabetic patients. *Diabetologia* 1988;31:68.

91. Verity, L. S. and Ismail, A. H. Effects of exercise on cardiovascular disease risk in women with NIDDM. *Diabetes Res Clin Pract* 1989;6:27-35.

92. Ronnemaa, T., Marniemi, J., Puukka, P., and Kuusi, T. Effects of long-term physical exercise on serum lipids, lipoproteins and lipid metabolizing enzymes in type 2 (non-insulin-dependent) diabetic patients. *Diabetes Res* 1988;7:79-84.

93. Schneider, S. H., Kim, H. C., Khachadurian, A. K., and Ruderman, N. B. Impaired fibrinolytic response to exercise in type II diabetes: effects of exercise and physical training. *Metabolism* 1988;37:924-929.

94. Poirier, P., Catellier, C., Tremblay, A., and Nadeau, A. Role of body fat loss in the exercise-induced improvement of the plasma lipid profile in non-insulin-dependent diabetes mellitus. *Metabolism* 1996;45:1383-1387.

95. Rubler, S. Asymptomatic diabetic females. Exercise testing. *NY State J Med* 1981;81:1185-1191.

96. Bottini, P., Tantucci, C., Scionti, L., Dottorini, M. L., Puxeddu, E., Reboldi, G., Bolli, G. B., Casucci, G., Santeusanio, F., and Sorbini, C. A. Cardiovascular response to exercise in diabetic patients: influence of autonomic neuropathy of different severity. *Diabetologia* 1995;38:244-250.

97. Estacio, R. O., Regensteiner, J. G., Wolfel, E. E., Jeffers, B., Dickenson, M., and Schrier, R. W. The association between diabetic complications and exercise capacity in NIDDM patients. *Diabetes Care* 1998;21:291-295.

98. Regensteiner, J. G., Sippel, J., McFarling, E. T., Wolfel, E. E., and Hiatt, W. R. Effects of non-insulin-dependent diabetes on oxygen consumption during treadmill exercise. *Med Sci Sports Exerc* 1995,27:875-881.

99. Regensteiner, J. G., Bauer, T. A., Reusch, J. E., Brandenburg, S. L., Sippel, J. M., Vogelsong, A. M., Smith, S., Wolfel, E. E., Eckel, R. H., and Hiatt, W. R. Abnormal oxygen uptake kinetic responses in women with type II diabetes mellitus. *J Appl Physiol* 1998;85:310-317.

100. Radice, M., Rocca, A., Bedon, E., Musacchio, N., Morabito, A., and Segalini, G. Abnormal response to exercise in middle-aged NIDDM patients with and without autonomic neuropathy. *Diabet Med* 1996;13:259-265.

101. Seneviratne, B. I. Diabetic cardiomyopathy: the preclinical phase. *Br Med J* 1977;1:1444-1446.

102. Ahmed, S. S., Jaferi, G. A., Narang, R. M., and Regan, T. J. Preclinical abnormality of left ventricular function in diabetes mellitus. *Am Heart J* 1975;89:153-158.

103. Raev, D. C. Which left ventricular function is impaired earlier in the evolution of diabetic cardiomyopathy? An echocardiographic study of young type I diabetic patients. *Diabetes Care* 1994;17:633-639.

104. Poirier, P., Bogaty, P., Garneau, C., Marois, L., and Dumesnil, J. G. Diastolic dysfunction in type 2 diabetes men without hypertension or coronary artery disease: importance of the Valsalva maneuver in screening patients. *Diabetes Care* 2001;24:5-10.

105. Vanoverschelde, J. J., Essamri, B., Vanbutsele, R., d'Hondt, A., Cosyns, J. R., Detry, J. R., and Melin, J. A. Contribution of left ventricular diastolic function to exercise capacity in normal subjects. *J Appl Physiol* 1993;74:2225-2233.

106. Sahn, D. J., DeMaria, A., Kisslo, J., and Weyman, A. Recommendations regarding quantitation in M-mode echocardiography: results of a survey of echocardiographic measurements. *Circulation* 1978;58:1072-1083.

107. Rakowski, H., Appleton, C., Chan, K. L., Dumesnil, J. G., Honos, G., Jue, J., Koilpillai, C., Lepage, S., Martin, R. P., Mercier, L. A., O'Kelly, B., Prieur, T., Sanfilippo, A., Sasson, Z., Alvarez, N., Pruitt, R., Thompson, C., and Tomlinson, C. Canadian consensus recommendations for the measurement and reporting of diastolic dysfunction by echocardiography: from the Investigators of Consensus on Diastolic Dysfunction by Echocardiography. *J Am Soc Echocardiogr* 1996;9:736-760.

108. Poirier, P., Garneau, C., Bogaty, P., Nadeau, A., Marois, L., Brochu, C., Gingras, C., Fortin, C., Jobin, J., and Dumesnil, J. G. Impact of left ventricular diastolic dysfunction on maximal treadmill performance in normotensive subjects with well-controlled type 2 diabetes mellitus. *Am J Cardiol* 2000;85:473-477.

109. Hilsted, J., Galbo, H., and Christensen, N. J. Impaired responses of catecholamines, growth hormone, and cortisol to graded exercise in diabetic autonomic neuropathy. *Diabetes* 1980;29:257-262.

110. Kitzman, D. W., Higginbotham, M. B., Cobb, F. R., Sheikh, K. H., and Sullivan, M. J. Exercise intolerance in patients with heart failure and preserved left ventricular systolic function: failure of the Frank-Starling mechanism. *J Am Coll Cardiol* 1991;17:1065-1072.

111. Roy, T. M., Peterson, H. R., Snider, H. L., Cyrus, J., Broadstone, V. L., Fell, R. D., Rothchild, A. H., Samols, E., and Pfeifer, M. A. Autonomic influence on cardiovascular performance in diabetic subjects. *Am J Med* 1989;87:382-388.

112. Diabetes mellitus and exercise. *Diabetes Care* 2001;24:S51-S55.

113. Effects of ramipril on cardiovascular and microalbuminuria outcomes in people with diabetes: results of the HOPE study and MICRO-HOPE substudy. Heart Outcomes Prevention Evaluation Study Investigators. *Lancet* 2000;355:253-259.

114. Hansson, L., Zanchetti, A., Carruthers, S. G., Dahlof, B., Elmfeldt, D., Julius, S., Menard, J., Rahn, K. H., Wedel, H., and Westerling, S. Effects of intensive blood-pressure lowering and low-dose aspirin in patients with hypertension: principal results of the Hypertension Optimal Treatment (HOT) randomised trial. *Lancet* 1998;351:1755-1762.

115. Ligtenberg, P. C., Hoekstra, J. B., Bol, E., Zonderland, M. L., and Erkelens, D. W. Effects of physical training on metabolic control in elderly type 2 diabetes mellitus patients. *Clin Sci* 1997;93:127-135.

116. Grundy, S. M., Benjamin, E. J., Burke, G. L., Chait, A., Eckel, R. H., Howard, B. V., Mitch, W., Smith, S. C. J., and Sowers, J. R. Diabetes and cardiovascular disease. A statement for healthcare professionals from the American Heart Association. *Circulation* 1999;100:1134-1146.

117. Hilsted, J., Galbo, H., Christensen, N. J., Parving, H. H., and Benn, J. Haemodynamic changes during graded exercise in patients with diabetic autonomic neuropathy. *Diabetologia* 1982;22:318-323.

118. Hilsted, J., Galbo, H., and Christensen, N. J. Impaired cardiovascular responses to graded exercise in diabetic autonomic neuropathy. *Diabetes* 1979;28:313-319.

119. Kahn, J. K., Zola, B., Juni, J. E., and Vinik, A. I. Decreased exercise heart rate and blood pressure response in diabetic subjects with cardiac autonomic neuropathy. *Diabetes Care* 1986;9:389-394.

120. Roy, T. M., Peterson, H. R., Snider, H. L., Cyrus, J., Broadstone, V. L., Fell, R. D., Rothchild, A. H., Samols, E., and Pfeifer, M. A. Autonomic influence on cardiovascular performance in diabetic subjects. *Am J Med* 1989;87:382-388.

121. Rubler, S., Gerber, D., Reitano, J., Chokshi, V., and Fisher, V. J. Predictive value of clinical and exercise variables for detection of coronary artery disease in men with diabetes mellitus. *Am J Cardiol* 1987;59:1310-1313.

122. Paillole, C., Ruiz, J., Juliard, J. M., Leblanc, H., Gourgon, R., and Passa, P. Detection of coronary artery disease in diabetic patients. *Diabetologia* 1995;38:726-731.

123. Chipkin, S. R., Frid, D., Alpert, J. S., Baker, S. P., Dalen, J. E., and Aronin, N. Frequency of painless myocardial ischemia during exercise tolerance testing in patients with and without diabetes mellitus. *Am J Cardiol* 1987;59:61-65.

124. Wei, M., Gibbons, L. W., Kampert, J. B., Nichaman, M. Z., and Blair, S. N. Low cardiorespiratory fitness and physical inactivity as predictors of mortality in men with type 2 diabetes. *Ann Intern Med* 2000;132:605-611.

125. Hu, F. B., Stampfer, M. J., Solomon, C., Liu, S., Colditz, G. A., Speizer, F. E., Willett, W. C., and Manson, J. E. Physical activity and risk for cardiovascular events in diabetic women. *Ann Intern Med* 2001;134:96-105.

PART XI

# Conclusion

## Chapter 30

# Expansion and Globalization of the Frontiers of Cardiopulmonary Rehabilitation

Jean Jobin, PhD, François Maltais, MD, Paul Poirier, MD, Pierre LeBlanc, MD, Clermont Simard, PhD, Canada

## Introduction

In cardiopulmonary rehabilitation, desired outcomes should not be measured exclusively at the end of a prolonged intervention. On the contrary, the evaluation process must be integrated into the intervention itself, and within the inter-relation with the person being treated. Desired outcomes must be integrated to the awakening of the "rehabilitatee", to his self control and to his novel reintegration into society and his environment. If it is true that cardiopulmonary rehabilitation is a determinant in the recovery of functional autonomy and health status and search for a better quality of life, it is also important to understand that the role of the "rehabilitator" cannot be assimilated and reduced to that of a care giver or a curator. He must be an educator/re-educator, a pedagogue and a companion. Education and integral development of a person will last a life time, and no matter what her or his capacities/disabilities are, these can always be improved.

## Challenging Acquired Paradigms

The traditional conventional medicine, has a narrow vision of the healing process which is easier to associate with a more natural type of medicine. Although we do not wish to get much further into these polemics, we think that it is worth mentioning that rehabilitation sciences are more in agreement with knowledge, values, and beliefs of the health sciences as opposed to the more conventional medical approach. We think it is in much better harmony with the new developing integrative medicine as described by Sullivan (chapter 9). As

discussed in the chapter 1, the conventional mechanistic medical paradigm addresses a disease while integrative medicine addresses a person suffering from a disease. It is somewhat disturbing to hear some medical experts talk about cardiopulmonary rehabilitation which in their hands, already looks stereotyped in knowledge and beliefs despite being recently included within health services. One must be more open to the broad needs of the individual affected by cardiovascular or pulmonary diseases.

Despite the fact that it may be difficult or even impossible for some of us to challenge acquired paradigms, one must take all means to adapt and to offer the most efficient and safe rehabilitation interventions to those who need it. One must put aside fragmented or stereotyped visions of the disease in order to adopt a broader view of the human being, making himself in a state of readiness toward the actual needs of the patient as a person. How can we awaken politicians, researchers, professors, scholars, and even more front line-practicing clinicians, to this new paradigm? This is one challenge to cardiopulmonary rehabilitation for the coming years.

## The Three Dimensions of the New Cardiopulmonary Rehabilitation Paradigm: Specificity, Normality and Wholesomeness

Even though cardiopulmonary rehabilitation experts should be aware of the importance of the dose-response principle in their interventions with individuals having a cardiopulmonary deficiency, their action must be taken in the light of a broader perspective. The dose-response principle deals mainly with the specificity part of the action. To have a comprehensive rehabilitation process, one must however add the concepts of normality or normalcy and wholesomeness to the action. Specificity not only concerns the diseased organs but also adjacent systems whether they are central or peripheral, which may be affected directly or indirectly by the disease. During the past decade, for instance, the impact of chronic heart failure and chronic obstructive pulmonary disease on peripheral skeletal muscle have been brought to our attention (1,2). The end result is that one cannot look at the effect of exercise or of any other intervention on the cardiovascular or pulmonary function alone to measure the impact of our intervention. Furthermore, the new concept of ergoreflex (3,4) implies that there is a two way communication between the heart-lung systems and skeletal muscle. Thus we must now look at musculoskeletal exercises as another potential way to impact the cardiovascular and respiratory responses to exercise in people with cardiac as well as pulmonary diseases (4). Normalization deals with the general health status, and over all fitness of the individual. In his search for his new self balance, the person with a cardiovascular or pulmonary disease is trying to get as close to a normal functioning as possible. Within the limits of the left over abilities and capacities, rehabilitation should aim at getting him or her as close as possible to that goal. Wholesomeness includes all the dimensions of a person along with the physical, social, spiritual and cultural environment in which he is an active part. The rehabilitation process must respect the personal values of the person being rehabilitated as well as set goals within the limit of these values. Whenever necessary it must teach new values.

In the same vein, one must realize that rehabilitation largely overflows the traditional world of medicine. As Benaziza (5) recently emphasized in "Policies on Physical Activity and Sport for All: An Efficient Means to Promote Health and Development", physical activity may be considered as a cure:

"An appropriate practice of physical activities and sports constitute a simple, fun, and low cost cure, accessible to all." (ad lib translation)

## Cardiopulmonary Rehabilitation and the Notions of Disability/Handicap

We must get acquainted with the new paradigms that are likely to develop interactive links between the individual and his physical and psychosocial-cultural environments. As Fougeyrollas (6) mentions:

". . . It must be recognized that the realities experienced and the personal factors of each different body are just as fundamental as environmental solutions with their own limits. . . . It is toward this delicate balance that a systemic conceptual perspective, which situates all of the variables involved, must maintain. It consists of a continually changing open game, within which personal factors are as essential as the environmental factors".

The concepts of disability and handicap as defined by Fougeyrollas (7) must orient future actions in cardiopulmonary rehabilitation. In this paradigm, disabilities are usually the consequences of diseases or of actions on diseases (drug and surgery side effects, etc. . . ) while handicap are, at least partially, created by the physical and psycho-socio-cultural-spiritual environments which impose demands that can't be met. For instance, my heart failure condition has decreased my work capacity such that I have a disability and can't climb 3 flights of stairs. I have an appointment on the sixth floor of a building. If there is no elevator or escalator, I experience a handicap and can't go to my meeting. Here, with the proper physical environment or facility I would still be disabled, my work capacity would not have been changed, however, I would not have any handicap, and could go to my meeting. For example, what could be done to minimize the potential handicap related to ambulatory oxygen (in public transportation, etc.) in chronic obstructive pulmonary disease (COPD), which is the disability? Why do we have to wait so long to begin rehabilitation of patients with COPD that their state of disability is so advanced? One of the limitations in inducing the rehabilitation process may be the time the patient needs to adapt to his disease, to accept it and stop denying. Cardiopulmonary rehabilitation must be oriented toward minimizing the possibility to get to the point of handicap, in addition to its action on risk factors through secondary prevention.

Those issues tell us that multi and inter-disciplinarity are at the heart of the cardiopulmonary rehabilitation process. Rehabilitation is a complex matter that cannot be put in the hand of only one body of knowledge let alone one discipline. Rehabilitation teams must be composed of health, medical, educational and psychosocial sciences people acting in a complementary manner. Who would have thought, a few years ago, that skeletal muscles were so important to the person in a cardiac as well as pulmonary rehabilitation process (8-10), and that peripheral circulation would become of interest in COPD rehabilitation (11).

## Rehabilitation of the Aged

Despite the progresses made by biomedical sciences over the past decades, we must learn to comply with the ever increasing number of people affected by chronic diseases (12,13). As a greater percentage of the population gets older, thanks to biomedical advances, we are faced with an ever growing number of people suffering from chronic diseases and decreased autonomy. Despite the impact of secondary prevention, rehabilitation may be through its socio-economic benefits (14,15), the most efficient means to control the rising cost of health services that are heavily related to the increase in disability in older persons (16).

## Integration of Cardiopulmonary Rehabilitation to the Treatment of the Disease

The integration of cardiopulmonary rehabilitation to the treatment of the diseases became the obvious theme for the Second Québec International Symposium on Cardiopulmonary Rehabilitation after an in depth reflection based on the introductory (15) and concluding (17) chapters of Advances in Cardiopulmonary Rehabilitation published after the first Symposium by Human Kinetics.

What can be said to justify the actual role of cardiac and pulmonary rehabilitation in health services throughout the developed countries of the world? How can we still accept that it is an alternative service being offered to so few patients and taken by even a lesser number despite the evidence of its numerous benefits (4,17), low cost (14) and in some instances proof that it may lower overall health systems cost (4)? Why don't we integrate rehabilitation within the treatment process of the disease instead of a service only offered to the wealthiest or the most educated people? How can we rectify some of the myths (4) associated with cardiopulmonary rehabilitation, such as the high risk of exercise in cardiac patients or that rehabilitation has no impact on mortality? Unfortunately, these myths are still very much alive in the medical-allied health care

professional communities as well as the lay public and they often prevent physicians and allied health care professionals from integrating rehabilitation into their treatment strategies.

Many papers included in this book will be of great value to the world of cardiopulmonary rehabilitation and to its development. However, the Editors want to emphasize the perspective brought by Christian Préfaut in chapter 2. Although the main theme of this Symposium, "Cardiopulmonary Rehabilitation Integrated to the treatment of the disease", appears innovative to many, Préfaut demonstrated very elegantly that rehabilitation was a long time ago an integrated part of medicine and health services. Did we need Hippocrates to remind us of our duties? Similarly, chapter 9 by Sullivan underlines the potential role model of the new concept of integrative medicine for the new cardiopulmonary rehabilitation paradigm.

## Globalization of Cardiopulmonary Rehabilitation

In developing countries, where the prevalence of cardiopulmonary diseases is ever increasing, the situation has become alarming. Some societal choices have to be discussed, reevaluated, and criticized. For instance, one should be disturbed by the deconstruction-reconstruction of physical education and the consequences that will soon need to be supported at least partially by the developed countries (18). The disengagement of societies and governments toward physical education in schools in both developing and developed countries, like the Province of Québec for instance, will undoubtedly increase the number of people with chronic diseases and thus the proportion of disabled and non autonomous citizens, inflating the number of people in need of rehabilitation. Young adults, instead of being "has been" will become "never was" in good physical shape. What can be done to improve rehabilitation services in the developing world?

Furthermore, research must be a major interest in cardiopulmonary rehabilitation in this new Millenium. The recent Symposium sponsored by the American College of Sports Medicine (19) on the dose-response issues in physical activity and health is worth mentioning in this context.

Dose-response is one of the issues which underlies some of the myths behind the reluctance of the medical community to adopt cardiopulmonary rehabilitation as an integrated tool in treating cardiovascular and pulmonary diseases (4). Many types of interventions used and developed for use in cardiopulmonary rehabilitation lack the proper evidence based data. This is why, the third Québec International Symposium on Cardiopulmonary Rehabilitation has chosen the following overall theme:

"Evidence Based Interventions: Science to the Art of Cardiopulmonary Rehabilitation".

This event will be held in Québec City, Canada, on May 11-13, 2003. More than 500 participants worldwide will discuss with the 26 internationally renown guest speakers on this issue as well as on ways to preserve the art component of cardiopulmonary rehabilitation, to keep the person at the center of its action, taking into consideration all its dimensions as well as its own psycho-socio-cultural-spiritual environments. The 2003 preliminary program is available at: **www.ulaval.ca/symp-rehab**.

## About This Book

This book features selected papers presented by guest speakers at the Second Québec International Symposium on Cardiopulmonary Rehabilitation held in Québec City, June 6-8, 2001. However, 60 more original research papers were presented during this event. These were published in abstract form in a supplement of Clinical and Investigative Medicine (20).

## References

1. Jobin J, Doyon JF. Peripheral Muscle Limitations to Exercise in Patients With Conestive Heart Failure: Implications for Rehabilitation. In Jobin J, Maltais F, LeBlanc P, Simard C. *Advances in Cardiopulmonary Rehabilitation.* Champaign, Human Kinetics, p. 90-104, 2000.
2. Maltais F., Jobin F, LeBlanc P. Peripheral Muscle Dysfunction in Patients with Chronic Obstructive Pulmonary Disease. In Jobin J, Maltais F, LeBlanc P, Simard C. *Advances in Cardiopulmonary Rehabilitation.* Champaign, Human Kinetics, p. 90-104, 2000.
3. Piepoli M, Ponikowski P, clark AL, Banasiak W, Capucci A, Coats AJ. A Neural Link to Explain the "Muscle Hypothesis" of Exercise Intolerance in Chronic Heart Failure. *Am Heart J* 137 (6):1050-6, 1999.
4. Jobin J, Maltais F, Poirier P. La réadaptation cardiorespiratoire: l'intervention sous-utilisée. *Le médecin du Québec*, 36 (4): 97-111, 2001.
5. Benaziza, H. Politiques en matière d'activité physique et de sport pour tous, un outil efficace de promotion de la santé et du développement. In: Simard C., Thibault G., Goulet C., Paré C., Bilodeau F. (eds). *Le Sport pour Tous et les politiques gouvernementales—Sport for All and Governmental Policies.* VIIIᵉ Congrès Mondial du Sport pour Tous—VIII World Sport for All Congress. AGMV Marquis Québec. p. 118. Juillet 2001.
6. Fougeyrollas P., Beauregard L. An interactive Person-Environment Social Creation. In: Albrecht G.L., Seelman K.D., Burry M. Handbook of Disability Studies. *SAGE.* pp. 172-194. 2001.
7. Fougeyrollas P, Bergeron H, Cloutier R, St-Michel G. "The handicap creation Process: Analysis of the Consultation. New full Proposals." *ICIDH International Network.* 4 (1-2): 5-37, 1991.
8. Noël M., Doyon J.F., LeBlanc P., Maltais F., LeBlanc M.H., Simard C., Jobin J. Can Electromyography Be Used as a Non Invasive Tool to Detect Muscle Abnormalities in CHF and COPD patients: A Preliminary Study? Chronic Heart Failure. *Clin Invest Med* Suppl. 24 (3): S63. Québec. June 2001.
9. Allaire J., Simard P.M., Maltais F., LeBlanc P., Whittom F., Doyon J.F., Simard C. Jobin J. A new Evidence of Peripheral Skeletal Muscle Oxidative Damage in Patients with COPD. *Rehabilitation.* October 2000.
10. Jobin J., Doyon J.F. Le muscle périphérique des insuffisants cardiaques. *Rev des Maladies Respir* 2001;18: S27-S31.
11. Maltais F., LeBlanc P., Whittom F., Simard C., Bélanger M., Breton M.J., Simard P.M., Marquis K., Jobin J. Oxidative enzyme activities of the vastus lateralis muscle and the functional status in patients with COPD. *Thorax* 2000; 55:848-853.
12. Maltais F., Simon M., Jobin J., Desmeules M., Sullivan M. J., Bélanger M., Leblanc P. Effects of oxygen on lower limb blood flow and $O_2$ uptake during exercise in COPD. *Medicine & Science in Sport & Exercise.* 2001; 33(6) 916-922
13. Camirand J., Aubin J., Audet N., Courtemanche R., Fournier C., Beauvais B., Tremblay R. Enquête québécoisee sur les limitations d'activités 1998. Québec Insitut de la statistique du Québec. pp. 516. 1998.

14. Delahaye F., Gevigney G. Épidémiologie et histoire naturelle de l'insuffisance cardiaque. *Rev Prat.* 47: 2114-2117, 1997. Oldridge N, Economic Evaluation of Cardiopulmonary Rehabilitation. In: Jobin J., Maltais F., LeBlanc P., Simard C. *Advances in Cardiopulmonary Rehabilitation.* Champaign, Human Kinetics. pp 211-26, 2000.

15. Jobin J., Maltais F., Simard C., LeBlanc P. Current and Future Issues in Cardiopulmonary Rehabilitation. In: Jobin J., Maltais F., LeBlanc P., Simard C. *Advances in Cardiopulmonary Rehabilitation.* Champaign, Human Kinetics. pp. 1-5. 2000.

16. Guillemette A., Cormier F., Allie R. Caractéristiques sociodémographiques et économiques des personnes avec incapacité. In: Camirand J., Aubin J., Audet N., Courtemanche R., Fournier C., Beauvais B., Tremblay R. *Enquête québécoise sur les limitations d'activités* 1998. Québec Institut de la statistique du Québec. pp. 143-165. 1998.

17. Maltais F., Jobin J., Simard C., LeBlanc P. Cardiopulmonary Rehabilitation in Clinical Practice: The Underused Intervention. In: Jobin J., Maltais F., LeBlanc P., Simard C. *Advances in Cardiopulmonary Rehabilitation.* Champaign, Human Kinetics. pp 303-306. 2000.

18. Hardman K. Physical Education: Deconstruction/Reconstruction. ICSSPE/CIEPSS. Sport Science & Phys Educ; 2001; 31: 26-31.

19. ACSM. Dose-Response Issues Concerning Physical Activity and Health: an Evidence-Base Symposium. *Medicine & Science in Sport & Exercise.* 2001; 33(6): S345-S641.

20. Jobin J., LeBlanc P., Maltais F., Poirier P., Simard C. *Clin Invest Med* Suppl. Vol 24, No 3: S1-S64, 2001.

# About the Editors

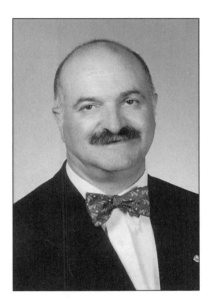

**Jean Jobin**, **PhD**, professor of medicine at Laval University in Québec, is director of the Cardiopulmonary Rehabilitation Research Laboratory at the Institut de cardiologie et de pneumologie de l'Université Laval at Laval Hospital.

Dr. Jobin is a certified program director of the American College of Sports Medicine's (ACSM) Certification for Exercise Specialists in French at Laval University; he is a fellow of the ACSM and of the American Association of Cardiovascular and Pulmonary Rehabilitation, a member of the Canadian Association of Cardiac Rehabilitation and the Canadian Cardiovascular Society. He was president of the scientific committee of the Québec International Symposium on Cardiopulmonary Rehabilitation in 1999 and 2001. He was an editor for the book, *Advances in Pulmonary Rehabilitation*.

Dr. Jobin jogs daily, is an alpine skier, and enjoys carpentry. He, his wife, and children live in Cap-Rouge, Québec.

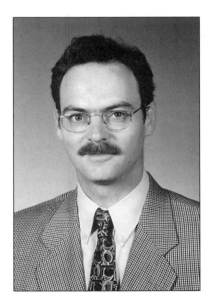

**François Maltais**, **MD**, is a respirologist at the Pneumology Center at Laval Hospital in Québec. He is adjunct professor of medicine at Laval University and medical director of the Pulmonary Rehabilitation Program at Laval Hospital.

A member of the Québec, Canadian, and American Thoracic Societies, Dr. Maltais is certified in internal medicine and in pulmonary medicine. He has been awarded numerous research grants from private and public foundations, including the Medical Research Council of Canada (MRC), to investigate such topics as peripheral muscle dysfunction, strength training, and exercise training in COPD, among many others. Having completed a two-year research training program in respiratory physiology, Dr. Maltais' research is devoted to the study of exercise and muscle physiology in chronic lung diseases. He was vice president of the scientific committee of the Québec International Symposium on Cardiopulmonary Rehabilitation in 1999 and 2001. He was an editor for the book, *Advances in Pulmonary Rehabilitation*.

Dr. Maltais enjoys mountain biking, downhill skiing, and golf. He lives with his wife and children in L'Ancienne-Lorette, Québec.

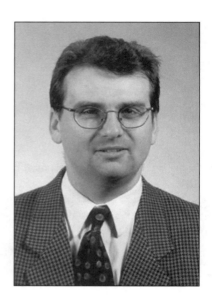

**Paul Poirier, MD**, is a cardiologist at Laval Hospital in Quebec, holding certifications from both the American College of Cardiology and the Royal College of Physicians and Surgeons of Canada. He is program director of the cardiac rehabilitation program of the Quebec Heart Institute.

A member of the American College of Sports Medicine, Dr. Poirier is widely known and well published. His is first author of a chapter about the heart and obesity in the cardiology textbook, *The Heart*; and he authored a discussion of exercise in the management of obesity in *Cardiology Clinics* (2001).

In his spare time, Dr. Poirier enjoys reading, outdoor activities, and spending time with his family. He makes his home in Ste-Foy, Quebec.

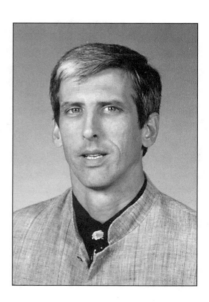

**Pierre LeBlanc, MD**, is clinical professor in the department of medicine at Laval University, where he is in charge of teaching respiratory physiology. He is a member of the American Thoracic Society and the Canadian Thoracic Society. Dr. LeBlanc has published highly significant and often quoted research concerning mechanisms of breathlessness during exercise in cardiorespiratory patients. He was an editor for the book, *Advances in Pulmonary Rehabilitation*.

Dr. LeBlanc is an avid cyclist and enjoys cross-country skiing. From 1975 to 1976, he was a member of the Canadian track and field team. He, his wife, and children live in Cap-Rouge, Québec.

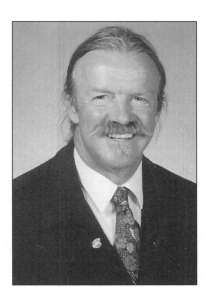

**Clermont Simard, PhD**, is professor of Physical Education and Special Populations at Laval University. He founded the International Federation for Adapted Physical Activity in 1976, for which he was specially honored by Spain's University of Lleida in 1999.

Dr. Simard is a fellow of the ACSM; was president of the Québec International Symposium on Cardiopulmonary Rehabilitation in May 1999; was president of the Motor Adaptation Foundation; and is president for the Rehabilitation International 21st World Congress in 2008. His many years of research have focused on adapting physical activity to populations with special needs, the impact of disuse on muscular metabolism and function, the aging process and physical activity as they affect quality of life, and on means of helping older adults live more autonomous lives. He was an editor for the book, *Advances in Pulmonary Rehabilitation*.

Dr. Simard and his wife make their home in St.-Nicolas, Québec.

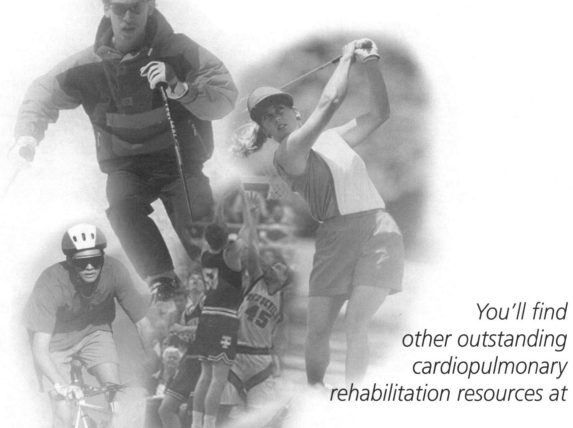